BORN WITH THE GREAT PHYSICIAN

BORN WITH THE GREAT PHYSICIAN

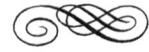

ASHTON A BOHANNON

The information in this book is not a substitute for professional medical advice. Readers carry the full responsibility for their health and well-being. Ashton Bohannon cannot be held liable for any misinterpretation or misuse of information.

Scripture quotations taken from the Amplified® Bible (AMP), Copyright © 2015 by The Lockman Foundation. Used by permission. lockman.org

Copyright © 2024 by Ashton Bohannon
All rights reserved. No part of this book may be reproduced in any manner whatsoever without written permission except in the case of brief quotations embodied in articles and reviews. First Printing, 2025

This book is dedicated to my son,
Gianni Andrew Bohannon.

Gianni, you were given to me by a loving and gracious God. After I'd undergone two hospital, surgical, cesarean births, God allowed me to birth you at home without any interventions. God has protected you from the very first day of conception. He was with you, helping you to grow throughout my pregnancy, and He is still with you, growing you today. He will never leave you or forsake you. I am eternally thankful for our perfect, healthy, homebirth. I learned so much about God's love and protection through my pregnancy with you and your birth. Together we had the divine protection of the Great Physician.

Your name was given to me by God.
Your name speaks to your future.

Gianni: God is Gracious

Andrew: Strong & Masculine

Contents

Dedication   v
Preamble   ix

1. The Witness: A Beautiful Homebirth with Jesus   1
2. Coparenting with Christ   31
3. Informed Consent, Boundaries, and Birthing Freedom   61
4. The Power of a Godly Decision   86
5. The Weapons of our Warfare: Faith and Confession   112
6. Demolishing the Spirit of Fear   138
7. Prophecy and Prayers of Protection   160
8. Attachment, Breastfeeding, and Circumcision   182
9. The Intentional Birth Plan   209
10. The Weapons of our Warfare: Prayer and Oil   234
11. Development and Dedication   254
12. The Importance of Names   280
13. Medical Witchcraft   302
14. Dreams, Visions, and Trances   329
15. The Sons and Daughters of God   360

| 16 Adoption and Infertility | 388 |
| 17 Embodying Christ | 411 |

About the Author   435

Preamble

Believing the word of God without hesitation or doubt has many advantages. One distinguished advantage is the safeguarding of a believer's divine rights to health and healing. Divine healing has been purchased for the Church through the blood of Jesus Christ. Divine healing and health are available to each believer as an inheritance. The divine health inheritance can be accessed at any given time through the combined knowledge and faith of the believer.

Knowledge and faith in our divine covenant rights as God's children helps us to walk supernaturally through life. Parents have been entrusted with authority as the gatekeepers of their children. A parent's faith can be used as a barricade to protect children supernaturally when the parent understands and implements his or her divine covenant rights on behalf of their children. This mediation process allows children to thrive and prosper as partakers of God's kingdom before they arrive at the age of accountability.

Three components make up humanity. Three components are also included within the divine health and healing inheritance. Jesus Christ: the all encompassing, compassionate Physician and Healer has provided for the physical, emotional, and spiritual health of His Church. The state of wellness and health are core elements of the covenant relationship between humanity and God.

Transgression of God's perfect law allowed sickness to abound in the earth even when this was never God's intention for humans. Jesus lived and died to redeem us and to conquer the curse of the law. As a sacrifice for the sins of humanity Jesus made a way for us to be forgiven and restored to perfection and health when we put our faith and trust in Him. Through Jesus's sacrifice alone, we are perfected and cleansed of our sins. Jesus bore the punishment for our sin, so we could be made whole. Isaiah 53:5 teaches, "But He was wounded for our transgressions, He was crushed for our wickedness [our sin, our injustice, our wrongdoing]; The punishment [required] for our well-being fell on Him, And by His stripes [wounds] we are healed.

As parents submit their lives and their children's lives to Him, beautiful things are decreed and established. Parents are capable of raising children to know the truth, ensuring they will never stray or depart from it. God has partnered with us through Jesus Christ's atonement to ensure that we are strong, whole, and healthy. God strengthens individuals and the family through His plan.

Psalm 92:12–13 says, "Those who do what is right will grow like a palm tree. They will grow strong like a cedar tree in Lebanon. Their roots will be firm in the house of the Lord. They will grow strong and healthy in the courtyards of God." Parents who plant children in the courtyard of God, protect the children, and allow them to grow and develop into healthy, thriving participants in the kingdom.

In the Old Testament the Egyptians could not cross the Red Sea with God's people. Consequently, they drowned in the water. When the New Testament Church of today hears the Word, and receives the Word, they will embody health and healing, even when the world is suffering from a psychological, spiritual, and physical sickness epidemic. The Church will thrive, prosper, and persevere in all things, and we will be seen walking through the waters unbelievers drown in.

1

The Witness: A Beautiful Homebirth with Jesus

Postmodernists believe there are multiple modes of knowledge and information and no absolute moral or universal boundaries. The postmodernism worldview assumes there is no absolute truth. Within a postmodern perspective, people have their own subjective truth and are free to decide what is true and what is false. Truth and lies are separated based on individualized life experiences and personalized perceptions of the world.

A postmodern philosophy contributes to people having no fixed identity. To form a healthy identity we need to have an understanding of right from wrong. God designed people to learn from their parents, intending for parents to guide and educate children in appropriate behaviors and cultural practices. This is achieved through modeling, love, and intentional instruction.

Postmodernism has significantly influenced child-rearing practices. Postmodern parenting philosophies contribute to children who growing up in homes without structure, boundaries, and parental instruction. Research has consistently shown these children will suffer due to the lack of security and safety within their world.

The prevalence of child-led parenting in America is giving rise to health issues effecting the lives of many, because children need the guidance and protection of their elders. Proverbs 13:24 explains, "He who spares his rod [of discipline] hates his son, but he who loves him disciplines diligently and punishes him early." From the moment of conception, humans require support due to their inherent immaturity and lack of innate understanding of right and wrong.

It is important to recognize that children are unable to discern truth for themselves until their cognitive development has progressed. All children require parental guidance; without it, they will be unhealthy and struggle to survive and thrive in society. Transgender children, delayed potty training, and significant behavioral issues can be traced back to child-led parenting practices that emerge from a postmodern worldview.

As God-ordained spiritual leaders, mothers must protect their children. Without a mother's love and assistance, children are vulnerable to the attacks of the enemy of our souls. For a short period of time in their children's lives, the parents must take their authority and leadership position to guarantee children receive the lessons, and an impartation of God's kingdom.

The postmodern mindset affirms people are to be their own god and ruler because no supreme ruler exists. A lack of understanding regarding authority and leadership leads many individuals to mistakenly assume they hold the highest position of power when, in fact, they do not. When people do not submit to proper authority and help from a superior, they are easily deceived and led of course by their human limitations.

Just as a child depends on the guidance of a parent, humanity similarly relies on the guidance support of their Creator. Humanity is ill equipped to properly navigate a supernatural spirit world apart from God. Without a supernatural guide, we are prey to the demon spirits living with us on the earth. A realization of the human condition and our spiritual vulnerability without God needs to resonate within us before we can rely on God as our source. We must realize we are in imminent danger in the world without a Savior and a Protector.

Once we are aware of our personal immaturity and the lack of protection, we have without God, we will submit ourselves to His leadership fully because we know it is a requirement to be healthy, survive, and succeed. Healthy people do not want to be orphans. They want to be apart of a family. Respecting God as a Father is the beginning of health and wisdom.

Many people let postmodern beliefs shape their thoughts and behaviors. By believing in the lie that no absolute truth exists, people become wandering, lost, vagabonds separated from their Father. As people separate from their Father, they live without a true purpose and are exposed to the corruption of the demonically ruled world. Like children without parents, vagabonds are ill-prepared to survive much less thrive. Ephesians 4:18 tells us, "They are darkened in their understanding, alienated from the life of God because of the ignorance that is in them, due to their hardness of heart."

Vagabonds wander from place to place without a home and they don't have a vision of where they are going. Vagabonds cannot see or properly understand what is happening around them, because they are living in survival mode. Without spiritual help and vision, life is difficult, and people are inherently weak instead of strong. As self-reliant, rebellious people, vagabonds attempt to survive alone, even when they were never created to live apart from their Creator. Revelation 3:17 says, "For you say, I am rich, I have prospered, and I need nothing, not realizing that you are wretched, pitiable, poor, blind, and naked."

On the journey through life, vagabonds connect with the wrong people, are in the wrong places, and enter wrong relationships. Everyone they meet and everything they do is completely outside of God's will. Without a clear spiritual identity stemming from intimacy with God, they are separated from their intended purpose and will never arrive at their God-given destination.

Genesis 4:12 says Abel became a vagabond, when he refused to submit to God's plan of salvation. Cain was separated from his intended identity and his spiritual family. "When you till the ground, it shall no longer yield to you its strength; you shall be a fugitive and a vagabond on the earth [in perpetual exile, a degraded outcast]."

Cain responded to God's consequence, saying "Behold, You have driven me out this day from the face of the land, and from Your face I will be hidden; and I will be a fugitive and a vagabond and a wanderer on the earth."

Vagabonds are disconnected from their heritage. Heritage is broadly defined as the history, traditions, buildings, or objects that a country or society has had for many years as an important part of their character. Our heritage serves as the foundation of our identity. Without a clear understanding of who we are and why we do what we do, we live a life devoid of meaning.

Heritage influences everything about our lives from the food we eat to the way we communicate with others and the language we speak. Heritage impacts the clothing we wear and the ways we behave and interact with the world around us. A person's heritage must be imparted and taught by those in their community. Without effective transmission and leadership, individuals may struggle to understand the reasons behind their identity and behaviors. Leadership within a culture plays a crucial role in instilling heritage in the younger generation.

In all nations of the world are large and small cultural identities. People within a nation share commonalities and beliefs. They share a big cultural understanding of who they are as a group, but within the small community, minute differences impact how we behave and respond. Our family heritage, the small cultural identity we share with close family members, is equally as important as cultural heritage.

A family heritage establishes social norms and guidelines and teaches right from wrong at an interpersonal level. Children learn to behave and to interact with others through their family. Children learn who they are and what they are expected to do from their inner-knit family. Family heritage shapes aspects of life, such as our perceptions of ourselves, our sense of belonging, and our medical history. It guides who and what we are.

Becoming a son or a daughter of God is a strong-rooted identity. As children of God, we know who we are and what we are on the earth to do. We receive customs and norms from our Father God, and we refuse to participate in things when we identify them properly as foreign and unhealthy behaviors. Our health, our finances, life trajectories, and general well-being is primarily influenced by our family identity as Christ followers and kingdom citizens. Christians aren't subject to the same diseases, disorders, and problems as unbelievers, because it isn't a part of their heritage and family projection.

The Christian's spiritual heritage is a collection of family heritage and cultural heritage, shaping our values, beliefs, and experiences, while connecting us to others in our family who share our spiritual roots. As we identify with our heritage as Christians, we are enabled to act, think, and live the Christian life successfully. We learn how to properly relate to the world from our Christian families' perspective. Knowing who we are in Christ and who we are in the kingdom of the Lord is the foundation of everything else in our lives.

The broad Christian family is a large family operating from a macro level. Believers from all over the world share in the heritage of God. Christians learn the norms and customs of God's family through the lens of the Bible. On a macro level, all Christians behave and believe in similar ways if they are following the precepts in God's Word. All Christians of all races, genders, and other groups throughout the world will share commonalities because of their connection to the Bible and to God. They will have a large-scale cultural identity.

However, within the family of God are smaller groups of closer-knit families. These smaller families are composed of local churches, communities, or other close-knit relationships among believers. These micro-family Christian relationships influence our interactions with others. Our micro interactions are established through our consistent, close contact with one another, like a small family unit living within a larger society.

To have a comprehensive understanding of Christian heritage, we must understand both the macro and the micro perspective relating to culture and family. The macro perspective helps us to understand who we are through holistic or broader analysis, and the micro examines the smaller, more personalized components of our lives. Both macro and micro perspectives help us to study complex human relationships and behavior.

Both the macro and the micro forms of analysis permit us to draw proper conclusions and understanding of who we are and why we do what we do. For instance, Americans share many beliefs, customs, and behaviors. This collective, large-scale cultural understanding of Americans is the macro-analysis of American culture. Americans, although diverse in their ethnic or racial background, share many commonalities and behavioral norms. Americans operate under American laws, and they believe many common things, such as the right for all to vote, succeed, and prosper.

Knowing the overarching themes found in American thought, behavior, and societal norms allows us to analyze ourselves as individuals and understand why we think the way we think and why we do the things we do. Once we see who we are from a macro-societal perspective stemming from the American culture at large, we can analyze the smaller families and cultures represented within American culture. Some American families homeschool and others choose public schooling. Some American families live on one income and some live on two. Some Americans live in cities and some live in rural communities. These smaller details are the micro-analysis perspective of American culture impacting who we are.

In America, many states have their own cultures, and within these cultures are smaller community cultures. States like Texas have very different cultural norms than other states, such as Maine. If you were to visit different communities within these states, you would also find cultural differences. Some cities adopt certain cultural customs and behaviors. Even the homes built in many towns represent the people and the culture in the area.

Within the Church, denominations and larger groups form their own religious culture. However, the local church branch, even of those denominations, may vary in their operations because they have their own small community cultures. A Pentecostal Holiness church in Texas will not be the same as a Pentecostal Holiness church in New York, because of the people in the churches. Even with the overarching themes of Christianity as the macro root of the Church, the families and people within those churches will vary greatly in their behaviors and customs.

As Christians, we must know we are a part of the global body of Christ and share the macro view of the Christian faith. However, we are influenced by our local and interpersonal relationships. Understanding who we are, and why we believe what we believe gives us a strong vision of our mission. We need to know clearly and confidently that we are to behave in certain ways and are to perform certain things because we have a strong heritage and identity through our macro and micro interactions with other believers. Without a personal analysis of our behaviors, mindsets, and relationships, we will not be able to clearly see who God wants us to be.

The church culture we join is important in determining our future and choices. Churches operating in divine healing and health will teach on it and will produce spiritual children who operate in divine healing and health. Likewise, churches that promote unhealthy doctrines, such as cessationism, the belief that spiritual gifts are not valid today, will breed spiritual children with a spiritual deficiency. The same is true for finances, or any other teaching combined with interpersonal learning. People learn, whether good or bad, from those they spend time with.

The spiritual people we interact with are the primary ones we learn from and the people we will become like. Like the nuclear family, a local church family influences our lives more than the mainstream culture and macro-Church. Children share the characteristics, good and bad, of their parents. For leaders in the church, this is very important to understand, because spiritual leadership and parenting will produce spiritual children—either good or bad—because of the leaders' and parents' choices and mindsets.

However, the larger Christian faith also plays a large role in our identity as Christians. For instance, as we understand who fathers in the faith are, we will understand who we are. When we read the Bible, we are reading the testimonies of those who have come before us as the Church. We can learn from the mistakes and the victories of our ancestors at large, and we can make choices today that will impact the next generation of believers. We know we have commonalities with all Christians because we are a part of the large cultural family of God.

If we are going to help our brothers and sisters and our spiritual children or grandchildren, then we should honor those who are in authority over us as spiritual leaders. As we interact in our local church body, we are interacting with the members of our personal "household" within the larger "household" of God. Some people in the house will hold authority over us, and others will be beneath our leadership and care.

Not all members of the household have the same position but must still be respected accordingly. A pastor should never be lowered into the position of "friend" to the congregants, thus reducing his or her leadership. When we are pastoring, we are not friends to our sheep, we are protectors and are a spiritual guide or parent. If we allow those who are immature in their understanding to dictate the house, we are as wrong as a father or mother who allows their children to run their home.

Many people do not understand honor and respect. This is an increasing problem with our American generation of people who do not follow parents' authority and proper instruction. One of the biggest problems of the move to equalize children to their parents in the home is the failure to translate the respect and honor of those in authority positions, such as leaders in the Church, or God Himself. Not everyone in the church is the same, and not everyone should be given equal access to lead and guide others.

First Timothy 3:1–7 teaches, "The saying is true and irrefutable: If any man [eagerly] seeks the office of bishop (superintendent, overseer), he desires an excellent task (work). Now a bishop (superintendent, overseer) must give no grounds for accusation but must be above reproach, the husband of one wife, circumspect and temperate and self-controlled; [he must be] sensible and well behaved and dignified and lead an orderly (disciplined) life; [he must be] hospitable [showing love for and being a friend to the believers, especially strangers or foreigners, and be] a capable and qualified teacher, Not given to wine, not combative but gentle and considerate, not quarrelsome but forbearing and peaceable, and not a lover of money [insatiable for wealth and ready to obtain it by questionable means].

"He must rule his own household well, keeping his children under control, with true dignity, commanding their respect in every way and keeping them respectful. For if a man does not know how to rule his own household, how is he to take care of the church of God? He must not be a new convert, or he may [develop a beclouded and stupid state of mind] as the result of pride [be blinded by conceit, and] fall into the condemnation that the Devil [once] did. Furthermore, he must have a good reputation and be well thought of by those outside [the church], lest he become involved in slander and incur reproach and fall into the Devil's trap."

Introspection allows us to determine who we are in the body of Christ. It helps us to have a balanced and honest perspective of ourselves and our position in the Church body. God will elevate and promote people, but we must never promote those who are ill-prepared to lead others in God's house. Who is in charge matters. God does care who is given a position as an overseer. And when there is a failure to properly implement this in our houses of worship, problems will develop because children or immature members are allowed to make adult decisions.

The way we grow up as believers is through wisdom and knowledge of God and His Word, combined with obedience and honor of those who are put in church positions above us Spending time understanding who we are in our relationship with the Lord permits us to decipher and change anything we have learned that does not properly represent the culture of God. God will show us when we need to alter our beliefs and behaviors so we can be conformed into righteousness and lead others along that path.

Christians should never accept all behaviors of everyone around them simply because someone is in our family. Some family members have unhealthy behaviors. We need to be willing to confront them, when necessary, instead of normalizing them, simply because we love the person. Confrontation of sin is loving, even if the person doesn't initially understand. If we are more mature than another, we can help them by respectively leading them to the truth.

Many times, leaders have been given positions that they should not hold. A man or woman who is put into a position of authority prematurely will cause problems for others in the house. If there are more mature believers underneath a child, they will be able to quickly identify a problem, and in these situations, we cannot afford to submit to irresponsible behavior of a spiritual child who has been given the responsibility of a spiritual leader. We must know how to recognize a child in a leadership position just as much as we are to recognize an elder in one.

Demonic forces recognize those who are God's children, and they know when we carry authority in the spirit. Consider Acts 19:5, when the evil spirit responded to the sons of Sceva saying, "Jesus I know, and Paul I know; but who are you?" The spirits recognized that these men were not in the family of God and did not carry spiritual authority. As people from other cultures can recognize and determine the heritage of another who does not share their culture, demons identify those who are not a part of their culture. Demons know when we are born of God and carry God's power and spirit. They also know when we don't.

Through the blood of Jesus, we share in the bloodline and biological family of God. The children of God are a part of a larger culture, noticeable to all who do not share the culture norms and values. When we are descendants of God, we share His characteristics, His nature, and His behaviors. We carry the resemblance of God that the devil and demons recognize. We represent something "different" within the general mainstream culture.

Children of the devil embody the characteristics of the devil. As people who live contrary to the Lord's teachings and culture, the devil's children are recognized by their behaviors and their appearance of evil. Like any spiritual family, children of the devil will pass on their evil to others. They want others to participate and normalize their deeds, so they can reproduce evil and form new families. The devil is the father of all who practice evil, and we must be able to recognize when someone is outside of God's family and doesn't share our cultural faith heritage.

Before joining God's family, I was incredibly sick. I suffered emotionally, physically, and spiritually because I had not committed my life to God. I suffered physically with endometriosis, and I suffered psychologically due to a trauma background and a diagnosis of extreme mood disorder. My behavior and characteristics were not godly. They were noticeably problematic and chaotic, and any discerning person or spirit knew who I was and what I carried with me.

We must be able to recognize who others are and where they are in their faith journeys. We need to be introspective of our lives and our associations so we can behave in ways that are mature and responsible, ensuring God's house is in order. It would have been foolish for me to become a leader shortly after my salvation, because I was a child in the faith without proper understanding. I needed a season of learning and development to prepare me to be a leader in the ministry.

The capacity to discern an individual's developmental age and comprehension serves as a protective mechanism. Through our observations we can identify whom to follow and whom to mentor and lead. Children may not understand the implications of bad associations, improper leadership, or the failure to submit to proper authority, but we as adults should. The people and connections we are joined to impact us and shape the trajectory of our spiritual lives. Thus we should give them attention.

All seeds take time to grow. Both healing and illness typically require time to fully manifest themselves. Jesus taught that we receive healing upon salvation; however, our healing often unfolds gradually as we grow in our relationship with Christ. Similarly, sickness also develops over time. Initially, when a person falls ill, they enter an incubation period during which the disease has not yet fully taken hold.

It is essential for us to assess whether those around us belong to God's family and to evaluate their spiritual development and overall health. The ability to discern between good and bad fruit, as well as to recognize the various stages of development within that fruit, serves as a preservative measure. Matthew 3:8 says, "So produce fruit that is consistent with repentance [demonstrating new behavior that proves a change of heart, and a conscious decision to turn away from sin];"

The severity of my sickness began to manifest when I was a teenager. Before that time, I was living in the incubation stage of disease because I had been in contact with many infections, but the symptoms were not evident until some time had elapsed. The psychological and biological changes my body underwent as a teenager brought forth the need for intervention, because time had elapsed and the seeds of sin, and the normalization of sin through my cultural influence, began to take root in my life. For most children the extreme symptoms of their disease will not manifest themselves upon initial contact with the diseases in their surrounding environments.

The culture we set our children in both at a societal level and an interpersonal one will shape their identities. Over time children develop mental schemes of normal/abnormal customs. All of us eventually reach the age when we can cognitively make a different decision, but as children we are at the liberty of those we need to instruct us.

As a child I needed guidance and help. I needed spiritual assistance to guide me into the truth and onto the right path. This is the primary reason I am so passionate about kids' ministry, because I believe children must have spiritual help to survive the enemy's assaults. If left spiritually unprotected, children will take the appearance of the world and the enemy. Children need to be intentionally set on the path of life. They have to be cultivated to life.

My mother tried to find counselors and doctors to help me. She believed the professionals were the best choice for my health, and I know she tried her best to get me the help I needed. For many years, doctors suggested birth control and talk therapy as an answer to my issues. Professionals, counselors, doctors, and others weren't helpful because they wanted to treat a spiritual condition as solely a physical one. I didn't need worldly solutions to spiritual problems. I needed a spiritual remedy that could solve physical problems.

My severe and increasingly prevalent issues were never directly addressed, only indirectly addressed. My problem did not stem directly from my period, biological issues, or my childhood trauma. I could have persevered through all of those things if I had not been ignorant of understanding in my relationship with God and the things of the spirit. I am absolutely convinced I would have been healed sooner if I had been taken to the Great Physician.

Without a firm understanding of God and His healing power, I lived apart from God and in a humanistic way. The impact of my friendships further caused me harm. As I associated with those who were unhealthy because of their childhood traumas and sin, I caught other sicknesses. Often, when we are sick, we spread disease to others without intending to. Parents or children who are experiencing personal health issues typically do not intend to transfer their struggles onto others in their lives. However, through their close relationships, this transmission often occurs unintentionally.

Humans are connected to their environments. We cannot understand human life without an analysis of the society in which the person lives. Likewise emotional, physical, and spiritual diseases are interconnected and cannot be understood properly outside of one another. We must understand and believe all diseases need to be first understood in the realm of the spirit. It is foolish to believe that we can prevent, address, or diagnose a disease without considering the entire being.

People are three parts, and we must consider all three parts to treat their health conditions. Holistic healthcare takes the whole person into consideration. Holistic health focuses on the connection between the spirit, the mind, and the body because these elements are interconnected.

Holistic medicine is also known as integrative medicine, and to be integrative means to be unified and combined. Without an integration of the whole essence of a person, medical professionals will never properly treat health issues, because it is impossible to ignore an entire component of the person. Only an integrative approach allows practitioners to see both the macro and micro elements, the spiritual, physical, and psychological elements that are interfering with an individual's health.

Most medical professionals have been trained as specialists. Specialists look at one aspect primarily and fail to connect with the whole person. But, where there is limited understanding of the necessity for holistic health, there is a failure to address and heal the person as an integrated individual. And without the integrated, holistic approach, true healing will never occur. Fragmented practitioners make people worse, not better, because they don't see the full picture.

Puzzles make no sense to us when we see them as individual pieces. Puzzles only become complete when the pieces are put together in a unified manner. As we put the puzzle pieces together, we begin to see the full picture. Practitioners who work in a holistic way will always be better at their jobs than those who are not holistic, because they are looking at more parts of the puzzle to figure out the preventive healthcare needs or a condition.

To my understanding, my midwife during my third birth was not a believer, but she was a holistic practitioner. This permitted her to understand the person as a whole being, and it allowed her to respect my beliefs as a Christian. The closer we are to understanding that we are three parts—spirit, mind and body—the better we will be as professionals, even if we do not fully rely on the spiritual. My midwife accepted the spiritual component to my identity, and even if she personally didn't ascribe to my faith, she respected that it was an important component influencing me.

If we want to find the solution to healthcare problems today, we need to search for the ultimate solution. Healthcare properly attended too will search the spirit to understand the physical and the emotional aspects of a man or woman. Only when we are holistic and integrated is the puzzle complete. The spiritual part of us is the basis of who we are. When practitioners acknowledge the whole picture, they begin to understand the truth. One puzzle piece will never make sense, but 100 pieces put together as one big collection does.

Sickness and disease trap people and cause them to feel as if there is no way out. When people feel they are cannot be healed from their infirmities, they lose their hope. Sickness and disease cause misery. If there is going to be any healing at all, a person must first know there is a way out of their trouble, and the only way out is through a relationship with Jesus. As we understand that a spiritual problem is influencing all other problems, we will begin to have hope in finding our solution to every aspect of human life. Proverbs 13:12 says, "Hope deferred makes the heart sick, but when the desire is fulfilled, it is a tree of life."

I healed so much when I understood a devil was behind my parents' divorce. Not only did it heal my anger and pain towards my dad, but it also healed my self-blame. Realizing the endometriosis and the mood disorders didn't have to control my future gave me hope of being a mother and bearing children and becoming a person who was not psychologically weak two weeks out of the month.

Without realizing an enemy was behind these things, and I needed to resist them, I would never have been free from my infirmities. I had to see the spiritual roots to my problems to be healed of anything I was experiencing.

When I was 17, doctors tried to put me on blood pressure medication. At the time, I was already on birth control, and I was overweight because ate unhealthy food as a coping mechanism. I didn't want to believe I was doomed to sickness. I wanted to believe I could live life without medications, and I knew the doctors' treatment plans were making me worse because I had been "treated" for five years and nothing was better, it was worse! This resistance to accept sickness led me to look for a solution outside of the medical world.

I had no spiritual basis to rebuke the doctors and their medications. I just had a personal belief that I could become healthy if I tried hard enough, so I became obsessed with working out, nutrition, and holistic health. I quit taking the medication and became consumed with fixing my own health through diet, exercise, and natural healing remedies. I believed if I ate the right foods, worked out excessively, and "balanced" myself with nature I would become whole and well.

While it did help me physically, it also led me into witchcraft because I began to worship nature instead of God. As I became more balanced in my physical health, I became less balanced in my spiritual health. I believed horoscopes, the sun, the moon, plants, water, and other parts of the earth could help me heal. I became obsessed with rocks, stones, crystals, and other earth elements because I thought they had healing properties. This mindset also led me into heavy marijuana use, and for a while, I thought marijuana was sent from the earth to help people to heal from their psychological trauma.

Romans 1:25 tells us, "Because [by choice] they exchanged the truth of God for a lie, and worshiped and served the creature rather than the Creator, who is blessed forever! Amen."

For a while I felt better than before, so I was reinforced in bad behavior. The seeds of sin in this season had not yet matured and grown. My physical health was better even though my spiritual health was worse. After experiencing more trauma, I started coping with my newfound religion, combined with excessive drinking and marijuana, because I had stopped binging on food. During this same period, I was attending college and began to learn about philosophy, sociology, and psychology. I started to doubt God more than ever before. As I became more separated from spiritual truth, my psychological and spiritual health deteriorated.

The further I walked away from God and His truth the worse everything became. I invited more spirits into my life, and I walked deeper into the depths of Satan. As I alienated myself from God and worshiped His creation, I became sicker. Even with a better outward "body" than I had ever had before, I was sicker than I had ever been. As Jesus said, we must look at what is on the inside, not the outside, to see what is truly pure.

I tried to make myself healthy on the outside to change the inside. I wanted to use the outward appearance of health and wellness as my basis for my inner wellness, and it didn't work. I couldn't change my inner spirit and emotional states by controlling my physical woman. I needed inner changing before I could enjoy the outer beauty I worked for. True health and purity cannot come from the outward and go inward. It comes from an inner healthy spirit, and then it will manifest itself outwardly.

God never intended for His creation to go into the depths of the sea, walking in the ways of Satan. God wants to give us a chance to walk through the waters, even when those same waters will destroy those who don't fear Him. Nehemiah 9:11 says, "You divided the sea before them, so that they passed through the midst of the sea on dry land; You hurled their pursuers into the depths, like a stone into mighty and raging waters."

I reached a point where I was very aware of evil spiritual forces surrounding my life. I was suicidal, and I realized I needed help to fight off the forces that surrounded me. I was engulfed by evil, and I was tormented day and night. I felt no and no rest. I was tossed around like a ship in stormy waters, terrified day and night. The waves, the storm, and the sea surrounded me, and I felt hopeless and helpless. Then I called out to God to save me because I knew without God, I would be shipwrecked or drowned and had no hope.

Before I was healed, I couldn't do participate in school or work because of my periods. I was doing things I couldn't believe I was doing, and I didn't even recognize myself. I behaved irrationally; I was led by my emotions and was even more out of control around my period. I got to the point where I was suffering so immensely, I finally gave in and went back to the doctor. I was diagnosed with premenstrual dysphoric disorder (PMDD) combined with endometriosis. The doctors put me back on birth control and tried to prescribe an antidepressant.

I also underwent surgery to remove some of the lesions from the endometriosis. I was still trying to eat healthy, do acupuncture, work out, and pursue a holistic lifestyle, but I was very unwell. Despite many interventions, something missing in my life, and I knew I was not being healed. I realized no human, including myself, could save me. I knew what I was experiencing was spiritual. I knew I had to have spiritual help to experience true health.

When I was in college, I stood in the parking lot of the school and told myself I was going to figure out what was wrong and use the information to help others. To this day, I can testify that the problem in my life was improper instruction inspired by Satan. Until I realized I had a choice to be saved and to opt out of the world's system, I was controlled by it. But once I realized Jesus was real and could deliver me from all manners of affliction I began to heal because I decided to reach out to my Savior and my Creator.

The first time I went to church as an adult, I knew God's Spirit was stronger than any of the spirits around me. I knew there was really a Redeemer, a Savior, and a Helper who could stop the storm. I knew Jesus was my only hope. The picture of a man or woman drowning in the sea because the waves and the storm engulfs them perfectly depicts my life before I reached out for help. Jesus walking on the water, completely unfazed by the surrounding storm grabbed me and saved me from the waves and the spirits trying to take my life.

Things in my life changed when I desperately went to God for help. I was the problem, not Him. I chose to journey into places I didn't have any business being in. I got myself deeper into the storm and into the darkness by not following spiritual truth. Jesus didn't save me because I deserved it or because I was worthy of His love or His help. He saved me because I admitted I was a vessel, unprepared for voyage without Him in my boat, and I asked Him to help me.

After becoming a believer, I needed help to understand the Bible. It took some time to learn more about God and His Word through studying the scriptures and spending time in God's presence. But even with my ignorance, God always provided me with help. He always showed up and gave me what I needed when I needed it. Jesus is the healer, and when you hang out with Him, you begin to be supernaturally healed. If we want to be healed, we can hang out with Jesus, and He will show us the path to healing. He will give us the help we need to be well.

It took me a few years of studying, connecting, trusting, and loving Jesus to see my healing manifest fully. My inability to see myself as a new creature in Christ kept me from healing entirely. I needed more revelation and to renew my mind and understand who I was in Christ because I had no idea what God had provided for me in my new spiritual identity. I was very sick, and I believe when we are severely wounded, it often takes us more time to heal than when we are only slightly damaged.

Like a patient in ICU compared to a patient who has a broken foot and simply needs a cast, there are levels of sickness and disease. Satan wants to take our health and our vitality, destroy our vigor, and ultimately, he wants to kill us. Jesus can restore even the worst-off person, barely hanging onto life. He will bring that person back to fullness of life, and He will restore him or her to health without a trace of trauma, pain, dysfunction, or disease. He is the best Physician there ever has been and ever will be. He is the One who created the human body, and He knows how to remedy our conditions, regardless of the severity of our disease.

I doubted God's love for me time and time again for years because I didn't *feel* like someone He could love. I had to learn to put my feelings into the backseat because my feelings were wrong, and God was right. I started Christianity as a newborn. I did not know anything, except I loved my Father God, and I needed His help. I took the medicine God gave me, and I walked out of faith, believing I was in good hands. Faith in God and His ability to help me healed me. My belief in the goodness of God allowed Him to work on my behalf.

I began the process of learning and separating myself from any feeling, idea, philosophy, person, or behavior God said to sever because I realized it was for my betterment to do so. As I choose to believe God more than humans, and even more than my own self, I rejected the concepts of postmodernism. I leaned fully onto the truth of God's Word, and I rejected the lies of Satan that were trying to mold me into humanistic understanding.

When we first start our spiritual walk with Christ, we must fully rely on God like a toddler relies on his or her parent. Like a patient in the ICU relies on the hospital staff. To heal, survive, and thrive in God's care, we must first realize we need Him to live and succeed.

To be healthy, we need to understand our total reliance on God. We can't survive without the assistance of God. I used to boast about my personal intuitiveness and my connection to my feelings. I even got a degree in counseling so I could talk to others about their feelings, because at one time I believed feelings would lead me and others into truth. But the more I tried to trust my own self, to trust in my feelings, the more lost I became. Not until I started to trust God and His truth, not my own, was I able to see clearly or to heal. True healing comes from reliance on God, not self.

1 Timothy 1:19 explains, "Keeping your faith [leaning completely on God with absolute trust and confidence in His guidance] and having a good conscience; for some [people] have rejected [their moral compass] and have made a shipwreck of their faith."

Feelings don't lead people into truth, and we can't live by our feelings if we want to be healthy. When Jesus told Satan that man doesn't live by bread alone, but by every word that proceeds from God, He was saying, "Do not live by your feelings." Even our appetite for food shouldn't control us more than God controls us. God must be our compass, providing us with direction in all things. We must submit our flesh to God's direction and plan, and we must refuse to allow our flesh or any evil spirit to determine the direction of our ship.

Whom we keep on our ship and whom we allow around us does impact our future. Jonah's rebellion to God caused other men on the ship to experience turmoil. Jonah's disobedience to God hindered his own life and the lives of those around him. Conversely, when Paul was on the ship with his crew, his positive influence kept the men on board safe from harm. Paul fed the men with the Word, and they were assured of their safety and given hope.

Healing is possible when we decide to cast away all the evil associations, customs, beliefs, perspectives, worldviews, and influence, willingly choosing to live on the words of the Great Physician. Healing is possible when we shun all forms of evil. To fully experience the blessing, the goodness, and the healing of the Lord, we must want to be healed, and we must choose to be healed by spending time with the Healer, intentionally adhering to His treatment plan and remedies for health. We must stop allowing things or people into our hearts if they carry sickness. We need to watch whom we have with us and where we are going, and we will always know the truth if we stay connected to God and allow Him to direct us.

Heritage doesn't mean we don't associate with anyone or anything outside of our faith community. To be healthy we must mingle with others, even those who do not share our culture identity. However, we must realize who we are, and we must be willing to assert who we are, not change who we are as we interact with those outside of our family or community. When we associate with people or spirits outside of our culture, we must stand firm in our identity and heritage and not allow their beliefs to change ours because we are proud of the people we are.

The reason many people do not experience the fullness of their supernatural healing and provision from God is because they still rely on the world's healing and provision. By receiving the culture and heritage of the outside world, they allow their spiritual roots to be compromised. We cannot remain on two ships that are heading in two separate different directions. It isn't possible to be strong in our identity, while being contaminated by another identity. We must choose the direction we are going to travel in. We must know the boat we are on and know who is on our boat. We must know the direction the boat is going, and we must remain on the voyage with Christ.

Throughout my third pregnancy and childbirth experience, Jesus was an ever-present source of support. He provided guidance on what actions to take, whom to consult, and whom to disregard. His presence offered clarity and direction, and He served as my sole advisor during this profound journey. Recognizing that God was all I needed empowered me to embrace my identity as a child of God with confidence. My complete reliance on Him provided a profound sense of security. I was confident that I would reach the other side safely, regardless of the circumstances, because I trusted the One accompanying me in the boat.

When I became pregnant with my son, Gianni, my spiritual understanding had significantly advanced. Gianni's pregnancy was supernatural. The Lord told me I was pregnant a day after I conceived. Then, before I got my first positive pregnancy test, I asked the Lord for a sign to confirm that I was pregnant, and He gave me three separate signs.

The first sign came when I was in church one week after I conceived, and I saw a sign on the back of the bathroom stall advertising pregnancy help and support. The Spirit illuminated the sign for me. I saw a light circling the picture. The Lord gave me the second sign as I rode in the truck with my family one afternoon. I asked God to show me a light blue truck—a very specific request—before we got home if I was pregnant. As we turned onto the back roads leading to our house, I saw an antique light blue truck parked outside of a gas station.

The third sign came when I was in a bookstore with my kids, and my middle child picked up a book called *I am a big sister!* When I saw her holding it, I knew the Lord was confirming that she was going to be a big sister. When I got my positive test right after that, I was not surprised. The Lord had already told me I was pregnant four times.

My spiritual roots in Christ influenced my physical and psychological health, and influenced and shaped my life's trajectory. My spiritual identity told me about my baby before medical science could.

I scheduled my first pregnancy appointment with an obstetrician, since I was used to having my children in a hospital. When I went to my first appointment, I saw a different doctor than I'd seen with my other two. I told my new doctor my medical history of two cesarean births, and I planned to try for a v-bac with my third baby. She told me I was "lucky" to get her because most doctors wouldn't allow me to have a vaginal birth after two cesareans, but she would!

The doctor also asked why I had two previous cesarean births, and I told her they were due to my baby's size, and high blood pressure with my second. In the first two pregnancies, I didn't watch what I ate or work out. I was very healthy when I got pregnant with my third. I was determined to eat healthily and to work out from the start this time, because I understood it would help me to have the birth I wanted.

When my husband and I were about to leave the doctor's appointment, the doctor told me I needed to eat ice cream every night to help with my nausea. Leaving the appointment with my husband, I didn't feel right about the situation. In the spirit, I knew this lady was trying to harm me. I had never had a doctor insist I eat ice cream. Even though the doctor seemed nice, I felt something was off in the spirit. I scheduled my next appointment for four weeks later, but I ignored the doctor's advice to change my diet to eat ice cream.

A week before I was to go back to the doctor, I got a phone call informing me my doctor was no longer practicing there, and I would be assigned a new doctor. The new doctor reviewed my medical history and said the other doctor noted I would be having a third cesarean birth. When I told the new doctor about my discussion with the previous doctor, she said she didn't see anything about a vaginal birth and vaginal births after cesareans weren't allowed.

If I had adhered to the medical communities' requirements, my third birth would have been a cesarean birth. I would have gained too much weight, been induced into a diabetic condition, and I would have been forced to have my baby their way, not God's way. I would have believed I could not have my baby vaginally. I would have been coaxed into a bad decision for my health and my child's health.

I am thankful to have the Spirit of the Lord as my guide. Without my spiritual identity and the help of the Great Physician, I would have relied on the hospital and an obstetrician. The first doctor's plan was clear; she wanted me to gain weight so I would develop gestational diabetes and would have to have a cesarean birth. But she was cunning enough to pretend to support my birth plan. The new doctor wasn't much better, because she told me I couldn't have my birth the way I wanted. She informed me that a cesarean birth was my only option, even when this wasn't true.

When I went home, I researched birth centers and midwives for home births. One birth center wouldn't take me either because of my cesareans. Sometimes, the right decision requires effort, work, and substantial time; just because it seems challenging doesn't mean it isn't the right choice. I kept looking and found a midwife who would partner with me to have a home birth. She was ordained by God to be my midwife. God gave me her to use for my birth, and I know she was the woman who was supposed to help me.

When I first talked to my midwife, she told me multiple babies were being born in our small county, and she usually didn't have anyone in that county. She agreed to take me as her last client, because I would be near the other moms, otherwise she couldn't have. She could only take on a limited number of moms because her services are personalized and she works by herself, with the help of one or two other assistants or doulas.

My midwife's office was not in a hospital or in a medical building. Her office felt more like a home than a doctor's office, and I felt serenity there. From the first appointment to the very last, I always felt comfortable when I went to my appointments. I was treated as an equal in the relationship. All my interactions with my midwife brought me peace because God's plan for my life was permitted and respected, not resisted and trumped.

During my first appointment, my midwife spent an hour learning who I was and what I wanted from my pregnancy and birth experience. She cared about me as a person, and she looked at every aspect of my identity, my spiritual, physical, and psychological. She also emphasized diet and full body care. My midwife operated from an integrative, holistic model. She looked at me as a whole person, and she saw the whole puzzle that made me who I was.

My midwife never forced me to do anything, but she held my hand by providing me with medical information as I decided what was best for my baby and I. During all my appointments throughout my pregnancy, my midwife spent an hour listening to me. She ensured I felt heard and answered my questions. She provided me with information instead of instruction whenever a decision needed to be made. I was granted informed consent and the autonomy to make personal choices as a fully mature adult capable of making decisions.

My midwife recommended I have a doula because of my traumatic birth experiences. Doulas are professionals who help in childbirth, but their role is separate from midwives. Doulas provide emotional and physical support to moms before and during childbirth. Others in my life also thought I should have a doula. And although I didn't really feel like I wanted or needed a doula, I eventually heeded the advice.

The first two doulas I talked to didn't click with me. I went against my spiritual intuition and hired a "Christian doula" even when I wasn't fully confident in her. A month before I had Gianni, my midwife scheduled a home visit for me, where she would come and see our house and help us to prepare for the home birth. She requested that my doula be there, and my doula didn't show up.

I decided to fire my doula three weeks before my birth. I talked to my midwife during my home visit, and since I was only a few weeks away from going into labor, she suggested I talk to someone she knew whom she thought she would be a good fit for me. This doula wasn't taking new clients, but she agreed to help me.

I got along very well with my doula, even though I only talked to her for a few weeks before Gianni was born. I had a connection with her, enjoyed talking to her, and she agreed to be at my birth if she was available. She spent a few hours talking to me on the phone before I went into labor and once while I was in labor. She didn't charge me for anything she did; she said she was just going to help me. What a serious blessing.

Doulas can cost up to $5,000, and my doula was one of the best. She had a lot of experience. She was also in medical school to be a midwife, so she had more medical training than the average doula. The Lord provided me with the midwife and a doula I was supposed to have at my birth. He gave me the two people who were going to encourage me, believe in me, help me, and guide me into a beautiful, healthy birth, and I am forever thankful for them. I know I had the two women present at my birth I was supposed to have.

The days before I went into labor, I talked to my doula about the feelings of fear that rose up in me toward the end of my pregnancy. My midwife was right birth trauma can lead to feelings of doubt, fear, and insecurity in subsequent pregnancies. I wondered if I would be able to have my son, because I was always told I couldn't have a home natural birth, because of my past. My doula told me to believe in the birth I wanted to have and to trust my body to do what it was supposed to do. She told me it was possible for me to have the birth I wanted, and she helped me to push away the spirit of fear.

In this very late stage of my pregnancy, I realized just how much fear had impacted my first and second births. I let fear make the decision for me both times before. But as I stood in my bedroom on the phone with my doula, I decided this time fear wouldn't control my birth. Doctors weren't going to tell me what I could and couldn't do. I wasn't going to back down to anyone who tried to keep me from doing what I knew God wanted me to do. I was going to use my faith, and I was going to go forward.

The last few days before I went into labor I talked to God. I meditated on His goodness in my life, and I refused to doubt. I knew God would bring my son into the world safely at home, and I held onto God's provision for me. I reminded myself that the Lord is good, and His mercy endures forever.

God gave me a few verses to encourage me as I trusted Him in the days leading to my birth. I went into labor at about 8 p.m. on Tuesday the 28th. My contractions weren't very strong, and they didn't keep me from sleeping or from doing my normal duties the next day. I woke up on the 29th and did my usual workout, homeschooled my kids, and just took it easy. As the day went on, I got more uncomfortable.

Our family ate dinner, and then I took a nap because I knew I was getting close to having Gianni. When I got up from my nap, I sat in the bath for a little while because my midwife said it would help me with the discomfort. Then I tried to go back to sleep for a while. Around 11 p.m. I began to get very uncomfortable. I couldn't stand or move around on my own. I asked my husband to stay with me, and he became fully involved in the labor process.

My husband put our kids to bed, and then stayed by my side. He called the midwife because my contractions were close. My midwife told me she was on her way, and she stayed on the phone with us. When my midwife and my doula got there, they asked me if I wanted to try to stand up. My husband, my doula, and my midwife helped me to get out of the bed and stand. About a minute after I stood, my son was born, and my husband caught him in our bedroom, right beside the bed. They handed him to me, and my husband and I sat together holding our son.

Gianni was born at 2:39 a.m., weighing 9 pounds 0 ounces. I was able to hold him and bond with him from that moment on. My husband took him a few times so my midwife and doula could help me get cleaned up and do routine after-birth necessities, but I got to hold him even when they were cutting his cord. I never lost sight of my son or felt he was being kept away from me in a nursery. I never was unsure of what was being done to him.

My pregnancy and my birth was intentional, managed, and coordinated by the Great Physician. God allowed me to birth my baby at home safely while my other children slept in their beds. God ensured I had the right people and was in the right place when I needed care. My midwife and doula helped to clean the house and started some laundry for us. They left around 6 a.m. My two older children woke up around 7 a.m. and came into our bedroom to meet their baby brother.

My favorite part about my birth was that my kids were never separated from me. They were all home during my labor, my delivery, and my postpartum recovery. Even though my older kids were asleep, they were home, and they were safe and never were disturbed in their regular bedtime and activities. God knew more than anything else I didn't want my children to be away from me. I wanted them all close to me so I knew they were safe. He gave me the birth experience I wanted.

I had so much joy and peace after Gianni was born. I was more content than I had ever been. I felt so empowered and close to the Lord. I was thankful to God for seeing us through, protecting us, and making my birth beautiful. I was thankful to have a husband who I was able to bond with and lean on. I was thankful that I got to decide what I wanted to do with my son, and no one could control me. I was thankful my whole family was under the roof of our home, where we were safe and comfortable.

The Lord orchestrated my pregnancy and my baby's delivery. He healed my spirit, my physical body, and all my emotional wounds, starting the very first day I counted on Him as my Physician. Until this day He has never left my side, caring for my health. He has also taken my children into his care. Jesus serves as their pediatrician and is their primary doctor.

My mature understanding of my spiritual heritage influenced who was in my life and what happened in my life. Without my strong spiritual roots, I would have been in an entirely different situation with different people, and I would have made different decisions.

Knowing who we are Christ is everything. Having a family we belong to shapes our entire lives. When we understand who we are and where we are going, we will not be led astray by people, spirits, or anything that tries to get us off course. God will show us clearly when we need to exit relationships or when we need to enter them. He will guide us into all truth by keeping us focused on the path He has for our lives.

More than anything else, we need to know who we are in Christ. Knowing our spiritual roots and heritage is a requirement to walk by faith, not by sight. Know whom you belong to. Know who is in your boat. It will change everything about your life and your voyage on the earth! I promise!

"A woman, when she is in labor, has pain because her time [to give birth] has come; but when she has given birth to the child, she no longer remembers the anguish because of her joy that a child has come into the world." (John 16:21)

2

Coparenting with Christ

We expect medical services in the modern American healthcare model to benefit the well being of society and individual families alike. Although medicine and medical professionals can be helpful, many scenarios exist that cannot be fixed, explained, or manipulated by humans and science alone.

At times, human systems fail, and in these times, supernatural assistance is critical or otherwise humanity has no hope. Despite science's best efforts, many diseases and other medical concerns cannot be treated, prevented, understood, or stopped with the help of modern medicine, and in many cases, human intervention makes issues worse, not better.

Parents often rely on pediatricians and other child-centered professionals to help them make decisions for their children. Competent parents want their children to be safe, protected, and cared for. For many years, people have assumed that licensed medical professionals are knowledgeable and qualified to give all the needed guidance and recommendations that parents need. Many Americans have relied on large institutions such as the healthcare system, the public school system, and the food and drug administration to guide their decisions with their children.

Numerous parents have falsely trusted that occupational professionals' services are all encompassing and sufficient. However, as we look to the services provided by occupational professionals, we can't ignore the supernatural influence and spiritual components that impact the soul and the physical body. The human makeup and experience has three components. These components are the spirit, the body, and the soul.

The soul is the emotional and psychological realm of the human. The soul is the mind, emotions, and the personality of a person. The physical makeup is separate from the soul/mind. The physical body is the outer shell that houses the soul and the spirit. The spirit is the essence of who we truly are, and it influences both the soul and the body. The spirit is the part of us that can be sanctified and set free and is the part that connects us to God and to the spirit world.

First Thessalonians 5:22 teaches us, "Now may the God of peace Himself sanctify you completely and may your whole spirit and soul and body be kept blameless at the coming of our Lord Jesus Christ." When we begin searching for pure health and wellness, God can illuminate and then eliminate the spiritual, physical, or psychological elements that are harming health outcomes. God will first illuminate problem areas and then He will uproot sickness in disease in the lives of those who are looking for healing and help. God is the light, and when the light enters a person, then the darkness must flee.

Evil spiritual entities and forces desire to influence and control situations of the soul/mind, the body, and the spirit. Even when people are unaware of demonic or angelic influence in their situation, there are often spiritual forces present that want to help or hinder growth and healing. Blindness is one of the tactics the enemy frequently uses to ensure that people remain in captivity. Without vision to see the problem clearly, individuals are unable to pursue, achieve and receive the things that God wants them to receive.

To facilitate our healing without hindrance, it is essential to engage with our faith and explore the supernatural realm. This involves having an interaction with God and recognizing the spiritual dimension inherent in both vision and healing. Second Kings 6:17-18 explains, "Then Elisha prayed, Lord, I pray You, open his eyes that he may see. And the Lord opened the young man's eyes, and he saw, and behold, the mountain was full of horses and chariots of fire round about Elisha. And when the Syrians came down to him, Elisha prayed to the Lord, Smite this people with blindness, I pray You. And God smote them with blindness, as Elisha asked."

Spiritual vision and the spiritual gifts come from the Lord and flow through God's people. God's divinely appointed leadership role operating through Elisha enabled him to perceive what his servant was unable to see. First Corinthians 12:28 says, "So God has appointed some in the church for His own use]: first apostles (special messengers); second prophets (inspired preachers and expounders); third teachers; then wonder-workers; then those with ability to heal the sick; helpers; administrators; [speakers in] different (unknown) tongues."

God gives ministers the gift of healing to help His church and bring new people into the kingdom. Spiritual leaders are tasked specifically to target their faith towards the sickness and disease of others who need healing so that they can become well. Healing miracles encourage praise and worship, and through miracles of healing, many people see Jesus and offer praise and thanksgiving to God.

If someone lacks the ability to see, hear, or they need help receiving their healing, then they are to go to the leaders of the church for assistance. James 5:14–15 instructs, "Is anyone among you sick? He must call for the elders (spiritual leaders) of the church and they are to pray over him, anointing him with oil in the name of the Lord; and the prayer of faith will restore the one who is sick, and the Lord will raise him up; and if he has committed sins, he will be forgiven."

The friends who lowered their friend through the roof to receive healing knew that their friend needed to meet with Jesus (Mark 2:3–5). These friends interceded for their friend when he could not get there himself. They helped their friend get near the Healer. At times, people need help from others to receive healing or miracles. During other times, however, a person must act in faith for himself or herself as in the story of the man at the pool of Bethesda (John 5:8).

During my third pregnancy and childbirth experience I relied on my faith to safeguard both my life and the life of my son. My faith was instrumental in ensuring God's plan for us was fulfilled. The journey of motherhood is both transformative and profound, as a mother's faith temporarily becomes the faith of her child. Motherhood is a ministry, as it involves guiding our children toward Jesus, enabling them to receive His blessings.

God promises pregnant women protection during their labor and delivery. First Timothy 2:15 says, "But women will be preserved (saved) through [the pain and dangers of] the bearing of children if they continue in faith and love and holiness with self-control and discretion." He grants mothers the autonomy to exercise their faith, or to forgo it, and this choice profoundly impacts every aspect of their lives and their children's lives. Before our children take their first breath alone they are fully dependent upon us spiritually, physically, and psychologically for their health and development. Mothers can lead their children to Jesus, or they can lead their children away from Him.

The supernatural realm influences health outcomes. There are angels of healing as there are demons of sickness. Angels are ministering spirits. The Bible speaks of an angel who stirred the waters in the pool of Bethesda. This angel was assisting humanity with healing in obedience to God. This angel worked for God and helped to heal people who needed to receive healing. John 5:3–4 tells us, "In these porticoes lay a great number of people who were sick, blind, lame, withered, [waiting for the stirring of the water; for an angel of the Lord went down into the pool at appointed seasons and stirred up the water; the first one to go in after the water was stirred was healed of his disease.]"

Demons are fallen angels harming humanity instead of helping them. Engaging demonic entities has detrimental effects on our well being in the same way a God appointed angelic visitation can be therapeutic aiding in healing. Mental, physical, and spiritual ailments frequently have their origins in these malevolent influences. Children exposed to unclean demonic spirits, even in utero, will experience adverse impact on their development. Devils frequently go after children and a child's only protection is the faith of their parent.

Matthew 15:21 explains, "After leaving there, Jesus withdrew to the district of Tyre and Sidon. And a Canaanite woman from that district came out and began to cry out [urgently], saying, "Have mercy on me, O Lord, Son of David (Messiah); my daughter is cruelly possessed by a demon."" This Canaanite woman's choice to bring her daughter to Jesus saved her daughter's life. Driven by faith, she earnestly pleaded with Jesus for her child's protection. Her story in scripture demonstrates to us that Jesus will heal and respond to a mother on behalf of their child if they come to Him in faith. A mothers faith in Jesus will protect her children from demon interference.

He answered, "I was commissioned by God and sent only to the lost sheep of the house of Israel." But she came and began to kneel down before Him, saying, "Lord, help me!" And He replied, "It is not good (appropriate, fair) to take the children's bread and throw it to the pet dogs." She said, "Yes, Lord; but even the pet dogs eat the crumbs that fall from their [young] masters' table." Then Jesus answered her, "Woman, your faith [your personal trust and confidence in My power] is great; it will be done for you as you wish." And her daughter was healed from that moment Matthew 15:24– 28.

When a person is sick spiritually, it is called sin. When a person is sick behaviorally and emotionally, it is a disease of the soul, and when a person is unwell with a physical disease it is a physical problem that manifests as disease of the physical body. Yet in all three scenarios, people need supernatural healing from Jesus, who is the greatest physician there ever was or will be.

Sickness, disease, and oppression are works of the devil's kingdom and are a result of sin entering the world. When the devil is involved, he produces pain, torment, captivity, and destruction. We know that the devil is behind sickness and disease, because the scriptures verify this. Job 2:7 says, "So Satan departed from the presence of the Lord and struck Job with loathsome boils and agonizingly painful sores from the sole of his foot to the crown of his head."

Born again believers do not have to tolerate or perpetuate the enemy's lies, as he insinuates that sickness and disease come from God. God does not get glory from keeping people sick. The Bible does not verify this, and in fact, the Bible says the opposite. God gets glory when supernatural healings occur. God gets glory when the supernatural presence of God sets the captives free. Matthew 4:24 says, "News about Him [Jesus] spread as far as Syria, and people soon began bringing to Him all who were sick. And whatever their sickness or disease, or if they were demon possessed or epileptic or paralyzed- he healed them all."

God is opposed to sickness and disease because sickness is a work of the devil. The following verses continue to verify the root cause of sickness and disease. "And there was a woman there who for eighteen years had an infirmity caused by a spirit (a demon of sickness). She was bent completely forward and utterly unable to straighten herself up or to look upward. And when Jesus saw her, He called her to Him and said to her, Woman, you are released from your infirmity! Then He laid [His] hands on her, and instantly she was made straight, and she recognized and thanked and praised God" (Luke 13:11–1).

Jesus spent much of His time on earth healing the sick. Jesus was opposed to sickness and disease, and His ministry focused on delivering people from it. Jesus also instructed His disciples to perform the ministry work of healing. Matthew 10:1 tells us, "And he called to him his twelve disciples and gave them authority over unclean spirits, to cast them out, and to heal every disease and every affliction."

Before sin entered the world, no sickness or disease existed, and we will find no sickness or disease in heaven. Satan has tried to steal the health and vitality of believers from the beginning of time, and he is working today in the world, still attempting to steal the health and wellness of the body of Christ and humanity at large.

If you have ever been to a hospital or have been sick, then you know the longing and the heartache of wanting to be well and whole. Sickness and disease steal many things from people, such as joy, peace, hope, money, and even human life. The Lord would not declare Himself as a healer, and then change His mind and begin to afflict people with sickness and torment. Numbers 23:19 tells us, "God is not a man, that He should lie; neither the Son of Man, that He should repent: hath He said, and shall He not do it? or hath He spoken, and shall He not make it good?" God said He is our healer, and He is a man of His word. God never sends sickness to His church. In Exodus 15:26 God said, "I am the Lord who heals you."

Because sickness and disease are scripturally demonic, the Church is obligated to resist and rebuke it. Devils of sickness and disease afflict people and keep them in bondage, but they can be stopped when the Church intervenes. People need to be set free, and they need to hear the good news that there is hope and healing available, and nothing is too hard for the Lord.

In Luke 4:18–19, Jesus said, "The Spirit of the Lord is upon Me, Because He has anointed Me to preach the good news to the poor. He has sent Me to announce release [pardon, forgiveness] to the captives, And recovery of sight to the blind, To set free those who are oppressed [downtrodden, bruised, crushed by tragedy], to proclaim the favorable year of the Lord [the day when salvation and the favor of God abound greatly]."

This generation of Americans, who have more tangible healthcare access than ever before, are presenting as less well than any other generation. Children are not exempt from the health concerns in America. Many American children suffer from physical, psychological, and spiritual problems. When we examine the medical system and its guidelines, recommendations, and treatment plans, we can see that this healthcare system lacks an element.

God's healthcare system is the only one that works every time without fault or error. God's healthcare plan has been around for thousands of years, and God hasn't changed His policies. Yet, many people, especially in first world nations, have chosen to walk away from God's healthcare system and lean onto the hand of man, because of the increase in technology and human strength. Jeremiah 17:5 tells us, "Thus says the Lord, 'Cursed is the man who trusts in mankind And makes flesh his strength, And whose heart turns away from the Lord.'"

In countries where healthcare isn't very accessible, people cling to the supernatural power of God for help with medical problems. In countries without doctors or industrialized medical care, people would be without any hope or help without the supernatural. The recent movement in some American churches to downplay the Holy Spirit's power and desire to heal and protect believers is truly a first-world luxury that is not an option for everyone in the world. Much of America has become over reliant on doctors, medications, and procedures. Many have gone as far as to willingly participate in cosmetic and unnecessary medical procedures, hoping to achieve physical aesthetics or lifestyle preferences.

Today, many Americans cling to the medical world when they need to cling to God. The Church can help bridge the gap and can draw people to the truth of Christ by members' personal examples. Demonstrating the power of God through the working of signs and miracles within our lives and the lives of others will bring people to Christ. John 2:23 explains, "Now when He was in Jerusalem at the Passover feast, many believed in His name [identifying themselves with Him] after seeing His signs (attesting miracles) which He was doing."

Christians need to inventory their lives and ask the Lord if they have become overly indulgent with their healthcare needs and expectations. We need to determine if our trust is in God or if it is in the world. Inventorying our lives and removing problem areas is incredibly liberating, because it draws us closer to our Creator. The Church has been warned about overindulgence and trust in the world, people, or in things. The sin of idolatry is an unbalanced and immoderate attachment to something besides God. Jonah 2:8 tells us, "Those who cling to worthless idols turn away from God's love for them."

We need to reprove the idolatry of modern healthcare today more than ever. The ever-increasing medical knowledge and advancement will tempt many to rely on humans and medicine instead of God. If people succumb to the temptation to turn away from the Lord and put their trust in people and things, they will become worse and worse. Putting trust in anyone or anything outside of God is dangerous because idolatry gives the devil an open door into our minds, bodies, and spirits.

Judges 10:14 warns us, saying, "Go and cry out to the gods you have chosen. Let them save you when you are in trouble." Americans choosing to turn away from the Lord will continue to experience a decline in their health. The Church's responsibility is to present another way to stop the healthcare crisis in America. As the Church does this, God's will prevails, and more adults and children can access God's promises of health and healing.

Many people are trying to heal the symptoms of disease without discovering the root cause. They do not discern the spiritual component impacting their health because they lack spiritual light. Within all of us there is a longing for wellness. Instinctively, many people know they are unwell and need help. Yet within the medical system, one diagnosis often leads to another diagnosis, and the merry-go-round of sickness becomes a revolving door, where many people never get healed.

For instance, today, people are treating mental disorders in children, such as transgenderism, with hormone-blocking drugs or body altering procedures and surgeries. These procedures and medical interventions cause lifelong problems and irreversible damage to the physical body, and they involve complications that cause more disease. In an attempt to "heal" oneself outside of God through medical interventions many will unfortunately discover themselves worse.

In the humanistic realm people search for help through their food and dietary choices, talk therapy, modern medicine, exercise, meditation, or through the elimination of toxin exposure, to name a few practices. However, without God's helpful insight and involvement, certain things will prevail, despite human interventions, because the roots of these problems are spiritual. Some people eat well and take care of their physical bodies, and they still suffer with a crippling physical disease or diagnosis. Some take their antidepressants and go to therapy, and they still battle to be well and whole.

The devil and some worldwide wicked leaders are attempting to steal the future and the lives of humanity, especially the lives of young people. Without the Church's intentional effort, adults and many children will not have a chance to be well and will be handed over entirely to the devil's captivity. We have the light and the world does not. If we choose to hide the light many will never see it. Believers must take their authority and act in multiple domains as commanded by God. Our foremost priority as the body of Christ should be to strengthen our communities and positively influence the lives of those whom God loves, aiming to bring salvation and liberation from all forms of demonic oppression.

Positions of authority, power, and influence exist in a variety of occupational spheres, including but not limited to healthcare, government, education, food sourcing, church leadership, and entertainment. There is a place for each one of us, and believers must commit themselves to proclaim the truth of God in their personal sphere knowing the reward is great. We must always remember our choices impact our lives and the lives of others both now and in future generations. James 4:17 tells us, "So whoever knows the right thing to do and fails to do it, for him it is sin."

Children should be a primary focus of our efforts, as it is vital to demonstrate to them a superior healthcare system through Christ.

In addition they need to be warned about sin and about the consequences of following the world's system, so they can make an informed decision about their future. God is merciful to children, and even if a child's parents decide to pursue foreign gods, Yahweh will still protect and save the willing and discerning children. For children to be saved, they must be presented with the truth. Adults in a child's life who help to create the culture impact children when they advocate and set Christian societal norms. By creating policies, cultural norms, laws, ethical expectations, and other influential systems Christians can impact the next generation of Americans living within their communities.

As believers teach, protect, and guide children, they are leading the next generation into developing successful adult lives. These children will in turn pursue truth for themselves and replicate truth for their children. The children who are taught the ways of the Lord will commit to justice and truth, impacting the world for God in their generation and the next. God gives a strong warning to those who hinder or cause children to go off course. In Matthew 18:6–14, Jesus said, "But whoever causes one of these little ones who believe in and acknowledge and cleave to Me to stumble and sin, that is, who entices him or hinders him in right conduct or thought, it would be better for him to have a great millstone fastened around his neck and to be sunk in the depth of the sea."

The future of our country is largely determined and established through the works of our hands. Although God is sovereign and knows the beginning from the end, He has given us an assignment and a purpose to fulfill. The choices of the founders of America continue to influence our culture and society as we know it today. Likewise our choices of today will continue into the future. Until Jesus Christ returns for His church the actions of the Church populus are the only determent of the establishment of the Antichrist system.

Ignorance and lack of proper guidance contribute to irresponsible and foolish decisions. The enemy knows this, and so he works hard attempting to keep children from receiving proper instruction. Satan attacks young people who are just starting out in the world, so he can influence and shape their minds and their worldview by creating strongholds.

Strongholds are inaccurate systems of thought. They are philosophies impacting human behavior through the internalization of lies. Strongholds can be personal/individual or they can be cultural/group based. Social norms of societies are regularly rooted in satanic worldviews. Social norms will produce group conformity even when these systems are inherently wrong.

God's standards of righteousness, truth, and justice, may or may not be liked or normalized within a society or other group of people. The normalization of a behavior endorsed by a large group does not necessarily constitute truth. In the Book of Exodus, many of God's people engaged in the worship of a golden calf, prompting outrage from Moses. He recognized the act as ungodly, and indeed, his stance was affirmed by God. The group of people in this instance were the majority, but they were participating in sin. Group conformity is good when the norms are built and established on truth. However, when societal norms are ungodly, group conformity poses a significant threat to the minds, bodies, and spirits of humanity.

Cultural strongholds embedded within the minds and hearts of the majority of a society reproduce incorrect systems of thought within the youth and young people being raised in the society. Through a mixture of ignorance, immaturity, and poor socialization, Satan attempts to build strongholds and fortified places of the mind beginning in childhood. When he is successful he harms and captures young people into believing and living out lies before they have been given a chance to know and experience God's truth. Passion and compassion should motivate us to acknowledge this reality and strive to establish truth within our communities and culture, thereby creating a safe environment for children to grow and thrive.

Childbirth and child rearing norms and social practices within cultures and groups infiltrated by demonic strongholds will harm health outcomes. Women within a society and culture advocating for certain customs may or may not be in alignment with the word of God on these issues. Young women benefit greatly from a relationship with an older, seasoned, believing spiritual mother because spiritual mothers can help guide younger women on the path of righteousness and holiness. A strong, compassionate, loving, and mature spiritual mother guides a younger woman into the understanding of the Lord. Spiritual mothers fight back against the Devil by ensuring the next generation is intentionally instructed into God's systems of thought which will produce righteous decision making.

The devil wants to put the wrong people and the wrong voices around young people so he can control their destiny and prevent them from walking in a relationship with God. Many ungodly women scream the loudest and use their voices and their platforms for destruction. Proverbs 18:17 tells us, "The first one to plead his case seems right, until another comes and cross-examines him. Women of God have a responsibility to push back against this and to use our voices, our wisdom, and our experience to bring positive change to the world. When we cross examine evil we will break strongholds and prove that the devil is a liar to anyone willing to listen.

Young women can receive instruction on how to conduct themselves as wives, homemakers, and mothers when they partner with a spiritual mother. Spiritual motherhood is a gift from God to impart the word of God to the younger generation. Titus 2:4–5 explains, "Older women are to teach the young women to love their husbands and their children. They are to teach them to think before they act, to be pure, to be workers at home, to be kind, and to obey their own husbands. In this way, the Word of God is honored."

When a woman discovers she is pregnant, it is a time of excitement and celebration. God's hope is that women receive support, encouragement, and accurate information about what to expect for their bodies and for their babies. Godly women who have walked in faith themselves can help younger women to make wise and sound conclusions, and these wise decisions will produce a continuation of wellness and wholeness. Hebrews 6:12 says, "Imitate those who through faith and patience inherit the promises of God." Even in a society where the devil has begun incorporating cultural strongholds, spiritual mothers and fathers can prevent the normalization of evil within the next generation by living out, preaching and teaching the truth.

The average woman who participates in America's healthcare system for her pregnancy will be coerced, manipulated, and taught what to think and how to behave by those who do not fear God. The devil has strongholds within the American medical system. The world's system has its own rules, expectations, and demands that women are expected to follow. For instance, when a woman has a baby in the hospital, she is told to not co-sleep with her baby, and instead, she is instructed to lay her baby in a bassinet. This choice is made for the woman and not with the woman.

A pregnant woman in America will also encounter extensive fear-based testing, monitoring, and checking, often without consent. Many procedures, such as checking for dilation during the weeks leading to labor or during labor are done because the doctors want to control the pregnancy. Women are told they will be checked for dilation instead of being asked if they would like to see if they are dilated. Women are given instructions instead of being asked if they would like to participate in a test or procedure.

This control commonly continues from pregnancy through children's lives. Countless parents unknowingly give over their parental rights and authority during pregnancy, and they never fully regain them. As Americans we have inalienable rights and within the eyes of God we have even more. Knowing and asserting our rights as Americans and as Christians is just as important today as it was during the American Revolution. Thomas Jefferson, the third President of the United States noted, "The price of freedom is eternal vigilance." Let us never forget our freedom wasn't free and if we are going to keep it we the people must choose to.

Pregnant American women are overly monitored and controlled because of an underlying assumption of sickness and disease. Currently, the obstetric model of care is the normative birth model built on of allopathic medicine, which pathologizes both pregnancy and birth. Due to their surgical training and knowledge of high-risk births, most doctors in this model will treat women as sick patients who need their help.

Women are told what is best for them and for their babies, throughout their entire pregnancy, and they receive a deceptive method of informed consent. Most American doctors of today do not want women make sound decisions based on their own conscience because they want them to make decisions based on their bureaucratic system's rules and guidelines. James Madison, the fourth President of the United States, famously stated, "The conscience is the most sacred of all property." When anyone tries to violate our rights, take our most prized property/our conscience, whether it is in medicine or any other field, we must perceive it as a threat and act accordingly.

John Hancock, one of the founding fathers of the United States, is noted saying, "Resistance to tyranny becomes the Christian and social duty of each individual. Continue steadfast and, with a proper sense of your dependence on God, nobly defend those rights which heaven gave, and no man ought to take from us." Realizing the system is corrupted and operating through the violation of human freedoms and choice should be enough to advocate for a demolition or a reformation of the medical system. Christians have a duty to resist when our resistance is tied to God's truth and justice.

Doctors and all other medical providers who willingly violate the rights of women do not realize the danger they are in personally if they choose to participate in the decay of the American healthcare system. The failure to protect the freedoms of others will become the failure to have your personal rights protected if the Antichrist system is allowed to continue to grow in strength. Thomas Jefferson noted, "It behoves every man who values liberty of conscience for himself, to resist invasions of it in the case others."

The fear of pathology as opposed to the fear of God is normative in the mainstream model of care, even when women are healthy and are experiencing a healthy pregnancy. This stronghold in the minds of many has become a social norm and custom relating to pregnancy and childbirth. Satan uses fear to manipulate both providers and patients through pathologizing a woman's pregnancy wrongly assuming and treating the woman and her baby are sick and in need of medical care.

Within the obstetric model of care, doctors expect women to come to an excessive number of pregnancy appointments to be treated and monitored for a surplus of potential problems. The obstetric model perceives women as inferior, potentially unwell, and ill-equipped to make the best decisions for their bodies and their babies. The psychological perception and lens that govern the obstetric model of care perceives danger because it is enmeshed with the spirit of fear. Consequently, it causes fear-based decision making for physicians and patients alike.

In the United States, most women are told how to birth, where to birth, and even when to birth, through procedures like inductions and cesareans. In the hospital, women who have been given an epidural cannot get up and must birth while lying down, as opposed to standing up. Many doctors do not want women to birth in standing positions, even if they prefer that method and have not received an epidural. Although women can find doctors and midwives to accommodate their rights and requests, many women are unaware of their rights and their choices. If a woman does not realize that she can decide what is best for herself and her baby, then she may not choose to birth in her preferred way, even if she is uncomfortable with the alternative option.

For thousands of years, women and their babies survived without the American healthcare system. In other countries, women birth babies every day without modern medical interventions. The coercing and pushing that is facilitated by medical professionals frequently comes without warning, and at times, women don't realize their rights, and the rights of their babies, have been violated until later. When people become accustomed to being victimized or have regularly had authority figures, such as doctors and medical professionals, determine their choices, then they lose their own autonomy and sense of control. Many of these common scenarios and services do not alarm them or raise red flags, even when they should.

In America the people are intended to rule and decide every aspect of their lives for themselves. Our country was established on representation. Medical professionals work for the people and thus should not determine the patient's care. Healthcare workers have been hired by the people not the other way around. As the consumer we need to know what we want and demand to get it, because we are paying for it and it is ours right to receive proper care or refuse to participate any further.

A system has become flawed when the consumer is not the dictator of terms determining the course of treatment and care. This is also one of the reasons the world leaders want to push for socialistic medicine and healthcare systems, because then we would not have a right to refute the services and treatments. Imagine if you went to order a smoothie and the cashier determined which kind you received. If you resist that smoothie you are shamed and in some scenarios even denied food service. When we order food from a restaurant we understand we are in control of what we receive and we as Americans should expect nothing less from our healthcare model and providers. Our health is far more important than a smoothie. If we are being denied proper treatment or ethical care it is mandatory to resist and demand better treatment.

In every society there are groups holding more power, wealth, or control over other groups. In America, licensed healthcare workers are an elite powerful group because they regularly influence, shape, and control another group of people. Leadership itself is a blessing from God, and leadership is not inherently evil. Leadership can be beneficial, and it can also be harmful, depending on who is in charge. Proverbs 29:2 says, "When the righteous are in authority and become great, the people rejoice; But when the wicked man rules, the people groan and sigh."

Recognizing when powerful men and women are corrupt, evil, and abusing their leadership position requires us to be informed and alert. Education, information, and knowledge about the rights, freedoms, and choices available are fundamental components people need so they have the confidence to defend themselves against injustice. Without proper education, understanding, and information, there is an unequal playing field. When a woman is uncertain about the necessity of a test, procedure, or recommended course of action, she may lack the confidence to speak up. She may not have any assurance as to what her alternative is or what her legal rights are. In these situations, women are vulnerable to abuse of power.

In an egalitarian medical relationship, all parties hold equal power, knowledge, and wisdom. The provider is responsible to ensure that the woman is informed and equipped to make wise and sound decisions. Women need to be presented with all their options and need to know that they have the right to say no. Women need to be able to choose what they truly want for their pregnancy and their baby. Providers are to respect, honor, and value the choices and needs of the woman and her child during her pregnancy. It is not ethical for a medical provider to assume a position of dominance and power over another person's life.

Women may face feelings of divided loyalty because they believe they should trust their doctor, but they also feel that something is off instinctively and spiritually. When a woman lacks confidence, she may consent to treatment reluctantly and under pressure, as opposed to accepting treatment willingly and cheerfully. A lack of confidence and knowledge leads to an inferior pregnancy and birth experience because women are following the doctor's recommendations, instead of following their own needs and God's leading.

It is possible for women to successfully assert themselves in their interactions with medical professionals' refuting their recommendations. However, standing against a doctor requires knowledge and insight, and a woman needs to be informed and equipped with wisdom and personal discretion to make that decision. For this reason, many women who have given birth before making different decisions relating to their pregnancies, births, child-rearing practices, and their children's healthcare. The knowledge of being violated in previous pregnancies, or the natural wisdom that develops from birthing and raising a child can help women by giving them vision as they acquire knowledge.

Wisdom and knowledge are precious jewels, and when women have knowledge, then they have power. Proverbs 8:11 says, "For wisdom is better than pearls; And all desirable things cannot compare with her." God gives wisdom through His Word, through His people, and through the leading of the Holy Spirit. All three of these avenues permit God to speak directly to us and to provide a clear and straight path. When a woman has the Word of God, the Holy Spirit, and godly counsel, then she is guaranteed success.

Those of us who have experienced and seen the errors, problems, and abusive laws procedures or norms within society occupational boards or other areas of society must intervene because we despise injustice. Christians are to advocate for change, progress, and justice in all domains of their lives. We are to fight for those who cannot fight for themselves. We are mediators and the light in a dying and lost world. We are influential and essential to this planet and our choices impact our lives and the lives of others. If we do not let our light shine there will be darkness covering the earth.

Christian women have a motherhood ministry far exceeding their reproductive. Christian women engage in a motherhood ministry that extends well beyond biological reproduction. We embody the role of spiritual mothers throughout our lives, and God desires for us to share our knowledge, experiences, and wisdom to positively influence the younger generation. Throughout this book, I share personal stories relating to pregnancy, childbirth, postpartum, and child rearing. I know God will give each yearning heart specific instructions relating to their individual health and wellness—and the health of the children entrusted in their care.

For my first two pregnancies, I did not rely fully on the Lord, or trust the Holy Spirit, to guide me into all truth. I leaned too much on the people in my life. I trusted in the world's system and listened blindly to the doctors, because I was ignorant of God's love and God's provision for my health and my children's health.

Now, after the birth of my third child, I am stronger than I have ever been. My birth experience with Jesus, The Great Physician, was one of wellness for my spirit, my mind, and my body. Throughout my pregnancy and my birth, I allowed the Lord to determine my steps, and I silenced the voices that contradicted His leading and direction. I conquered the spirit of fear by challenging the enemy and his suggestions. Gianni, my third baby, was born at home in my bedroom, under the care of God first and a compassionate midwife second. My third birth was beautiful and perfect because a perfect and loving Physician orchestrated it.

I chose to step away from the conventional medical system and engaged the services of a private midwife. The midwife model of care emphasizes and recognizes menarche, pregnancy, and birth as a normal, physiological, and developmental processes. Women are given freedom and support to decide where and how to birth. Women decide the setting and the circumstances for their birth they feel comfortable and confident with.

Most midwives promote women's autonomy and personal decision-making, and they limit the overreliance on medical interventions, preferring holistic intervention, touch, and intuition. Midwives are reproductive justice advocates, and they have helped believers' birth since the book of Genesis.

Genesis 35:17 says, "When she was in severe labor the midwife said to her, "Do not fear, for now you have another son."

Genesis 38:28 tells us, "Moreover, it took place while she was giving birth, one put out a hand, and the midwife took and tied a scarlet thread on his hand, saying "This one came out first."

Exodus 1:15–21 explains, "Then the king of Egypt said to the Hebrew midwives, one of whom was named Shiphrah (beauty) and the other named Puah (splendor), 'When you act as midwives to the Hebrew women and see them on the birthstool, if it is a son, you shall kill him; but if it is a daughter, she shall live.' But the midwives feared God [with profound reverence] and did not do as the king of Egypt commanded, but they let the boy babies live. So the king of Egypt called for the midwives and said to them, 'Why have you done this thing, and allowed the boy babies to live?' The midwives answered Pharaoh, 'Because the Hebrew women are not like the Egyptian women; they are vigorous and give birth quickly and their babies are born before the midwife can get to them.' So God was good to the midwives, and the people [of Israel] multiplied and became very strong. And because the midwives feared God [with profound reverence], He established families and households for them."

In America today, the midwife model of care is less popular than the obstetric model of care. For many, the obstetric model may appear to be the best choice. This path is enticing in times of indecision and uncertainty or when a woman is facing a major life event, because it offers us with perceived control and certainty. *And no wonder! For Satan himself transforms himself into an angel of light* (2 Corinthians 11:14).

Many doctors and child specialists willingly fill parents with information and "knowledge" of what is best for children. People need help, and they look for answers, so the doctors try to give them what they seek. However, not all knowledge is created equal. From the beginning, in the Garden of Eden, the knowledge of good and the knowledge of evil both existed. Knowledge is not always helpful, and in fact, sometimes it is harmful. Where our information comes from is important.

The spirit of the Antichrist wants to use professionals, such as doctors, as pawns to the end-time Antichrist agenda. Evil spirits want to destroy our Christian society, weaken the Church, and prepare the world for the one-world government and one-world system as mentioned in the book of Revelation.

First John 4:3 says, "And every spirit which does not acknowledge and confess that Jesus Christ has come in the flesh [but would annul, destroy, sever, disunite Him] is not of God [does not proceed from Him.] This [non-confession] is the [spirit] of the Antichrist, [of] which you heard that it was coming, and now it is already in the world."

The spirit of the Antichrist wants people to be weak, dependent, and unable to resist world dominance and control. The devil wants people to rely on mankind, because a reliance on humans keeps people from depending on God.

In recent years, the mainstream United States' medical model has begun to change to a system of greed and control as opposed to patient protection and welfare. When a medical system becomes violent, because it is led by corrupt leaders, while operating primarily for profit, it is dangerous because the roots are enmeshed with sin. The pursuit of personal power, wealth, occupational reputation, and occupational relationships frequently triumph over truth and ethics for many providers. Things such as money laundering and unholy alliances within the workplace have become common occurrences for many, and consequently, providers are entangled in Satan's work.

Some have embraced the doctrines of their profession and unwillingly aligned their life with a doctrine of demons and a worldview that is anti-biblical. These individuals need to repent and be delivered.

When God liberated His people from Egypt, He freed them from authoritarian and abusive governmental leadership. In contemporary times, individuals must earnestly seek God and desire liberation from oppressive control and dominating systems of governance. When people willingly submit and cooperate, they permit Satan to reign and exercise dominion. However, we have an alternative. We need not succumb to malevolence.

First Timothy 4:4–2 says, "Now the Spirit expressly says that in the latter times some will depart from the faith, giving heed to deceiving spirits and doctrines of demons, speaking lies in hypocrisy, having their own conscience seared with a hot iron." The average obstetric provider contends on the medical arrangement that suits the medical profession's best interest, as opposed to supporting the best interest of mom and baby. Their own seared conscience leads to the desecration of another person's right to operate from good conscience.

An inflated sense of self-confidence, combined with a seared conscience, creates room for abuse of power, justifying the abuse. Patients are assigned the position of victim and are viewed as inferior, thus, unable to make wise decisions without their providers' help. A personal conflict of interest, combined with extensive medical training, impaired spiritual vision, or willful compliance enables violence against women and their children. The normalized standards that push moms-to-be into situations, outcomes, and health plans that ensure that the medical professionals' and the systems' own liability and name is protected, over the patients' rights and well being, are unjust and unholy.

The abuser/abusee dynamic that is present in many provider/patient relationships is a textbook scenario and is easily identified by those who know what they are looking for. An abusive provider's deluded self-concept and inflated ego will manifest itself in many ways. For example, providers often compare themselves to superheroes or as saviors. They assign themselves a place reserved for God alone. Nurses and doctors alike commonly make statements like, "Without me people would die. They need us! What would they do without us?"

The conscious or unconscious awareness of abuse does not justify violent acts and cannot be used as an excuse for occupational failure. Accountability is necessary for personal or societal change to occur. When someone does something that is wrong, he or she must be held accountable for it. The victim/abuser dynamic is classic and is seen in all forms of abusive relationships. The abusers justify the control because they see the abused person as weak, vulnerable, and unable to live without their help and control.

Abusers convince themselves that they are helping the victim because the victim is weak without their guidance, support, and overstep of boundaries. The victims have a weakened sense of knowledge, power, and authority and are unaware of their inner strength. People allow abuse to continue because they feel helpless and unable to make a different choice. Abusive providers in America hold power through both financial control and social status. They perpetuate violence against their victims by isolating outside involvement, violating personal privacy and autonomy, limiting independence, threatening and intimidating, minimizing, and victim blaming.

The Governments Overreach on American's Occupational Boards

Throughout the American workforce, strict regulations and requirements govern most careers. If business owners or employees won't conform to the standards of practice, ethics, or licensing and education requirements that are preestablished by industry leaders and the government, then they can be shut down or made unable to work. Standards of practice, rules, and regulation are needed to maintain order, but we must oppose the overregulation of industries spearheaded by wicked and ungodly leaders who have been inspired by demonic agendas.

During the COVID–19 lockdowns of 2020, many Americans saw just how much demonic leaders desired to control all industries. The medical profession was hit the hardest by this, and many people lost their jobs because they wouldn't comply with a forced vaccine.

All companies were urged to require vaccines, and a lot of hospitals would not allow doctors, nurses, or other healthcare workers to work without the vaccine. Other industries also threatened to fire employees who wouldn't comply. When rules and regulations of occupational boards begin to impose upon our God-given freedoms and the American Constitution, then Americans must refuse to comply to these guidelines and regulations. Americans need guidelines, but we also need to have our God-given freedoms, and to be represented fairly and equally. Wicked leaders should not control the entire trajectory of our country.

Numerous doctors, healthcare workers, scientists, and other professionals refused to get vaccinated during the COVID-19 pandemic. Many opposed the government's overstepping during the pandemic, and many didn't agree with the medical science behind the vaccine. Unfortunately, many licensed professionals lost their jobs.

Many others were stigmatized and received a bad name in their field for holding a different perspective than their peers.

Even with previously successful careers, good evidence, scientific studies, and personal or religious reasons to back their claims, many medical professionals were shut out of their chosen careers and occupations. The refusal to bow to the government's control caused many to lose the lives they knew before the COVID-19 pandemic. The fear of losing things in life often keeps people stuck in a system they know is broken. I believe many medical professionals know the system is not working properly, and they want to change it, but they are afraid to step out or stop practicing medicine. This fear leads to conformity.

The refusal to bow to an ungodly system of control and domination is a righteous decision. In the book of Daniel, four men who served the Lord refused to bow to a wicked government mandate. Daniel was one of the men who refused to stop praying to God, even when he was threatened. Ultimately, Daniel was arrested and thrown into a lion's den, being given a death sentence. God sent an angel to shut the lion's mouth and protected Daniel, because Daniel refused to bow to an idol. Daniel didn't listen to the government. Daniel listened to God.

Shadrach, Meshach, and Abednego also chose to denounce and rebuke idol worship. The wicked government of the day, the king, mandated that citizens bow to a gold statue. Shadrach, Meshach, and Abednego were thrown into a fire because they would not bow to a false god their government had created. God protected these men, like He did Daniel, because they boldly stood for Him alone. The standard of righteousness and holiness, and a refusal to bow to idols, should always triumph over the world's system. When believers choose to serve God alone, the Lord goes with them, protecting them supernaturally from all who seek to destroy their lives.

The commitment to genuine ethics and best practice within all occupational boards must guide us over all rules, mandates, ethics, laws, or expectations, even if this means we lose our jobs. Occupational boards, governmental leaders, laws, or mandates should never be allowed to reign over the commands and the laws of the Lord. Many professionals in various fields denounce God and the Bible and serve other gods. The spirits in the world that are at work in the lives of those who turn away from the Lord intend to normalize and mandate compliance from all in the land. These evil spirits will not stop taking ground unless they are forced to, and we are obligated to combat them with a refusal to comply.

The Church must be represented through a variety of positions, and we must maintain leadership roles in our society. Christians should be represented in politics, education, and in all spheres of government and public life. We must participate in shaping the culture and trajectory of the country by stopping the spread of unholy mindsets, mandates, and laws on local, state, and national fronts.

Each of us has a role to play in shaping the future of our country. The Church must be militant and united, in words and in deeds, to stop the enemy's advance. Philippians 2:2 says, "Make my joy complete by being of the same mind, having the same love [toward one another], knit together in spirit, intent on one purpose [and living a life that reflects your faith and spreads the gospel—the good news regarding salvation through faith in Christ]."

In the Bible, the midwives decided to obey God and His precepts over the precepts of the Egyptian king. The Lord honored and rewarded their compassion and protection of the babies in their care. Currently, in the United States, the midwife model of care is more closely aligned with the Bible and God's desire for human birth than the obstetric model of care. Many midwives permit women to follow the Lord's guidance, because they respect a woman's autonomy in making healthcare decisions.

By partnering with women, midwives partner with God, because they do not determine the woman's path and interfere with a woman's decisions. Midwives give women the freedom to listen to the guidance and recommendations of the Holy Spirit and scripture, while providing safety and support within the birthing process.

When I chose to birth my third baby at home, I rested in God's protection instead of the protection of the medical mandates and suggestions. After a woman has undergone two cesarean births, many providers do not allow for trials of labor for vaginal births. Although it is technically illegal for providers to require cesarean births from their patients, many providers eagerly recommend them. Even when providers know the risks, the ethics, and the law, out of a sense of self-interest and self-preservation, many do not support women's body autonomy and their desires to vaginally birth their child after a previous c-section.

The more c-sections a woman has had, the harder it may be for her to find a provider who will let her have a trial of labor and attempt for a vaginal, low-intervention birth. Women need to be informed before they have the first c-section about the potential long-term birth consequences and repercussions that could come from an unnecessary cesarean birth.

In addition, many home births are regulated by the state. Some states do not allow women to have a home birth if they are carrying multiple babies or if they are deemed unfit or unhealthy to birth at home. A former cesarean birth can be a reason to deem a woman unfit to have a home birth or a vaginal, low-intervention birth in future pregnancies.

My midwife partnered with me to give me freedom of choice before, during, and after birth. I legally pursued a home birth in my state because I was healthy with no problems presenting in my pregnancy. My midwife did not manipulate, control, or force me into testing, or procedures. Because I chose to give birth at home, I wasn't given medications that often cause side effects and problems for mothers and for babies. I wasn't told what I was going to do for vaccines, circumcision, breastfeeding, or co-sleeping. Birthing at home allowed me to be respected for what I wanted to do, and it gave me freedom, allowing me to birth and parent as a co-parent with Christ alone.

The Lord was with me, and He protected my baby and I throughout my pregnancy and postpartum period. I enforced my covenant rights as a believer, because I believed that my baby and I were safe and healthy in God's care. God's Word reassured me that I didn't need to fear problems, sickness, or disease.

My midwife partnered with me in these beliefs, and was encouraging and supportive in these truths. Her belief in my ability to have my son at home safely was helpful and provided me with the encouragement I needed on the journey. When another person partners with us in faith and positive expectation, it can bring forth positive things in our lives. This truth is one of the distinguishing things separating homebirths with midwives and hospital births with physicians.

Positive expectation brings positive results! Proverbs 23:18 teaches us, "Surely there is a future [and a reward], And your hope and expectation will not be cut off." When mothers and midwives believe together that babies can safely and healthily be born through low intervention practices, then it is more likely to happen. Conversely, when professionals or individuals look for problems, sickness, disease, and issues, they are believing and attracting those things into the lives of people. Job 3:25–26 says, "For the thing which I greatly fear comes upon me, And that of which I am afraid has come upon me. "I am not at ease, nor am I quiet, And I am not at rest, and yet trouble still comes [upon me]."

Challenges may arise when they are sought, yet blessings also spring forth when we place our faith and trust in God. Let no challenge stop you from the victory you have been given in Christ. I knew my family's insurance would not provide financial assistance for my child's birth. Our insurance did not cover any of the medical expenses of my pregnancy when the services were to be performed by a birthing center, at home, or through the assistance of a midwife. This could have stopped us from pursuing midwife care, but I refused to let money be a deterrent of God's plan for my life.

Our family chose to pay for our son's home birth, and doing so did cost us more money than it would have if we had chosen to use insurance through a doctor and a hospital. However, the financial cost for the ability to be in total control of my pregnancy was well worth it. I was afforded an exceptional birthing experience, characterized by superior care. A healthcare system that emphasizes choice is truly a blessing, and it is important to recognize that there are forces opposed to such options. Finances often impact women's provider choices. The enemy and the Antichrist spirit want us to go to an "easier, more affordable" socialist form of medicine so we will lose all control.

If a provider or birthing choice is not covered through insurance, then a woman should choose to do what is best for her and her family without financial pressure. To be truly liberated and free, a person must not be controlled by external pressures and scenarios. Instead, she must be led by a God who is bigger than anything that exists in the material world. Matthew 6:24 says, "No one can serve two masters; for either he will hate the one and love the other, or he will be devoted to the one and despise the other. You cannot serve God and mammon [money, possessions, fame, status, or whatever is valued more than the Lord]."

3

Informed Consent, Boundaries, and Birthing Freedom

In the United States of America due process laws exist to protect and safeguard Americans' rights to control and possess their own person. Liberty interest protects a person's right to consent in many spheres of life, giving them the right to do, or not to do, something, if it doesn't impose on governmental interests and law. To consent means to give compliance in, or approval of, what is done or proposed by another party. When someone gives his or her consent, he or she is making an agreement with another voluntarily. This voluntary agreement is based on a person's own free will and does not involve manipulation or coercion.

The liberty interest protection of the law provides American adult citizens with personal autonomy in matters relating to their own medical treatment plan and medical options. American adults are legally protected to refuse any unwanted medical treatment, if they decide they do not want to be treated. The American Supreme Court has long upheld the right of individuals to make medical decisions for themselves and for their children, except in situations where the individual or the parent is deemed incompetent and unfit to make a safe, informed, and wise decision.

Throughout history, many healthcare personal autonomy cases have been heard in courts across the country. There are and always have been many fiery debates and court hearings on the national and the state level regarding the medical issues involving children and women's health. Due to the age and the developmental level of children, children cannot consent legally to medical treatment and procedures. Parents are given legal responsibility to represent their children, and parents consent, permit, or deny healthcare procedures on behalf of the child.

In most cases, parents have their children's best interest in mind, and these laws protect and preserve lives. However, when parents are mentally unsound or choose to protect their own self-interests over the interest of their children, this is incredibly dangerous to children. Most parents want to protect their children and will make wise medical decisions to protect, help, and save their child's life, but unfortunately, some parents in the world do not make the best decision for the safety and protection of their child.

Deuteronomy 12:31 instructs us, "You shall not behave this way toward the Lord your God, for they have done for their gods every repulsive thing which the Lord hates; for they even burn their sons and their daughters in the fire [as sacrifices] to their gods."

False gods in the lives of people can take on many forms. Some parents worship money, and they put their children in dangerous and unsafe situations for money. Others worship drugs and become mentally incapacitated and ill, unable to care for themselves or others due to their addiction. Other parents abandon and abuse their children for sexual lust and a relationship with sexual sin. Sexual sin can result in child sexual abuse by a boyfriend or other acquaintance that is allowed access to a child, and it can cause a mother or father to abandon the child to start a life with someone new.

False gods are demons that want to destroy the lives and the minds of children and parents alike. Many children grow up traumatized, abused, and neglected as the result of their parents' relationship with false gods. Devils are given access to children through the parents' sins. These scenarios can take many forms and contribute to a plethora of situations, but they all leave children vulnerable to Satan's attacks because of the parent's refusal to serve the Lord.

Aborted children are those who have been sacrificed to false gods. Sin and demon worship are the reasons why many babies are murdered in their mothers' wombs. In the landmark case of 1973 *Roe v. Wade*, the court ruled in favor of abortion as a woman's right to privacy, establishing the right of a woman to terminate her pregnancy. The *Roe v. Wade* court ruling stated the constitutional right of a woman to an abortion should be protected before the gestational age of 24 weeks when a fetus is viable outside of the womb. After the ruling, women were given a legal right to kill their children due to their own personal reasons and desires. This case legalized the right of women to perpetuate an act of violence against their children with medical professionals' assistance.

In the mental health field, there are commitment laws that govern *the threat to life of self or the life of another*. When any American citizen threaten to harm themselves, or to harm another person, this law interferes, deeming the individual a threat to themselves and society. Authorities attempt to stop any individuals threatening harm to themselves or others through commitment laws because of the sanctity of life. If a mother confesses a desire to harm her own child, she should be immediately deemed legally unfit to make a proper decision on behalf of her child, forfeiting all rights to make welfare decisions regarding the child's life because of her mental incapacity.

It is ethical, fair, and just to apply the same standards of care for mental health and protection of life to women who are pregnant. A failure to apply the same standard is inherently biased and allows a subpopulation of society to receive rights other groups do not have.

All threats to human life need to be taken as a mental health crisis, enabling authorities to step in with the attempt to save another person's life. A failure to respond in this professional and compassionate way shows a lack of moral judgment as well as an unequal enforcement of proper procedure and law.

Bias is a prejudice in favor of or against one thing, person, or group, compared with another in a way considered to be unfair. The willful allowance of pregnant women's homicidal idealization, without proper crisis intervention, is harmful to women and babies alike and meets the formal definition of bias.

By providing a woman with a biased right to kill another human being who is living in her womb, without the law attempting to stop the murder, the authorities neglect their duty to protect, willfully refusing to act on the behalf of America's most innocent population. Women and babies alike are neglected through this failure, because women will personally suffer when they are not restrained from abortions.

Many women live to regret their abortions and suffer with psychological issues after an abortion. "Abortion is consistently associated with elevated rates of mental illness compared to women without a history of abortion" (Reardon 2018). Physical complications, as severe as death, have occurred because of abortions. Un-repented abortions are spiritually taxing and will count as murder during the judgment. Women need to be safeguarded and protected through love and compassion from having abortions, because abortions are not healthcare. Healthcare attempts to save lives and abortions aim to take them.

A mother's homicidal idealization towards her child needs to be addressed on behalf of the woman and the child. There must be an attempt to stop a woman from harming her baby per mental health protocol. Holding women accountable for homicidal idealization and behavior protects the rights and freedoms of all Americans, chiefly the unborn American.

Without the proper understanding and implementation of this kind of responsibility and accountability for American citizens and society, people inherently perpetuate victimhood mindsets and begin to lean towards communist and socialist forms of government. Both socialist and communist mindsets, policies, and customs must be rejected entirely if America is to remain a healthy and thriving nation.

Communist and socialist political, economic, and social systems are established as the result of a victim mindset and worldview. These systems exist because people fail to hold themselves and others as responsible agents relating to the choices they make and the outcomes of their lives. Personal autonomy, responsibility, and accountability are cornerstone components of a thriving society and political system such as the American republic form of government. In a republic government, citizens are representatives and are responsible for the outcomes of their lives, and they take responsibility for their choices. Republics give people power and decision-making capability, while holding people accountable for both good and bad decisions.

A sense of agency mentality is present within thriving political, economic, and social systems. The sense of agency mentality exemplifies the truth that change in circumstances comes from taking responsibility for the future and contributing to your life and the lives of those around you. A person with a sense of agency realizes through personal growth and accountability that great things can be achieved individually and socially. True empowerment is directly associated with a sense of agency mentality, because through wise decision-making and effort, there is hope for change and for success.

In direct opposition to a sense of agency, an individual who holds a victim mentality feels like an inactive participant in his or her own life. These individuals feel they are not responsible for the outcomes of their lives, and as a result, they become victims of life and life's circumstances. A victim mindset exemplifies the belief that there is no hope or confidence in positive change because positive change is viewed as impossible or uncertain. As a result, an individual with a victim mindset will have life dictated to them and are easily manipulated and controlled by others who realize the power that is available to those who harness it.

Victims are weak, vulnerable, and easy to control. Weakness, vulnerability, and a loss of autonomy and personal control are not characteristics that should be normalized among American women. God created women to prosper, succeed, and to dominate and conquer in life. Women were created to build and to accomplish, and women hold immense power. Proverbs 14:1 says, "The wise woman builds her house with her own hands but the foolish one tears hers down."

The abortion advocates prey on women, teaching and instructing women to be controlled by a trillion-dollar industry. Women are lied to and are told they are unable to build and succeed, while being used to contribute to the success of an immoral and successful industry facilitated and predominantly run by women.

We must learn to accept responsibility for our lives and our choices to maintain our American civilized society. Responsibility and accountability allow people to feel confident in their abilities to make good decisions. Accountability empowers people because it forces them to face consequences for both wholesome and bad decisions.

Holding someone responsible for a bad decision highlights and instills a sense of awareness. Without a conscious awareness of the need for good decision-making there is little hope for change in choices, because the person remains blind to his or her own influence in the outcome of his or her situation.

People learn lessons through poor decision-making as well as good decision-making. For instance, a wholesome decision leads to wholesome results. When people learn their good decisions are directly related to their success, then they are motivated to continue making wise decisions. As an active participant in their success, people become empowered and confident in their own abilities and choices. Through consistent, wise decision-making, there is hope for positive change even in unfavorable starting places.

The founding fathers understood the elements of responsibility, accountability, and individual empowerment. The underlying premise of our American republic is rooted in choice and control, where the people get to govern and represent themselves. In a republic, people take responsibility for their lives and the lives of their community and country through choosing representatives. The choice a person makes directly contributes to the outcomes of his or her life. In this system, there is an understanding of sowing and reaping. What you do affects what you receive.

Sowing and reaping is God's system He established for the earth. Genesis 8:22 says, "While the earth remains, seedtime and harvest, cold and heat, winter and summer, And day and night Shall not cease."

When there is a denial of sowing and reaping in people's lives there is chaos. Denial of sowing and reaping is correlated to a person becoming obstinate to the laws of nature God established.

When a person sows good decisions and makes wise choices, he or she will reap those decisions. Likewise, an individual who sows evil and unrighteousness will reap from their decision. Galatians 6:7 teaches, "Do not be deceived, God is not mocked [He will not allow Himself to be ridiculed, nor treated with contempt nor allow His precepts to be scornfully set aside]; for whatever a man sows, this and this only is what he will reap."

Freedom of choice is a right and a privilege that comes from our creator. Our American unalienable rights, mentioned in the United States Constitution, state that our rights have been given from God and not man. All people in America have the right to life, liberty, and the pursuit of happiness, because these are God-given rights to human beings. People are free to decide what they want to do with their lives. Blessing or cursing in this life and the next is directly related to the consequences of our human choices while we are alive and living on the earth.

Women may feel the desire to kill their babies, and many may choose to have abortions against the government's standard. Yet, if a woman confesses her idealizations or makes the decision to abort her child, she should be held accountable for it. Women need to be made consciously aware of the reality of their bad decision, so they are ultimately empowered to make the right decisions, which will lead them to true success and fulfillment in the long run.

God wants us to know that the person who sows will reap, and there is a direct blessing or cursing associated with choice and decision. When we fail to enforce consequences for poor decisions in our lives or others' lives, we enable people to not realize the impact of their choices on a personal or a societal level. The lack of enforcement of consequences hinders individuals from fully understanding God's design.

Galatians 6:8 says, "For the one who sows to his flesh [his sinful capacity, his worldliness, his disgraceful impulses] will reap from the flesh ruin and destruction, but the one who sows to the Spirit will from the Spirit reap eternal life."

Today, science confirms and supports that babies are separate beings from their mothers from conception. In fact, science has proven that babies and mothers have separate blood circulatory systems. The blood of the baby does not mix with the blood of the mother because of the separation process occurring within the placenta. The placenta is also separate and not a part of the mother's body, coming out upon the birth of the baby. Science shows babies and mothers are separate entities from conception onward.

Jeremiah 1:5 declares, "Before I formed you in the womb I knew you [and approved of you as My chosen instrument], And before you were born I consecrated you [to Myself as My own]; I have appointed you as a prophet to the nations." God established boundaries in the womb separating the mother and a child.

A refusal to acknowledge the separation of mother and child shows a person is living in a delusional state of mind, because science and religion both confirm this truth. Human beings are separated from one another, beginning in the womb, through our personalized DNA, the instructions for our development and creation.

God gives each person his or her own identity through specific coding and instructions threaded within the DNA. From conception, babies are unique humans with their own coding and instructions, and several scientific proofs show this separation, difference, and boundary that separate babies from their mothers.

Boundaries are unseen walls and lines that separate people or things from one another. They are personal property lines that divide and separate. Boundaries help people to identify where their rights end and the rights of another person begin. Boundaries protect, guard, and separate people, places, and things to bring order and protection. Boundaries separate personal rights, wants, needs, feelings, and thoughts from those of other people.

God established boundaries in the heavens and in the earth to bring security and order. In the beginning, God separated the heavens and the earth, and He separated the land from the water. From the beginning, God has used boundaries to divide and bring order to all life forms.

People who promote abortion do not have an understanding of proper and healthy boundaries. Abortion advocates ignore the lines separating a mother from her child, which are confirmed through scripture and science. These individuals do not differentiate the child as *separate* from the mother; instead, they view the child *as* part of the mother. Abortion advocates live in a delusional state of mind, believing the lie that a child is not a "self" of its own, because a child is one with the mother.

This is a mental health identity disorder called depersonalization/derealization disorder (DPDR). DPDR is an identity disorder causing delusional mental states in which people do not have a strong sense of personal self. Without a strong sense of self, a person cannot acknowledge the sense of self in others.

DPDR puts people into "an estranged state of mind that involves profound feelings of detachment from oneself, sense of self, and the surrounding environment, respectively" (Murphy 2023). Due to the inability to acknowledge one's own "self," the person does not perceive the "self" of another, because he or she lives in a state of delusion and lies about his or her own identity.

In these mental health disorders, boundaries are blurred and people cannot separate *the truth* from a lie. They cannot separate the rights, desires, needs, and presence of others because they cannot identify these elements within their own self. Through a state of delusion and confusion, these individuals are unsure of their own decisions because they lack a sense of self.

This is what enables them to perpetuate evil against others. They cannot see the other's rights, needs, desires, or choices or respect the other's separate, unique, and valuable self. Depersonalization of self and others leads to dehumanization, which is the deprivation of positive human qualities in another person. Dehumanization has led to many worldwide abuses and atrocities, abortions being among them.

Anyone who is under the influence and control of Satan lives in a delusional state of mind confused about his or her true identity. God created each person with a plan for his or her life. When people fail to find out who God is and who He created them to be, they are destined to live a lie and to live in an alternative state of mental, spiritual, and physical confusion. Mental health disorders related to identity have their roots and their foundations tied within the lies of Satan. In Matthew 4:6 Satan tried to attack Jesus' identity when he said, "And he said to Him, If You are the Son of God, throw Yourself down; for it is written, He will give His angels charge over you, and they will bear you up on their hands, lest you strike your foot against a stone."

When Satan gets people confused about their *identity*, he can tempt them to do things God has not created them to do. Mental health identity disorders deceive and enslave humanity into thoughts, beliefs, and actions that are against God and His plan by severing the individual from his or her Creator and his or her intentional, God-given design.

God ordained boundaries and identities to protect and preserve lives. Evil boundaries and identities harm and destroy lives. Satan inspires the separating and creating of boundaries that place human groups into "less or more" or "more valuable or less valuable." This enables people to be dehumanized and treated in horrible ways.

Acts 17:26 says, "And He made from one man every nation of mankind to live on the face of the earth, having determined their appointed times and the boundaries of their lands and territories."

God created people, and made boundaries to differentiate them, but God shows no favoritism and makes no room for abuse or injustice. Human life is sacred, and people matter to God. God created the babies in the womb, and He created the women who are carrying them.

James 2:1–4 teaches, "My fellow believers, do not practice your faith in our glorious Lord Jesus Christ with an attitude of partiality [toward people- show no favoritism, no prejudice, no snobbery]. For if a man comes into your meeting place wearing a gold ring and fine clothes, and a poor man in dirty clothes also comes in, and you pay special attention to one who wears the fine clothes, and say to him, "You sit here in this good seat," and you tell the poor man, "You stand over there, or sit down [on the floor] by my footstool, have you not discriminated among yourselves, and become judges with wrong motives."

The Bible has many warnings to humanity about treating certain groups as superior or inferior. When people treat others with partiality, they assume lesser, or greater, characteristics of certain groups, leading to higher instances of abuse. In cases of abortion, babies are classified as inferior to the mother and thus are dehumanized and violated in the womb. This is anti-biblical, and it is against the instruction and word of the Lord. Anytime a group of people is dehumanized and violated, abused, or mistreated, it is a work of the devil, and God is opposed to this work.

When the government operates from a sense of agency mentality and operates as a republic, the people will be empowered to make good decisions. In these types of social systems, people will suffer less from identity disorders like depersonalization disorder, and human life will be protected from crimes and violations of dehumanization and depersonalization. "Power and organizational hierarchies are ubiquitous to social institutions that form the foundation of modern society.

The mental health of Americans is related to the social and political system reigning the land. Born again believers who fight to end policies and laws such as abortion are working on God's behalf and freeing people from the lies and deceptions of the enemy. They are also making a positive impact on the mental health of our society.

For human kingdoms to prosper, they must be set up to model God's kingdom. Power and organizational hierarchies are not evil. In fact, God's kingdom is hierarchical. God established authority, power, and boundaries for a reason. God wants order on the earth. Power and organizational hierarchies help to establish boundaries, accountability, and responsibility, and bring order to the earth when they are modeled after God's righteousness and justice. America has been a thriving and successful country because it was molded and founded by God's laws and definitions of righteousness and justice.

Romans 13: 1–5 teaches, "Let every person be subject to the governing authorities. For there is no authority except from God [granted by His permission and sanction], and those which exist have been put in place by God. Therefore whoever resists [governmental] authority resists the ordinance of God. And those who have resisted it will bring judgment (civil penalty) on themselves. For [civil] authorities are not a source of fear for [people of] good behavior, but for [those who do] evil. Do you want to be unafraid of authority? Do what is good and you will receive approval and commendation. For he is God's servant to you for good. But if you do wrong, [you should] be afraid; for he does not carry the [executioner's] sword for nothing. He is God's servant, an avenger who brings punishment on the wrongdoer. Therefore one must be subject [to civil authorities], not only to escape the punishment [that comes with wrongdoing], but also as a matter of principle [knowing what is right before God]."

When an organization's hierarchical system becomes corrupted and fails to model after God's laws and precepts, there will be trouble. Proverbs 29:2 tells us, "When the wicked rule, the people mourn."

In recent years there has been a movement to destroy the United States of America through the establishment of wicked social norms, law, occupational standards, and other demonic agendas and doctrines. Many unbelievers have instituted social norms, laws, and policies against the traditional values and culture of our country.

The medical system is one system that has increasingly become infiltrated and manipulated through laws, systems, and occupational ethics and norms that are anti-biblical in nature. The infiltration of evil agendas has contributed to a decline within an American hierarchical system and has led to an inferior health model for many Americans.

Many physician/patient relationships enable an abuse of power facilitated by unhealthy separation of groups. Inappropriate boundary knowledge or implementation combined with secular training and education may create an atmosphere where doctors are perceived as superior, and patients are seen as inferior. These perceptions can easily lead to a coerced system of reluctant patient consent, taking away a person's autonomy and responsibility. The limiting of personal choice will then interfere with the sowing and reaping on behalf of the patient because the responsibility for health has been given to the authoritarian professional who is deemed to be more informed and powerful.

Many patients never learn to take responsibility for their own health and their own choices for healthcare. Countless Americans are thoughtlessly led through the system, being told what to do as opposed to being given choices and options for their own lives.

When medical professionals practice medicine using an unhealthy authoritarian style of leadership, they will harm and hinder their patients' long-term health and growth. Authoritarian leadership breeds emotional and spiritual sickness and disease. Some of the problems shown to be associated with authoritarian leaders are a lack of self-awareness, limited accountability, poor decision-making, and a refusal to challenge the status quo, even when a positive change needs to be facilitated.

Under a doctor's authoritarian leadership, many patients will consent to treatment plans or procedures grudgingly because they don't feel comfortable saying no to their provider. Patients may be afraid of being denied care and give into their providers' abusive demands out of fear and insecurity. Many authoritarian leaders in medicine refuse to see patients that do not follow their recommendations.

For instance many pediatricians refuse to see children who have not been vaccinated. These medical professionals would rather deny children medical service than allow parents to determine a preventive treatment plan for their children independent of the physician's recommendations. These providers deny women and their children their legal and their God-given rights, circumventing individual choice and freedom through occupational control, domination, and abuse of power.

Reluctant giving and coercion are anti-biblical concepts. As a leader, God never uses unhealthy forms of leadership to gain control. God instructs and provides information and then allows people to determine for themselves what they want to do. Decisions made reluctantly and rooted in coercion violate the individual. Reluctant and coerced decisions break true consent by imposing the will of the physician and denying the patients the right to choose for themselves. The authoritarian doctor will control instead of instructing the patient. He or she will deny service before allowing freedom of choice.

Medical professionals require patients to sign consent forms that can be held up in a court of law. Legally, the doctors and medical professionals cannot be held responsible for the negative consequences or repercussions for many of their professional actions and decisions once the patient signs the forms acknowledging the risks. In such circumstances, the patient remains accountable for their medical decisions, even if they were reluctantly influenced by the doctor's recommendations. Doctors who know the law and then manipulate the law for their own benefit, trying to avoiding the repercussions and consequences for their actions, should be removed from the medical profession. Any avoidance of consequences and responsibility on behalf of the doctors that leads to an abusive treatment model for patients should not be tolerated in the field of medicine.

It is always the professional's responsibility to ensure that he or she is handling patients with care and proper ethics. The leader should be held accountable for his or her interactions with those he or she leads. Patients need to be informed and knowledgeable about their rights, and they need to stand up when those rights are being tested or violated. Yet, all professionals should be held to a standard of care that protects the patients' rights even when the patients are unaware of their own rights.

Many Americans today do not know their medical or God-given rights, and they assume the doctors are treating them in an ethical manner. Toxic doctors frame the conversations and the interactions with patients through deceptive language and behavior.

When I was taking my children to their pediatrician for well visits, the nurses or doctors would come in with the legal paperwork and say, "Your child will receive these vaccines today." The nurses and doctors didn't ask me if I would like to get my child vaccinated, because they don't want parents to feel as if it is an option.

Many unhealthy medical professionals are fully aware of the deceptive language, the power differential, and the legal angle they are using to victimize people. Many providers have an intention to ensure that their view of the preferred treatment or healthcare plan is performed, because many believe they are better equipped to make the best decisions for people's health. These providers treat consenting adults as if they are children, undermining their autonomy to make decisions regarding what is best for their lives.

This abusive and twisted perspective of superiority is an overstep of personal autonomy and responsibility, allowing for a justification of an abuse of power. By keeping patients out of the driver's seat for their families' health, many medical professionals feel they are doing what is best for their patients, while perpetrating an unhealthy and abusive leadership style within a relationship.

Being in control of our own destiny and our own life is a gift from God. God gave us freedom when He created us. No person or spiritual entity has the right to take that away from us.

"Coercive power is the use of force (implied or otherwise) to achieve compliance" (Gibson, Medeiros, Giorgini, Mecca, Devenport, Connelly, Mumford 2014). When physicians and other professionals use their position of power, suggestive language, and other forms of manipulation to gain compliance and control of another person's health, they are violating a person's right to choose for himself or herself [the liberty interest]. These professionals intentionally cross another human being's boundary, even when they refuse to acknowledge it or when they choose to justify their behavior.

There is *societal* pressure to give into authority figures. Christians feel this pressure even when they feel a reluctance in their spirit. Christian citizens in particular want to follow order and proper authority, because they know most law and authority comes from God. Yet, whenever we feel a reluctance in the spirit, there is a reason for it.

God does not expect us to obey and to submit to all authority in all circumstances because at times when those in charge will be against the Lord's plans and commands. God warns His people of error and trouble, and He leads people away from problems through the inner knowing of the Spirit. If a professional or an authority figure is abusing their power and authority, the Holy Spirit will try to intervene and warn the believer to protect him or her. When a believer discerns something is off, the believer must listen to his or her spiritual discernment. We must trust our spiritual knowing more than we trust our physical surroundings.

The Bible is a book of power. God gives His people the power to overcome, the power to defeat the enemy, and the power to succeed. Acts 1:8 says, "But you will receive power when the Holy Spirit comes on you."

Rights are often stripped from individuals through the power of deception. Many con people use deception to get people to hand over their power and forfeit their rights willingly and unknowingly. A decision to consent to something, even when you are deceived into consenting, is still often upheld by the law. From the beginning, Satan convinced humanity to willingly consent and violate the commands of God through deception and manipulation of the law.

God's design for society and family is hierarchical. In the family, God is on top, the husband is the head of the family and leads the wife, and the children are under the parents. Individuals outside of the home, including extended family, are not to have an equal say in the family's affairs and decisions.

When a professional or extended family member oversteps and attempts to influence, control, or interfere with a family's decision-making process, that person is performing the work of Satan. Professionals and extended family members are free to make suggestions when they are willingly brought into a decision-making process by the family member, but if the guidance and the interference is done out of proper order, it is unbiblical.

Many parents are undermined because they let others have unbridled access to their life and the lives of their children. Unethical professionals and unhealthy family members often push to control the lives and destiny of the family. Yet, this pushing must be confronted and stopped, so God's system and expectations for marriage, parenting, and family can be fulfilled. The parents are responsible to stand against all attempts to control and dominate the decisions and the destiny of the family. In doing so, the family follows the proper hierarchy of God and allows God's design to manifest.

Anytime the order established by God is reversed or infiltrated, problems will occur. In recent years, some states have legalized a child's choices to have abortions or surgeries to change their gender when they are not developmentally prepared to consent to these procedures. In these wicked and demonically inspired scenarios, the providers place themselves and the child at the top of the pyramid while placing God and the parents at the bottom, ultimately reversing God's design for family and social life.

Satan intentionally reverses God's design. Today in society, we often see the providers controlling families from the top, followed by the child's self interest. Then the mother, the father, and God come underneath.

Satan has intentionally infiltrated God's design for marriage, family, and societal relationships. It is not a coincidence that God's plan for a healthy functioning family and society has been polluted and inverted in recent years. Through inverting healthy family design and healthy relationship patterns, Satan gains dominion over people and society alike. Individuals and groups are dictated and determined through cultural and societal norms or laws that are antibiblical and thus unhealthy, and everyone becomes increasingly unwell.

In an unhealthy family model, a grandparent will attempt to determine the decisions for their grandchildren, when the grandchildren's parents are capable to decide. In turn, these grandparents violate God's standard. This is also true for professionals outside of the home or family. Doctors can suggest and provide information to a mother or a father regarding their child's care, but they are not free to impose their own belief systems and ideas onto the family.

Many grandparents or professionals exert unhealthy pressure to force their grown children or patient's decisions believing it is normal behavior. I have heard testimonies of mothers who were coerced into allowing procedures such as circumcision because of external pressure. Whenever a parent is undermined and usurped of their God-given authority and power, the devil has had an influence.

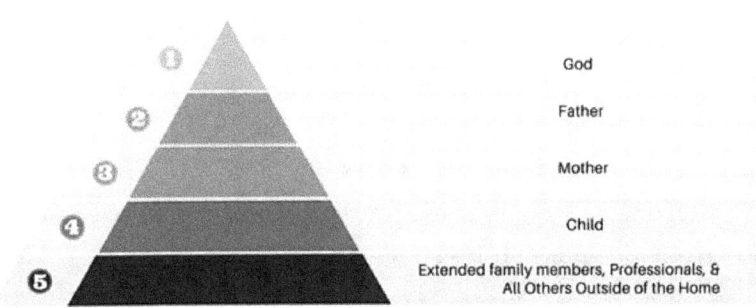

God's Family System

1. God
2. Father
3. Mother
4. Child
5. Extended family members, Professionals, & All Others Outside of the Home

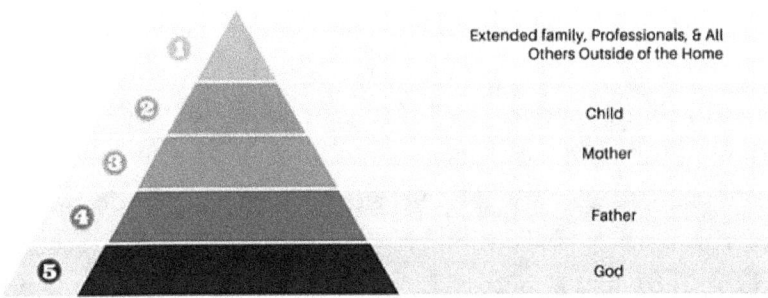

Corrupted Family System

1. Extended family, Professionals, & All Others Outside of the Home
2. Child
3. Mother
4. Father
5. God

Proverbs 25:17 instructs us, "Do not let your neighbor's house become an extension of your own life." Honoring the boundaries and the borders between individuals is fundamental in promoting health and respect. No authority figure, whether in society or within the family, has the right to control anothers life.

Parents are given a short window of time to train their children, but even parents must allow for personal choice and consequences, so their children can learn right from wrong. Parents who try to force their children to do the right thing through an authoritarian leadership style will find that their children are emotionally unwell and unprepared for life.

Boundaries are to be used to protect individual and family life. As followers of Christ, we are expected to not conform to humans or to allow anyone to impose themselves in a place where they don't belong. By asserting and establishing proper boundaries, believers can do the work of God and exalt his system for society, and marriage and family relationships.

When believers interact with others on the earth as imitators of God, they refuse to allow anyone to force, dominate, and control them. There must be a check and an accountability on all individuals who are willingly or unwillingly insubordinate to God's system and design for society, marriage, and family.

As believers, we are free from Satan's power and dominion, and a boundary separates us from the people of the world. Yet, Satan tries to violate our covenant and cross the boundary into the believer's life. For this reason, Satan is called a thief, because he attempts to gain access to things that are not his to gain access to. Satan wants to take things through violating boundaries.

Ephesians 4:27 teaches, "Neither give place to the devil." The body of Christ has a responsibility in their lives to restrict access to the devil. The Church must resist and stand up, holding firm boundaries with the devil and with the world.

God has a will that does not automatically come to pass. We must choose to take responsibility and cooperate with God and His will to see God's plan unfold. God allows us to consent to His plan and to choose what we want to do with our life.

In John 2:5 we read, "His mother said to the servants, 'Whatever He says to you, do it.'" The servants had a choice and decided if they wanted to listen to Jesus's instructions. When the servants decided to obey, they received their blessing, witnessing a supernatural miracle. Yet, the servants could have chosen to ignore the instructions of Jesus and experienced an entirely different fate.

Many Bible stories illustrate that we have personal responsibility apart from God. There are healthy boundaries between God and humans. There is always respect and choice combined with strong leadership and clear expectations from the Lord, but God never practices coercion or forces His will upon humanity. God allows people to consent in all things.

When Moses instructed the Israelites to put blood on their doorposts, he created a boundary, but the people were free to choose to obey or disregard the instruction. The blood on the doorpost boundary divided people into two groups, due to their personal choices. Exodus 12:12–13 says, "For I [the Lord], will pass through the land of Egypt on this night, and will strike down all the firstborn in the land of Egypt, both man and animal; against all the gods of Egypt I will execute judgments [exhibiting their worthlessness]. I am the Lord. The blood shall be a sign for you on [the doorposts of] the houses where you live; when I see the blood I shall pass over you, and no affliction shall happen to you to destroy you when I strike the land of Egypt."

We can refuse to comply with the work of the devil by refusing to do something. For instance, when the government legalizes abortion in many states, Christians must obey the "Do not kill or do not shed innocent blood" verses in the Bible, choosing to not do something that the government says we can do.

Then, there are situations where Christians must demand to not do something against the recommendations of the authorities if the authorities oppose God's standards and laws. For instance, when pediatricians or the CDC insist through coerced power that all pregnant women and young babies receive certain vaccines, on certain intervals, at certain times, the believer must not comply if the Holy Spirit has prompted them to not vaccinate their child.

Although public schools generally require vaccines for children to attend, Christian parents can exempt their child from vaccines on a religious ground. As a former school counselor, I was tasked with collecting religious exemption vaccine paperwork. Through my background in education, and my knowledge of my rights as an American citizen, I was equipped with the tools necessary to resist the coercion of the medical professionals and their personal preference to vaccinate my children. First Corinthians 6:19–20 teaches us, "Do you not know that your bodies are temples of the Holy Spirit, who is in you, whom you have received from God? You are not your own; you were bought at a price. Therefore, honor God with your bodies."

My daughter's pediatrician did not know about my background or my profession when she attempted to vaccinate my daughter. The nurse told me what shots my daughter would receive that day, and she attempted to have me sign the paperwork. When I told the nurse that my daughter would not be vaccinated, she got the doctor.

The doctor tried to convince me that I was making the wrong decision by not vaccinating my child. As I refused to compromise, and I instructed her that I was religiously objecting, she attempted to use religion as a means of making me comply to her personal preferences for my daughter's health by insisting the pope approved of vaccines.

When the religious manipulation failed, my daughter's pediatrician asked if I was going to send my daughter to public schools. My daughter was a few weeks old, but this doctor tried to induce a fear of the future into my heart by telling me my daughter would not be allowed to attend any public school in the area without these shots.

I politely informed her that I was aware of the religious exemption laws for education, and I didn't appreciate her not respecting my right to not vaccinate. After multiple failed coercion attempts, this pediatrician backed off. Yet, without intentionality and a strong refusal to participate in the unhealthy medical relationship, I would have consented to something that I was not comfortable with, due to a pediatrician's coercion.

This experience demonstrates the agenda of many medical professionals' self-interest and their refusal to respect another person's boundaries and rights given by God and the law. The pediatrician understood parents have a legal right to deny vaccinations on religious grounds for schooling, but she concealed this information from me to safeguard her own interests. She used deception was used as a tool to coerce me into following her will for my child.

Unfortunately, I also encountered coercion and deception with my pregnancies in the hospital setting. Two separate obstetricians at two separate hospitals coerced me through their language and the spirit of fear to have cesarean births, even when I was opposed to doing so.

I strongly expressed my desire to have my children naturally to both of my doctors. However, the medical providers used their "medical expertise" to shame me into believing I was wrong, insisting that I should trust their judgment more than my own. With my first pregnancy, I was given an ultrasound at 40 weeks, to measure my baby's size. This information was used to determine that I was to give birth through a cesarean. Despite the scientific evidence showing that ultrasound measurements for babies are unreliable and often inaccurate, my doctor convinced me it was necessary to have my son through a cesarean.

"Ultrasound estimation of fetal weight is a highly influential factor in antenatal management, guiding both the timing and mode of delivery of a pregnancy. Although substantial research has investigated the most accurate ultrasound formula for calculating estimated fetal weight, current evidence indicates significant error levels" (Milner & Arezina 2018).

My medical providers didn't tell me that I had to consent to a cesarean birth. My doctor framed our interaction, ensuring that I felt that I had to have my baby this way, for the child's protection. He brought in my paperwork, and asked me to decide on which date I would like to have my baby through a cesarean.

I was not presented with the full picture, and I did not know that I could say no. I was not informed about the errors in ultrasound weights, and I was not told about the potential consequences associated with cesarean births. Additionally important to note, many women have given birth to children bigger than my son was measured in his ultrasound. In fact, my third pregnancy was done at home with a baby of the same weight, proving I had not needed a cesarean birth for my first child.

However, as a new mother, days away from giving birth, I was easily manipulated and swayed to obey my doctor's orders. I did not know my rights, and I wanted my baby to be safe, so I trusted a doctor who negligently refused to present me with all the information.

In both my first and my second pregnancy, my doctors knew what they were doing, and I was not the first woman to be violated in this manner. Just like a domestic abuser or a rapist continues to abuse and violate woman after woman, doctors and many other professionals continue to violate women and children in the name of medicine. Any professional who violates a woman's rights and then attempts to cover himself or herself legally is still guilty in God's eyes. God designed humanity to choose for themselves. God designed a hierarchy for family and human relationships, and He designed sowing and reaping, but within God's perfect design, there is peace and order, never forced compliance.

Individuals and families need to be empowered in their decision-making abilities for the future of our American republic. Personal decision-making and accountability is God's system to keep people healthy and strong. Stripping and weakening humanity and human autonomy furthers the enemy's agenda and should be resisted at all costs. When we are not responsible and accountable for our choices, we are emotionally sick.

God's design for humanity is choice and consequence for choice. His plan is to allow sowing and reaping, seedtime, and harvest. God does not determine the outcome of people's lives. Instead, He gave that right to us!

Genesis 1:26–28 says, "Then God said, 'Let Us (Father, Son, Holy Spirit) make man in Our image, according to Our likeness [not physical, but a spiritual personality and moral likeness]; and let them have complete authority over the fish of the sea, the birds of the air, the cattle, and over the entire earth, and over everything that creeps and crawls on the earth.' So God created man in His own image, in the image and likeness of God He created him; male and female He created them. And God blessed them [granting them certain authority] and said to them, "Be fruitful, multiply, and fill the earth, and subjugate it [putting it under your power]; and rule over (dominate) the fish of the sea, the birds of the air, and every living thing that moves upon the earth."

4

The Power of a Godly Decision

Most women know from the time they are young girls that being a mother is a reward. Young girls model their mothers and enjoy playing with baby dolls. Psalm 127:3 says, "Behold, children are a heritage from the Lord, the fruit of the womb a reward."

Motherhood is a role unlike any other. Pregnancy and childbirth are a gift to women from our Creator. In James 1:17 the Bible explains, "Every good and perfect gift is from above, coming down from the Father of the heavenly lights, who does not change like shifting shadows." In the book of Genesis, Satan impacted human consciousness and thought through introducing lies and the temptation of evil. Satan used the tactic of faulty reasoning to lure humanity away from God's will and purpose.

Anyone who asserts themselves as a feminist and pro-women and simultaneously advocates for abortion has been misled. The pro-abortion movement states the beliefs and actions of abortion advocacy empower women. Yet, the popular narrative claiming that abortion is pro-women is falsehood. Permitting an act of violence against children does not empower women. Acts of violence are in direct opposition to women's God-given makeup. Women are designed to be nurturing, loving, and compassionate. God appointed women to protect and honor life forms.

The rights of humanity do not come from the government. Human rights are from God. God establishes absolute truth, and people can be deceived through philosophy, faulty education, unhealthy social norms and relationships, and even their own feelings. In the fallen and corrupted world, many things attempt to separate people from biblical thinking, believing, and behaving.

In Proverbs 14:34 we learn, "Righteousness exalts a nation, but sin condemns any people." Righteousness in this context means a group of people governed by just and godly principles. When leaders establish their leadership based on God's definitions of righteousness, the people will reap the benefits. When leaders have an established leadership based on wickedness and sin, the people will suffer. Leadership is important, because leaders can inspire and motivate, or they can tear down and demoralize groups of people.

The United States of America was founded on godly and righteous principles. Woven throughout the Constitution and the laws of American history, the founding fathers established a government that allowed people to worship God freely. The Founding Fathers used the Bible to create many of the laws and the norms of the country. The Bible has been an influential force in the success of America. The first President of the United States, George Washington, wrote, "While we are zealously performing the duties of good citizens and soldiers, we certainly ought not to be inattentive to the higher duties of religion. To the distinguished character of Patriot, it should be our highest glory to add the more distinguished character of Christian."

Because America's governmental leaders are voted in by the people, the governmental laws and social norms are a direct result of the choices of the American people. Christians must be represented through political candidates and involve themselves in politics to ensure their leaders are like-minded in their policies and the vision for the trajectory of the country. Christians make up a large margin of people within America. The Christian voice represented properly can secure and influence the vision and the future of the United States.

We are negligent if we fail to contribute to the politics of our country. When the Church opts out of politics, it results in wicked people's interests being represented and normalized. Then the rights and agendas of the wicked become exalted over the rights and agendas of the just.

In recent years, the loosely defined concepts of "choice and rights" have become cornerstone principles of a mainstream feminist advocacy group to legalize and create access to, abortion in the United States. Abortion was only normalized and legalized, because the wicked agenda of evil individuals became acceptable in the land, while the righteous agenda of pro-life Christians became secondary.

God does not want the interests and beliefs of the Church to be second to the rights and interests of immoral secular groups. Born-again children of God have an obligation to challenge and despise all evil agendas and theories. We must rebuke all evil, instead of allowing it to take hold within our country.

Theories are not absolute truth, and many theories exalt themselves against the word of God. Evil thoughts, agendas, and theories that are rooted in wickedness and sin can be stopped from infiltrating the United States of America when they are not the beliefs and norms of all people in the country. If the American Church votes and is militant and involved, the Church's agenda will take ground.

Many American policies and laws have state, local and federal government variations. Federal laws and standards are expected to be upheld by the entire country. Then, other laws and standards are selected individually through the state and the local governments. The American voting system encourages the variations present in the federal, state, and local levels to ensure that all people are represented in the environment in which they live and work.

In June 2022 the federal government overturned the *Roe vs. Wade* case that required all states to adhere to the federal law for women to have the right to an abortion. This overturning of the federal mandate to accept abortion directed the abortion issue back to the individual states. Before the overturning of this case, the federal government required the states to accept and legalize abortion, even when many people within the states opposed legalized abortion. Since the overturning of *Roe vs. Wade,* individual states have been strengthened, empowered, and protected legally to stop abortion in their state and local community.

Stubborn and rebellious decisions or laws established against God and His Word are the precursors to failure. When individuals or groups choose to be rebellious or callus to God and His precepts, then they are on the route to destruction. The route to destruction continuously leads to future problems in health, economics, and other critical fields.

However, there is a road that is full of peace, prosperity, and success. This road can be found, even when the starting place is a prison. Psalms 68:6 tells us, "God makes a home for the lonely; He leads the prisoners into prosperity, only the stubborn and rebellious dwell in a parched land." Disadvantages dissipate from our lives when we align ourselves with Christ. When we choose to remain close to Him and place our trust in His guidance, God will remove the obstacles in our path, granting us promotion, success, and assistance. This principle is applicable not only to individuals but also to communities and nations. Divine support is granted to those who align themselves with God.

Believers must advocate for righteousness and justice in our communities and our country, because our lives and the lives of the next generation depend on it! God will make a way for a country that chooses to honor Him. He will prosper and protect a country that loves Him and His laws and precepts. If America wants to remain prosperous, successful, and a light on a hill, then it must remain in covenant with God's laws and standards.

Matthew 5:14–16 tells us, "You are the light of [Christ to] the world. A city set on a hill cannot be hidden; nor does anyone light a lamp and put it under a basket, but on a lampstand, and it gives light to all who are in the house. Let your light shine before men in such a way that they may see your good deeds and moral excellence, and [recognize and honor and] glorify your Father who is in heaven."

A Christian nation, like the United States of America, is visibly successful because of the leadership, laws, and the policies that respect God's standards. Through our laws, our values, and our actions, we shine a light to the lost and dying world surrounding us. Our choice to do good to all people through moral excellence is the lure that continues to draw others to us as Americans.

The American Declaration of Independence, states that the American identity "holds old these truths to be self-evident, that all men are created equal, that they are endowed by their Creator with certain unalienable rights, that among these are life, liberty and the pursuit of happiness."

Somebody who chooses to obey God's laws because they are culturally taught to do so will inherently be happier, healthier, and more successful than the person who is taught culturally to disregard God and His precepts. Social norms and laws that honor God will benefit those who follow them, even when the individual does not know that he or she is in agreeance to God's plan for mankind and are benefiting from His Word.

Equally true, social norms and laws that are anti-biblical in nature will form roots of destruction. In places where evil policies, agendas, and leadership reign, chaos and devastation will fill the economy, the social structures, and the overall health of the people.

Advocating for righteousness and justice for all Americans begins with believing that God's Word is true and everything else is a lie. We must know that God's truth will help our culture and our society. Through this inner knowing we advocate for the truth of God, resting assured it will restore, and bring hope and healing to the lost and dying world. Second Timothy 1:7 says "For God did not give us a spirit of timidity or cowardice or fear, but [He has given us a spirit] of power and of love and of a sound judgment and personal discipline [abilities that result in a calm, well-balanced mind and self-control.]"

A sound mind enables people to make decisions that are godly, righteous and full of wisdom. The Church must influence the world to make sound decisions, because we have been given a sound mind that the world does possess. Without continually renewing the mind, people cannot attain a sound mind, and they will make fear-based, emotional decisions. Fear-based decisions always lead humanity into difficulty. Thus, the Church is responsible to lead the world into truth, because without God's light, the world cannot see, hear, or understand the way to go. Without the light, they will stumble and fall within utter darkness. They will be controlled by human emotions and fear.

Christians are called to be bold and confident in their beliefs, and they are called to stand courageously against evil. Part of standing up for righteousness and truth is refusing to be quiet or to back down when the Devil or evil individuals attempt to stop the Lord's will from coming to pass. A believer must know the truth and must refuse to compromise with the enemy's lies. The authority of the earth has been given to believers, and Jesus delegated us with the assignment to stand firm in the evil day, proclaiming His truth at all costs.

Second Corinthians 10: 1–5 says, "Now I, Paul, urge you by the gentleness and graciousness of Christ—I who am meek [so they say] when with you face to face, but bold [outspoken and fearless] toward you when absent! I ask that when I do come I will not be driven to the boldness that I intend to show toward those few who regard us as if we walked according to the flesh [like men without the Spirit]. For though we walk in the flesh [as mortal men], we are not carrying on our [spiritual] warfare according to the flesh and using the weapons of man. The weapons of our warfare are not physical [weapons of flesh and blood]. Our weapons are divinely powerful for the destruction of fortresses. We are destroying sophisticated arguments and every exalted and proud thing that sets itself up against the [true] knowledge of God, and we are taking every thought and purpose captive to the obedience of Christ,"

Paul wanted believers to know that thoughts and purposes that set themselves against God are to be rejected. He wanted the Church to know the enemy and the enemies' forces would come against Jesus and God's will through arguments, theories, beliefs, thoughts, and concepts that are in opposition to God's definitions of righteousness and truth.

Paul encouraged believers to be bold and fearless and to stand against all temptations of the flesh, including the temptation to be passive and cowardly. The fear of being accepted by the world is not a new fear, but we are specifically warned to resist this demonic spirit.

The pro-abortion propaganda instills feelings of fear and shame into women. These feelings are opposite to faith and confidence. Pregnancy is a time of a woman's life when women need to be encouraged and supported, not discouraged and undermined. Yet, the enemy uses people to bring his plans and purposes to the earth. Those who speak for the devil will use prophesies to demean, degrade, and destroy any woman who believes them. Women who believe evil spirits and abort their children believe an evil report or evil prophecy that has been spoken over their lives.

The Bible says in Numbers 13:30–32, "Caleb quieted the people before Moses, and said, "Let us go up at once and possess it; we are well able to conquer it." But his fellow scouts said, "We are not able to go up against the people [of Canaan], for they are stronger than we are. So, they brought the Israelites an evil report of the land which they had scouted out, saying "The land through which we went to spy it out is a land that devours its inhabitants. And all the people that we saw in it are men of great stature."

Satan strategically used the ten spies to instill doubt and unbelief into the people. Most of the Israelites believed the evil report spoken by the ten spies. But accepting the evil prophecy was detrimental to the people. Their unbelief brought great mourning, crying, and weeping.

Many women today believe the evil report about their baby and their future as it is given to them by those who speak for the enemy. Many women also mourn, weep, and cry over their decision to abort their baby. The evil spirits inspiring the evil report of unbelief bring the same sadness, heartache, pain, and suffering to people in the modern world as they did thousands of years ago.

Satan knows the way we view ourselves can influence our choices. It is not a coincidence that many abortion advocate considerations are formulated on the basis that women cannot or should not continue a pregnancy because they are not properly equipped to handle it. These same assertions of inadequacy impacted the minds and behaviors of the Israelites. The Israelites believed in the evil report of the spies because they viewed themselves as ill equipped to take the land God had given them. The Israelites looked at themselves and their limitations and consequently shrunk back in intimidation and fear, when they could have moved forward in faith in God.

Women who have aborted their children can receive forgiveness for their sin when they have a repentant heart. God pardons sin when people repent. Although women can receive the forgiveness of God, many women will continue to suffer from their decision all through their lives. Many women never get over the trauma of an abortion.

These women experience a lingering consequence that cannot be erased even when the Lord has pardoned the sin. The Israelites suffered a similar fate for their unbelief towards God. Numbers 14:22-23 declares, "Surely all the men who have seen My glory and My [miraculous] signs which I performed in Egypt and in the wilderness, yet have put Me to the test these ten times and have not listened to My voice, will by no means see the land which I swore to [give to] their fathers; nor will any who treated me disrespectfully and rejected Me see it."

Notions and assertions opposing faith, empowerment, and the ability to conquer and prosper are perpetually rooted in the lies of the enemy. When given the proper opportunity and the correct information, women can be successful against all natural odds if they choose to partner with God and His Word. Women can do all things with the help of God. God will give help and direction when a woman asks Him for it. In Numbers 14:24 God said, "But My servant Caleb, because he has a different spirit and has followed Me fully, I will bring into the land into which he entered, and his descendants shall take possession of it."

People should never give up the right to control their personal lives and destiny. Joshua and Caleb's decision to determine their fate allowed them to take the Promised Land when the rest of the camp died in the wilderness. Personal choice determined the outcome of these men's lives, showing us that God permits each person to choose and to receive based on their choosing.

Yet, in cases of abortion, people impose themselves upon another's rights. In doing so, they are demanding domination of another's destiny, instead of controlling their own destiny. Women have a choice to do as they please with their own bodies. They can choose to have sex, which they know can lead to pregnancy. Once pregnant, they can choose to raise the child or to put the child up for adoption; however, they should not be able to choose to murder the child, because the child is a separate human being from the mother.

Many feminists have rightfully advocated for the rights of women against the domination of men and sexist institutions. When men victimize women for their own gain, they are wrong and need to be stopped. Yet, the advocation for abortion is also an advocation to exert unhealthy control of another human being.

Abortion devours the vulnerable child for a type of "success" or gain. This contradiction in theory and behavior is hypocritical. Women who demand to be given respect and fair treatment by an advantageous group cannot rightfully justify controlling another person that they have an advantage over.

The assumptions that in some situations women can't be responsible and keep their baby have been constructed from the demonic doctrine claiming that human beings are not free beings acting from a sense of self-determinism and agency. A belief that a woman is disadvantaged and hopeless, and thus cannot succeed because she is oppressed and weaker than the system at large, stems from a deterministic worldview.

Determinism is a demon doctrine of philosophy and science that states that events in the universe, including human decisions and actions, are casually inevitable. In a deterministic view, all situations are determined by preceding events, natural laws, or sociological systems, and thus, people have little to no influence over their life, choices, or their future.

Determinism, as a theory, is demonic because it directly opposes the word of God. Consistently, the Bible emphasizes the human's free will and the human's right to act and determine his or her own destiny. People who are deceived by determinism often stop making good decisions in their lives, because they feel helpless to change life's outcome through good decision-making. A deterministic view limits humanity while exaggerating the intensity of external life circumstances. Determinism minimizes the authority, control, and power of humanity, and it reveres and establishes itself against God's Word.

Determinism theory when applied to an individual's circumstances allows the devil to dictate life for a person, because the person does not resist evil or demonic attacks, assertions, or claims to their lives. Those who are deceived by determinism accept the enemy's lies and allow evil to reign over everything that happens to them and to their loved ones.

When challenge, opposition, or heartache occurs, these individuals embrace adversity instead of rejecting it, because they view themselves as unable to overcome, change, or address the situation. Situations and outcomes are viewed as fixed or controlled, instead of free standing and able to be manipulated.

Some in the body of Christ have been blinded by determinism. For religious people, determinism leads them to blame God for the problems they face. Determinism also contributes to people losing their faith. First Timothy 4:1 warns us, "But the [Holy] Spirit explicitly and unmistakably declares that in later times some will turn away from the faith, paying attention instead to deceitful and seductive spirits and doctrines of demons."

For people to *turn away from the faith,* they must have *at one point been in faith.* Ministries that overly emphasize the "sovereignty of God," while minimizing personal responsibility, authority, and self-control, are being misled by a demonic doctrine. God does not control and *determine* all things.

If God were sovereign and controlling all things as some suppose, then we would be able to blame Him for all good and bad occurrences. A deterministic doctrine in the Church blames God for evil things such as murder, rape, sickness, and disease. It questions God's goodness and tolerates the enemy forces' attacks against humanity.

If a born-again believer gets diagnosed with cancer, then deterministic churches will say things like, "We don't know why God allowed this to happen to brother George" or "It must be God's will for George to go through this so he can learn something."

These approaches to disease are inspired by the devil. When the Church leaders should take their authority over the cancer and heal George, they instead blame God for making George sick and refuse to step into their God-given position of power and influence. This allows Satan to remain in control of the person's life, when the Church could have intervened and set George free from his disease.

Deterministic doctrines within churches present a gospel that is different than the one that Jesus presented to His Church. Second Corinthians 11:4 teaches, "For [you seem willing to allow it] if one comes and preaches another Jesus whom we have not preached, or if you receive a different spirit from the one you received, or a different gospel from the one you accepted. You tolerate all this beautifully [welcoming the deception]."

We are warned not to tolerate or choose to accept a demonic doctrine. God does not *determine* this for us. People determine their fate and others' fate by performing the good works and deeds we were instructed to perform while believing God and opposing the enemy. God knows what is going to happen, but He doesn't sit in heaven manipulating the fate and the future of humanity.

A deterministic mindset is unhealthy because it is a doctrine of demons. The deterministic doctrine that is present both inside and outside of the church spreads emotional disease and produces symptoms of dysfunction in the lives of those who expose themselves to it. The Church was warned in Second Corinthians 11:4 not to willfully welcome these kinds of demon spirits, but unfortunately some churches today spread this form of emotional sickness and disease from the pulpit.

Proverbs 23:7 says, "For as he thinks in his heart, so is he [in behavior-one who manipulates.]" If we believe in our hearts that we can or cannot achieve something in life, then this truth manifests itself outwardly. What we think about ourselves and others impacts our life choices and our life outcome. It affects the way that we do ministry. We can have a healthy view of self and others, or we can have an unhealthy one.

When someone is free to be anything, choose anything, and become anything, he or she isn't limited, confined, or unable to achieve due to set criteria. Most abortion advocates believe being a woman is an obstruction in life. Through a deterministic worldview, women are perceived as disadvantaged compared to men, and for this reason, abortion is believed to be necessary in certain situations.

However, Jesus didn't believe that women were less than men. Jesus gave power to all who believe, including women and children. The religious leaders of Jesus's day were opposed to men, women, and children sharing spiritual power and authority. Likewise, the leaders of many countries, nations, and religious groups today share the hatred of this truth found within God's Word.

Women and children who have been saved through the blood of Jesus have the same access to the Holy Spirit and Father God as men do. Women and children can receive revelation, authority, and power when they choose to believe in Jesus Christ and are baptized in the Holy Spirit.

Acts 2:17-21 teaches, "And it shall come to pass in the last days, God declares, that I will pour out of My Spirit upon all mankind, and your sons and your daughters shall prophesy telling forth the divine counsels] and your young men shall see visions (divinely granted appearances), and your old men shall dream [divinely suggested] dreams. Yes, and on My menservants also and on My maidservants in those days I will pour out of My Spirit, and they shall prophesy telling forth the divine counsels and predicting future events pertaining especially to God's kingdom]. And I will show wonders in the sky above and signs on the earth beneath, blood and fire and smoking vapor; The sun shall be turned into darkness and the moon into blood before the obvious day of the Lord comes—that great and notable and conspicuous and renowned [day]. And it shall be that whoever shall call upon the name of the Lord invoking, adoring, and worshiping the Lord—Christ] shall be saved."

The only demobilizing agent that can stop a person from overcoming through the power of God is unbelief. Doubting the things the Lord has written and spoken causes God's will to not come to pass in our lives. Jesus was restrained from performing miracles in Mark 6:5, because of the unbelief of the people. "And He could not do a miracle there at all [because of their unbelief] except that He laid His hands on a few sick people and healed them."

Faith in God's Word, even in small increments, can do the things that are otherwise humanly impossible. Faith in God allows us to do the unimaginable. Matthew 17:20 says, "And He said to them, 'You are unable because of your little faith; for truly I say to you, if you have faith the size of a mustard seed, you will say to this mountain, "Move from here to there," and it will move; and nothing will be impossible for you.'"

In abusive relationships, whether personal or institutional, one party attempts to intimidate and put down another party. This intimidation is used to instill anxiety and the skepticism of success, often through verbal abuse. Verbal abuse is a spoken or written language of doubt, unbelief, and criticism towards the victim, insinuating that he or she cannot do certain things, or there will be negative repercussions if they do not conform. Fear, doubt, and insecurity are weapons of conformity and control abusers use to keep victims from taking positive steps of action in a forward trajectory.

Fear, doubt, and insecurity are the weapons wicked leaders and the devil alike use. Evil leaders have been inspired to demean others personally or on a large-scale societal level. These elements manifest themselves in the relationship between abortion advocates, abortion institutions, and pregnant women. Abortion clinics and advocates attempt to con women into conformity through verbal abuse and notions of failure. Abortion advocates want women to know that if they try to go forward, then negative circumstances will follow.

Fear and insecurity say that people can't possess the land because there are too many giants; yet faith says we can, and we will with God's help. Joshua and Caleb were the only men who believed they could take the land when the rest of the spies doubted it was possible.

Many people look at their circumstances and doubt their own ability and the ability of others to move forward, even when God has provided a way forward. Numbers 13:33 explains, "There we saw the Nephilim (the sons of Anak are part of the Nephilim); and we were like grasshoppers in our own sight, and so we were in their sight." The perception held by the Israelites in the wilderness kept them from believing God and going into their destiny.

Believers must choose to be on guard, filtering all voices, thoughts, and feelings that come to us in life. Listening to God's perception of who we are and what we are capable of is the only foolproof way of success. Christians must choose not to accept the taunts, lies, and intimidation of our enemy, who desires to make us feel like we are invaluable and unable to achieve great things. Believers must always remember the favor for success, joy, prosperity and peace rests on us because we stand with God, even when the odds are stacked against us in the natural world.

The majority is often opposed to the Lord. The Bible describes times when entire nations, communities, and people were opposed to God and His work on the earth. When the majority, the leaders, or other groups normalize what is wrong, the believer must know the truth and refuse to compromise with evil. A group of people wanted to let Barabbas to live instead of Jesus, not because they loved Barabbas, but because they hated the truth. Even though the crowd knew Barabbas was evil, they still chose to crucify the innocent, who was Jesus Christ, the Son of God.

Today, many men and women side with abortion advocates because they do not follow God and God's truth. Because they hate God and God's precepts, they willingly accept evil and immoral behavior in others' lives. Even when people know abortion is murder and is a crime against humanity, they attempt to look the other way or justify evil deeds, because they do not want to stand with the truth and the justice of the Lord. Jesus's crucifixion exemplifies that some people hate truth and innocence and choose to side with wickedness and immortality. It is the same in all cases of abortion.

Now at the feast [of the Passover] the governor was in the habit of setting free any one prisoner whom the people chose. And at that time they were holding a notorious prisoner [guilty of insurrection and murder], called Barabbas. So, when they had assembled [for this purpose], Pilate said to them, "Whom do you want me to set free for you? Barabbas, or Jesus who is called Christ?" For Pilate knew that it was because of jealousy that the chief priests and elders had handed Jesus over to him.

While he was seated on the judgment seat, his wife sent him a message, saying, "Have nothing to do with that righteous and innocent Man; for last night I suffered greatly in a dream because of Him." But the chief priests and the elders persuaded the crowds to ask for Barabbas and to put Jesus to death. The governor said to them, "Which of the two do you wish me to set free for you?" And they said, "Barabbas." Pilate said to them, "Then what shall I do with Jesus who is called Christ?" They all replied, "Let Him be crucified!" And he said, "Why, what has He done that is evil?" But they continued shouting all the louder, "Let Him be crucified!"

So when Pilate saw that he was getting nowhere, but rather that a riot was breaking out, he took water and washed his hands [to ceremonially cleanse himself of guilt] in the presence of the crowd, saying, "I am innocent of this [righteous] Man's blood; see to that yourselves." And all the people answered, "Let [the responsibility for] His blood be on us and on our children!" So, he set Barabbas free for them; but after having Jesus severely whipped (scourged), he handed Him over to be crucified." (Matthew 27:15–26)

Pontius Pilate was a leader who believed he could absolve himself of responsibility for the death of Jesus. However, by permitting it to occur, he remained complicit in the sin of murder. Similarly, how many leaders in America condone abortion while attempting to distance themselves from the consequences? The reality remains that the spiritual and moral implications endure. There is no justification for the act of murder.

Moses was a murderer. Moses killed another person when he was angry. Exodus 2:11–13 tells us, "One day, after Moses had grown [into adulthood], it happened that he went to his countrymen and looked [with compassion] at their hard labors; and he saw an Egyptian beating a Hebrew, one of his countrymen. He turned to look around, and seeing no one, he killed the Egyptian and hid himself in the sand."

Moses rationalized his decision to kill the Egyptian, because he had compassion and emotional sorrow for another person. However,

Moses's emotional decision was wrong in God's sight, and it cost Moses many years of living in exile and bondage.

Some abortion advocates state they are showing compassion to women by allowing abortion, yet they are deceived by their emotions as Moses was. Compassion and empathy are emotions that can benefit us, but like all emotions, at times, they negatively impact our behavior. Emotions regularly contribute to bad decisions, and being led solely by emotion will cause people to sin. God designed us to live by His absolute truth and the Spirit of God, as opposed to living by our emotions.

Joseph refused to be led by his emotions despite many opportunities to lash out towards others. Joseph's brothers sold him into slavery when he was young. He also endured Potiphar's wife lying about him, which landed him in prison. Despite the mistreatment Joseph faced, he showed strength and wisdom, choosing to control his emotions and his decisions. Joseph trusted God with his life's outcome, and he rejected the feelings of victimhood.

By allowing God to deliver justice on his behalf, Joseph rose to a top position in government and in his family. Moses and Joseph were both permitted to help God's people and God used both in miraculous ways. Yet, Joseph could enjoy more of the fruit of his labor, because he consistently made the right decision and refused to be controlled by his emotions. Joseph dictated his emotions and did not let his emotions dictate to him. On the contrary, Moses let his emotions blind him within different portions of his life, and it impacted his future.

Although Moses was given an opportunity to bless God's people, his disobedience kept him from entering God's best for his life—the promise land. Deuteronomy 3:23–28 says that Moses said to God, "'Please let me go over and see the good land beyond the Jordan, that good hill country and Lebanon.' But the Lord was angry with me because of you and would not listen to me. And the Lord said to me, 'Enough from you; do not speak to me of this matter again. Go up to the top of Pisgah and lift up your eyes westward and northward and southward and eastward, and look at it with your eyes, for you shall not go over this Jordan. But charge Joshua, and encourage and strengthen him, for he shall go over at the head of his people, and he shall put them in possession of the land that you shall see.'"

The choices that Aaron and Moses made led them to not receive the blessing and the promise God wanted to give them.

From creation, Adam and Eve were given the choice to obey or disobey God's commands. The right to choose our destiny is incredible. God gives us the right to determine how close we get to His design for our lives, and to determine how far we go. God wanted Adam and Eve to remain in the Garden of Eden, but their choice changed the trajectory of their lives and the lives of their children. God forgave Adam and Eve for their sin, but they still suffered consequences for the sin.

We can be forgiven for sins when we repent, but those same sins can still affect the future of our lives. Consequences are the negative results of actions or choices that have been made against the direction or the will of God. Some mistakes are profound and eternal and lead us totally off course in life, where others only slightly detour us. To remain on the path of life, and to reduce the consequences of bad decisions, we must listen and obey all of God's commands, even when they don't make sense to our human mind or reasoning.

A GPS in our cars tells us when we miss a turn or choose to go off the most direct path. When we make a turn or head in the wrong direction, we can see our estimated time change, because we must be redirected. If there is an appointed time of arrival such as a business meeting, and we were redirected, then we may miss the meeting. In these times, even when a boss may forgive the absence, the meeting is over and we've missed information we should know.

God's flawless will is for humans to reach perfection. God intends perfection for His people. The more we aspire to become perfect as God is perfect, the closer we will get to our God-given destiny. Matthew 5:48 teaches, "Be perfect, therefore, as your heavenly Father is perfect."

Christians should desire to stay on course, to obey the word, and to do the things that God instructs them to do so they can reach their promised land. When making a choice, believers must determine the short term and the long-term consequences. We must accept that our choices have consequences for our lives and the lives of others, and some choices can be forgiven but not fully reinstated.

The pro-abortion propaganda is executed by Satan to target women at the soul level. Women innately desire to protect their children. When the devil uses the lie of financial lack and insecure finances in the time a woman is facing a pregnancy, he taps into a woman's desire to protect her child. This emotional trigger is linked psychologically to the belief a woman must provide and care for her child to be a good mother.

By targeting the woman's emotions in this way, the enemy tricks the woman to believe she cannot provide a good life for her baby, therefore she would be doing the baby a favor by aborting it. The woman's emotional desire to protect and nurture her baby is twisted and used against her instead of being used for her. This is the same kind of emotional compassion and human thinking or reasoning as occurred in Moses's killing.

Many days I have composed the pages of this book while holding my infant on my lap. I have had to delete a few words here and there because he was tapping on my keyboard with his little hand, but I wouldn't change the fact he is sitting with me! My longing to succeed financially has increased significantly from having my children, because they inspire me to be better and work harder.

I believe women who choose to keep their babies as opposed to aborting them will find creative ways to care for them, and these women show dedicated strength, wisdom, and ingenuity that is unmatched by childless women. Women who choose life are ultimately empowered and strengthened when they use their resourcefulness and find ways to be an awesome mom while contributing to the outside world too.

I continuously pray to God for help me as a mom and a worker for His kingdom. I have stopped writing my book to help my kids with their schoolwork, make dinner, brush teeth, and perform other mom duties for my kids. Of course, someone without kids wouldn't have these opportunities to do both, but I am thankful for the opportunities to be a mom and an author, teacher, and kingdom woman.

The Bible says whatever believers put their hands to for work will prosper. So, I believe with God's help, I will prosper. I believe I can do all things, because I am a woman called by God to succeed and prosper! Deuteronomy 30:9 promises, "The Lord your God will make you abundantly prosperous in all the work of your hand, in the fruit of your womb and in the fruit of your cattle and in the fruit of your ground. For the Lord will again take delight in prospering you, as He took delight in your fathers."

The next propagandist lies alleging that a pregnancy has come at the wrong time and there will be a better time for a child to be born are fundamentally and biologically false. A child conceived is unique, and there will never be another child identical to the one who has already been conceived in the woman's womb. Every human is exclusive, and even future siblings will never be the same as the child aborted or born into the world. This demonic lie allows for the life and the existence of the baby to be controlled by the woman and her desires, while dehumanizing individuality and purpose.

This calculated lie of Satan targets a woman's soul, aiming in the domain of "dreams, visions, and success." Dreams, achievement, success, prosperity, and growth are all elements God has put inside the man and the woman to help them move forward in their destiny and their life.

God constructed people to prosper and to succeed in life, and He places the desire for great dreams, visions, and success within the heart of people. Satan targeted Joseph in this manner when he was challenged to give up on his dreams for success because of his current circumstances. Satan wanted Joseph to believe the lie that he could not achieve the things God placed inside of him, because of his demonically inspired, vulnerable situation. But because Joseph knew who he was, and he was firm in his God-given identity, he was able to disregard Satan's lies.

The devil, not the Lord, wants to stop people from progressing and prospering. John 10:10 explains, "The thief comes only in order to steal and kill and destroy. I came that they may have and enjoy life, and have it in abundance [to the full, till it overflows]."

When the devil robbed Job of his earthly possessions given to him by God, he assumed that Job would curse God and stop serving Him. However, God knew Job would continue to trust Him and serve Him even during his temporary suffering and the loss of his possessions. God's love and protection of Job was certain, and He never stopped wanting Job to be successful and prosperous. Satan was the author of Job's misery.

The devil hated Job's prosperity, and he desired to take everything good away from Job and his family. The devil tried to inflict Job with financial problems, sickness and disease, and other losses to cause Job to walk away from God and God's provisions and blessings. Job 1:22 says, "Through all this Job did not sin nor did he blame God."

Job and Joseph both knew it was wise to not blame God for the calamity in their lives, even when they didn't fully understand what was happening.

The threat of stagnation in life is the devil's devious attempt to manipulate a woman's spiritual desire for success. Satan tries to convince women to feel they are not possibly able to fulfill the things they are called to do without an abortion. This strategic lie maintains that it is not an opportune time for this baby to come into a family. However, the story of Job and the story of Joseph can both teach us that any yoke of bondage placed on a woman from the works of the devil in our lives, is temporary and is not eternal, long lasting, or indicative of the future.

If either Job or Joseph had projected their future success based on their circumstances or of their past, neither of them would have been abundantly blessed by God in their future.

Current circumstances are not indications of future circumstances. God redeems people's lives from the pit. God gives us talents, dreams and visions, and He will fulfill them. God sets us on high when we consistently place our trust in Him. First Samuel 2:8 says, "He raises up the poor from the dust, He lifts up the needy from the ash heap To make them sit with nobles, And inherit a seat of honor and glory; For the pillars of the earth are the Lord's, And He set the land on them."

The Lord made us in His image as creators. He designed us to have and use our talents and our aptitudes. Christians must know we are within our covenant rights to hold positive expectations of the future, even in undesirable beginnings or circumstances, because the Bible testifies of these truths. If we do not know our true God-given identity, then the devil can steal our God-given future by tempting us to give up and make our own way apart from the Lord.

Habakkuk 2:2 says, "Then the Lord answered me and said: 'Write the vision And make it plain on tablets, That he may run who reads it. For the vision is yet for an appointed time; But at the end it will speak, and it will not lie. Though it tarries, wait for it; Because it will surely come, It will not tarry.'"

Isaiah 46:3–4 declares, "'Listen to Me,' [says the Lord], 'O house of Jacob, And all the remnant of the house of Israel, You who have been carried by Me from your birth And have been carried [in My arms] from the womb, Even to your old age I will carry you! I have made you, and I will carry you; Be assured I will carry you and I will save you.'"

God is our Father. Like any good father, God has promised to watch over us and take care of us all the days of our lives. When we put our faith and trust in God like a child puts their faith and trust in his or her parents, we won't worry about how we are going to be successful.

When I tell my kids we are going to take a trip to the beach, they don't wonder how we are going to get there. They get excited and start packing their bags, knowing they are going to the beach, because mommy and daddy said they are going! As children of God, we can rest assured that our Father will get us where we are supposed to go, even if we don't know how we will get there.

Joseph had a foreknowledge of his marvelous future, because God had given him his dreams. Joseph knew God was going to help him do great things in his life, but during a time, Joseph had to live by faith and not by sight, because the devil was trying to destroy his faith in his dreams coming to pass. The devil was working through Joseph's brothers to tempt Joseph to give up on his God-given dreams, so he wouldn't reach his true full potential.

Genesis 37: 19–20 says, "'Here comes that dreamer!' they said to each other. 'Come now, let's kill him and throw him into one of these cisterns and say that a ferocious animal devoured him. Then we'll see what comes of his dreams.'"

God's plan for Joseph was greater than anything Joseph could have imagined, even after his brothers abused him. In abusive situations such as rape, incest, or domestic violence, women must resist the temptation to become violent themselves and justify the harm of another person out of personal hurt and victimization. Abortion doesn't cancel or undo a rape or a violent situation. Abortion simply propagates more violence and abuse. Studies show that abused people either reject abuse or become abusive. The choice is theirs, but abortion is always an unhealthy choice.

Individuals responsible for violence and victimizing women are solely responsible for their decisions and will be held accountable for their actions as Joseph's brothers eventually were. God doesn't condone abusive situations. God shows us through His Word that He sees abuse, human suffering, and pain.

The Bible promises us that God will restore to us anything stolen from the enemy. Victims of abuse can know God vindicates and sees the evil that has been done to them. They can know they will be repaid if they wait on the Lord. Isaiah 61:7 declares, "Instead of your [former] shame you will have a double portion; and instead of humiliation your people will shout for joy over their portion. Therefore in their land they will possess double [what they had forfeited]; everlasting joy will be theirs."

It is wise to discern that God gave the earth to humans. People get to decide to do right or do wrong and determine the outcome of life's circumstances. When evil and wickedness are perpetrated, it is done through human hands because of sin and darkness in the man or woman's heart. Psalm 115:16 tells us, "The heavens are the heavens of Yahweh, But the earth He has given to the sons of men."

The devil's primary agenda is to inflict pain and suffering on a woman through abuse, and then convince a woman that God willed for the abuse to happen. He insinuates that sovereign God in heaven, "permitted the act of violence," because after all, "He is in control of everything" (determinism). This demonic doctrine positions a woman against God when the woman needs to embrace God and receive His power, His strength, and His vindication for her abuse.

If a woman believes Satan's lie about the origin of her abuse, she will believe she should vindicate the abuse herself, because God won't vindicate her from something He caused to happen in the first place. We must realize that God hates all forms of abuse and sin, and the Devil is behind any form of abuse. Satan knows when a woman takes matters into her own hands, she violates God's command and becomes ineligible to receive God's vindication on her behalf.

Romans 12:19 instructs us, "Beloved, never avenge yourselves, but leave the way open for God's wrath [and His judicial righteousness]; for it is written [in Scripture], "Vengeance is Mine, I will repay," says the Lord."

God is the perfect judge. God brought Joseph's brothers before him, and God humbled them before Joseph at the appointed time. Joseph's brothers were forced to face their own sin and to apologize to their brother whom they had abused and sold into slavery, because God was on Joseph's side and hated the abuse and injustice. Joseph didn't become abusive, hurt others, or vindicate himself. Joseph waited on God.

Satan uses people to perpetrate his plan and his evil motives, intending to destroy a woman's confidence, hope, and future. Like he did to Joseph, the Devil encourages people to harm others through abusive acts. These terrible, violent, and malicious actions are intentional and vile works of Satan as an attempt to pollute a person's destiny.

Through deceiving women into believing abortion is a justified act in response to abuse, the devil attacks a woman through abuse and trauma and then controls her next course of action, telling her to hurt her baby to avenge what has been done to her. However, when a woman chooses to perpetuate an act of violence upon an innocent baby, she, too, becomes guilty of murder. The woman becomes guilty of the same sin of their attacker and aggressor, guilty of the same sins of abuse and murder.

Deuteronomy 22:25–27 shows us, "But if in the field the man finds the girl who is engaged, and *the man forces her and lies with her,* then only the man who lies with her shall die. But you shall do nothing to the girl; there is no sin in the girl worthy of death, for just *as a man rises against his neighbor and murders him, so is this case.* When he found her in the field, the engaged girl cried out, but there was no one to save her."

Hurting a child is wrong in the eyes of God, and it is not justified by the Lord for any reason. Amos 1:13 says, "Thus says the Lord: 'For three transgressions of the people of Ammon, and for four, I will not turn away its punishment, because they ripped open the woman with child in Gilead, that they might enlarge their boarders.'"

Women who have experienced abusive and terrible situations can take heart knowing the Lord sees, punishes, and vindicates abuse. Women who wait on the Lord to avenge them will see the Lord's hand of deliverance. God will deliver them out of bad situations. He will restore what was stolen from sexual abuse or domestic abuse. First Peter 3:12 tells us, "For the eyes of the Lord are toward the righteous, And His ears attend to their prayer, But the face of the Lord is against those who do evil."

Evil people, who walk in darkness, marvel at the power and the light of women who choose to do things God's way. John 1:5 says, "The Light shines in the darkness and the darkness did not comprehend it."

Darkness does not comprehend light, and wicked people do not understand how women can overcome and face opposition and pain and still become victorious and successful. But the Lord has established and decreed that the women who put their faith in Him will overcome and achieve things a mortal person could never comprehend or imagine. They will be successful, even when they have been hurt and mistreated. Psalm 46:1 declares, "God is our refuge and strength, always ready to help in times of trouble."

Regardless of the leader, ruler, or political system, God's Word remains the same today as it did thousands of years ago. Absolute truth has been established since the beginning of time, and we get to decide if we are going to side with God or if we are going to exalt our own thoughts, desires, and beliefs over His Word.

God will always keep His Word and deliver the righteous from their enemies, oppressors, and the devil. By choosing to submit to the Spirit of God, women don't fight their battles alone. A righteous woman has the backing of heaven. God ensures we will not be ashamed; instead, the wicked people will be humbled and ashamed for their wicked deeds. Psalm 25:3 tells us, "Indeed, none of those who [expectantly] wait on You will be ashamed; Those who turn away from what is right and deal treacherously without cause will be ashamed (humiliated, embarrassed).

5

The Weapons of our Warfare: Faith and Confession

Knowledge of the Bible is foundational for everything in the Christian life. The scriptures provide us with absolute truth. Whenever people lack awareness of God's truth, they cannot submit to and apply that truth effectively. Jesus quoted the scriptures to the devil when He was tempted in the desert. Matthew 4:4 tells us, "But Jesus said, 'It is written, Man is not to live on bread alone, but on every word that God speaks'"

What we do not know can be exploited by our adversary, who is well-versed in the word of God. To effectively engage in and triumph over this spiritual warfare, it is essential that we possess a deep understanding and unwavering faith in God's Word. This knowledge will enable us to articulate scripture during times of trial and testing Learning about God through the Bible permits us to reject or accept His truth. However, the more truth we know and apply to our lives, the brighter the path we walk will be.

Matthew 13:10–12 teaches, "The disciples came to Him and asked, 'Why do You speak to the crowds in parables?' Jesus replied to them, 'To you it has been granted to know the mysteries of the kingdom of heaven, but to them it has not been granted. For whoever has [spiritual wisdom because he is receptive to God's Word], to him more will be given, and he will be richly and abundantly supplied; but whoever does not have [spiritual wisdom because he has devalued God's Word], even what he has will be taken from him.'"

The hearers and the doers of the word are exclusively permitted to stand against the evil spiritual forces trying to destroy humanity. Believers who renew their minds consistently receive information and help from heaven. Assistance from God permits us to be invincible to the enemy forces. Those who hear the word, receive it, and apply it to their lives will be enhanced and preserved, even during storms or trials, because they have supernatural assistance given to them.

Matthew 7:24-27 says, "Everyone therefore who hears these words of mine, and does them, I will liken him to a wise man, who builds his house on a rock. The rain came down, the floods came, and the winds blew, and beat on that house; and it didn't fall, for it was founded on the rock. Everyone who hears these words of mine and doesn't do them will be like a foolish man, who built his house on the sand. The rain came down, the floods came, and the winds blew, and beat on that house; and it fell- and great was its fall."

Articulating internalized scripture, along with the authority bestowed upon us through the name of Christ, enables us to invoke an anointing that liberates captives and restrains the forces of the devil. For illustration purposes, the scripture is likened to the law, Christ is the governmental system, and we are the police officers. A police officer who is unsure of the law is unable to arrest violators of the law, because he or she is ignorant of the offense or the trespass. However, a police officer that knows the law and uses the law to arrest offenders will stop crime.

To stop Satan or to free prisoners there must be both a combined authority and a knowledge of the law. Police officers must get permission from the courts to let prisoners walk free. Jesus is the only one who can forgive sin and pronounce someone as guilty or innocent.

Police officers aid the governmental system, but they are not in control of the system. Likewise, we are to assist heaven, and we are to free prisoners and to bind the devil with the help of the Holy Spirit, through Jesus Christ. Jesus Christ alone bestows us with our authority. Jesus decides who has authority, and He decides how much authority an individual is permitted to carry. He decides who is guilty and who is free.

Jesus perceived and resisted the devil's twisting of scripture. Satan knew Jesus was not ignorant of God's law, so he attempted to manipulate the law. When Satan twists scripture, he manipulates scripture to try to gain control and power. Satan lies and speaks half-truths. He often uses the scripture to try to manipulate and confuse humanity, and if people do not know who God is and what the scriptures mean, they can be deceived.

Jesus' knowledge of scriptures, combined with His personal relationship with His Father, protected Him from Satan's deceptive attack. Jesus responded to Satan saying, "It is *also* written."

Jesus's interaction with Satan shows us the significance of learning the whole essence of the Bible. Without knowledge and understanding of the Bible, we cannot appropriately enforce God's laws. However, Jesus also knew His Father's will and His Father's nature, and knowing God personally is equally as important as knowing the law.

Matthew 4:6–7 says, "The devil said to Him, 'If You are the Son of God, throw yourself down. It is written, 'He has told His angels to look after You. In their hands they will hold You up. Then your foot will not hit against a stone.' Jesus said to the Devil, 'It is written also, 'You must not tempt the Lord your God.'"

Biblical knowledge can only be attained through the study of God and His word. There is not a cheat sheet to memorizing and knowing the laws and ways of God. Knowledge of God and His character only comes through spending time in His presence. The Bible tells us we will not be given more spiritual knowledge unless we have first learned and applied the previous knowledge (Matthew 25:29). In other words, God will not continue to show us things, if we aren't receptive to His teachings.

The Bible warns us that worldly desires conceive problems. The natural human mind that has not been renewed by the scripture will birth trouble. James 1:13–15 says, "Let no one say when he is tempted, 'I am being tempted by God' [for temptation does not originate from God, but from our own flaws]; for God cannot be tempted by [what is] evil, and He Himself tempts no one. But each one is tempted when he is dragged away, enticed and baited [to commit sin] by his own [worldly] desire (lust, passion). Then when the illicit desire has conceived, it gives birth to sin; and when sin has run its course, it gives birth to death."

Maintaining control over our mind is a substantial part of receiving victory in life. As new creatures in Christ, we are commanded to lay aside our old selves, not to give into the desires of the human flesh. Self-control rejects access to Satan and denies the self from fulfilling worldly lusts. We can only attain self-control through the renewing of the mind. Our minds influence what we do. Thoughts influence behavior. As a man thinks, so is he!

Ephesians 4:22 tells us, "Regarding your previous way of life, you put off your old self [completely discard your former nature], which is being corrupted through deceitful desires."

Thinking is the precursor to behaving. If a person wants to change his or her behavior, then he or she must first change his or her thinking. Matthew 16:24 instructs, "Then Jesus said to His disciples, "If anyone wishes to come after Me, he must deny himself, and take up his cross and follow me." To spiritually thrive, we must choose to follow Jesus through a continual renewing of our minds. We must follow Christ and conform our minds into the image of Christ.

The Bible does not indicate a lack of storms or temptations. John 16:33 tells us, "I have told you these things, so that in me you may have peace. In this world you will have trouble. But take heart! I have overcome the world."

The Bible reveals that we will face opposition as we live in the fallen and evil world. Yet, our mindset during times of adversity makes the difference between those who become victorious and those who suffer defeat. A mind that has been renewed through learning scripture will respond to life differently than a mind that has not been renewed by God's Word.

Psychological knowledge and understanding of scripture are only part of the puzzle. Knowledge of scripture alone is not enough to understand God. Scripture teaches us spiritual knowledge, and insight is given and is accessed supernaturally from the Spirit. We cannot be given more spiritual knowledge without using the knowledge we have previously been given.

The kingdom of God works like a multi-part riddle, and to move forward, the previous riddle must be solved. If a person has been taught a spiritual truth and has not implemented that truth, then he or she will be unable to access more truth, even if the person studies more of the scriptures.

In a formal learning atmosphere, children must properly learn the material from first grade to move on to second grade. If a child were placed in second grade without learning the material from first grade, they would be lost, confused, and unable to complete their work. The child could be forced to listen to second grade lessons every day and would still not comprehend the lessons taught, due to his or her failure to comprehend the first-grade curriculum. To properly succeed in second grade, a child must first learn and implement their knowledge of first grade. Once the knowledge has been learned and applied appropriately, the child is able to hear and understand the material in a new grade.

Children need teachers to help them with their learning. Without a teacher, it would be hard for a child to learn and develop properly. Teachers permit children to move to a new grade once the previous grade has been mastered.

We cannot access spiritual truths outside of our teacher Jesus Christ. To learn about God and His kingdom, we must spend time with Jesus. We must interact with the one who is teaching us, while interacting with the curriculum being taught. A well-rounded student connects with his or her teacher, loves the class, and subsequently learns the curriculum. This student can be promoted to a new grade because his or her teacher verifies that the child is prepared to move forward.

As students grow in their development and their understanding, they are given more responsibility. A kindergarten student would not be trusted to lead and teach others like a tenth-grade student would be, because the older and more mature student can be trusted with more responsibility due to their development and their age.

Jesus gives us more information and authority in the kingdom as we show ourselves to be faithful. Authority and spiritual wisdom in the kingdom of God is not based on physical age, but it is based on spiritual maturity and responsibility. As we grow and progress in the kingdom knowledge, we grow and progress in our ability to lead and spiritually impact others.

When a believer undergoes a test, a storm, or a temptation, he or she will not be overtaken if he or she is connected to Christ and has been responsive to His teachings. Jesus always gives us the lessons that we need, at the time that we need them, so we can access and move onto the next level or grade. We must be willing to listen, and respond to the lessons we are given if we are going to continue to move forward spiritually.

If we sit in class, hear the lesson, and fail to respond, then we will fail our test when it comes. However, if we sit in class, hear the lesson, and appropriate the lesson, we will pass the test, and we will continue to move forward at our teacher's approval.

We limit or stop our destiny from being fulfilled when we fail to learn the lessons God has for us. To advance, we must hear and apply the information God gives us at the time He gives it. James 1:25 teaches

"But he who looks carefully into the perfect law, the law of liberty, and faithfully abides by it, not having become a [careless] listener who forgets but an active doer [who obeys], he will be blessed and favored by God in what he does [in his life of obedience]."

God has given us authority in the earth and in the spirit realm. Jesus rebuked the disciples in the boat for not using their God-given authority. The disciples cowered and froze in fear because they needed a deeper understanding of who was with them on the boat. The disciples' submission to fear was a response tied to the flesh and the old self but was primarily due to ignorance. The disciples needed a deeper revelation of whom Jesus was to be able to properly pass their test by using their God-given authority to rebuke the storm.

The disciples had been with Jesus, but they didn't fully understand Jesus' teachings. They had been in class, but they had not fully learned from the material. The disciples' response was one of shock saying, "What sort of man is this that the wind and the waves obey Him?"

This response indicates that the disciples were not confident who Jesus was, or in His lessons He was teaching, even though they were following Him. Luke 8:23–27 says, "And when he got into the boat, his disciples followed him. And behold, there arose a great storm on the sea, so that the boat was being swamped by the waves; but he was asleep. And they went and woke him, saying, Save us, Lord; we are perishing. And he said to them, Why are you afraid, O you of little faith? Then he rose and rebuked the winds and the sea, and there was a great calm. And the men marveled, saying, 'What sort of man is this, that even winds and sea obey him?"

The disciples were able to know and go deeper in their understanding of who Jesus was because of their encounter with Him on the sea. Before this encounter, they did not realize they didn't need to beg Jesus for help, because they had not learned and applied this teaching. Jesus must have already taught the disciples this lesson, because He was disappointed in their response during the test. Jesus rebuked the disciples because He had already taught them a lesson in the past, and they didn't process His teaching and apply it to their lives.

The lack of assurance about who Jesus was, combined with the lack of knowledge of the taught curriculum, contributed to the disciples' failure at the time of the test. If we experience a temptation or a storm, we don't need to beg Jesus for His help any more than the disciples needed to. In times of testing or temptation, we simply need more revelation and knowledge, through more time in class with Jesus. Through our learning of scripture and our time in class with Christ, we are equipped to pass our trails and tests.

God knows the storms that will come into our lives before they occur, and for this reason He tries to teach us the lessons we need ahead of time. If we know a student will need to learn subtraction in kindergarten, then we begin teaching him or her number recognition in preschool. Like any good teacher, Jesus will teach His students the information He knows they will need to be successful down the road.

Peter was evidently further along than the other disciples in his understanding of scripture, because Peter was able to go further than the other disciples. Peter had acquired more information, and more applied knowledge of Christ through his time and his effort in class with Jesus. We know that Peter and Jesus had a deep bond and relationship because John 13:23 tells us, "One of His disciples, whom Jesus loved (esteemed), was leaning against Jesus' chest."

Peter admired and loved Jesus. Peter had a relationship with his teacher, and he had a desire to learn and understand Jesus' teachings. Peter's combined relationship and desire for learning permitted him to move forward at a faster pace than his peers. Matthew 14:28–31 says, "Peter replied to Him, 'Lord, if its [really] You, command me to come to You on the water.' He said, 'Come!' So Peter got out of the boat, and walked on the water and came towards Jesus. But when he saw [the effects of] the wind, he was frightened, and he began to sink, and he cried out, 'Lord save me!' Immediately Jesus extended His hand and caught him, saying to him, 'O you of little faith, why did you doubt?'"

Unbelief stops the power of God from flowing through us. Doubt is our own carnal mind questioning God. Peter knew the truth because he had learned the truth, but after learning the truth, Peter doubted the truth. Doubt was able to stop God's power, showing us that it is possible for people to know the truth and then not receive from the truth because of doubt. We can overcome doubt through time and relationship with Christ. When we spend time with Christ, we learn His goodness, and we trust Him even more. The longer we walk with Christ and see His mighty acts and miracles, the more we rest and trust the things He teaches us.

Fear is separate from doubt. The Bible tells us that fear is a spirit and is an attack of Satan. Although fear and doubt often are experienced together, we need to understand the biblical distinction of the two. A submission to the spirit of fear will cause doubt as it did in Peter's life. Peter first submitted to the spirit of fear, and then he became afraid of the winds and waves around him. His submission to fear caused him to doubt his supernatural protection and provision.

We can overcome the spirit of fear with the spirit of faith, but to have the spirit of faith, we must have a deep revelation of God and His word. We must trust Jesus Christ and know He is with us. Romans 10:17 teaches, "So faith comes from hearing [what is told], and what is heard comes by the [preaching of the] message concerning Christ."

Doubt originates within the mind. When we consistently renew our minds through God's word and through our relationship with Jesus, we overcome the human psyche, and consequently we become eligible to overcome evil spirits. We can use our five senses to help us navigate the world in which we live, but they are not meant to control our entire existence. Spiritual sense experiences are just as real as physical sense experiences. Spiritual experiences with Jesus, our Teacher, should transform our minds, and influence our lives more than our physical senses do. Proverbs 28:26 tells us, "Whoever trusts in his own mind is a fool, but he who walks in wisdom shall be delivered."

Neuroplasticity permits us to change our brains through learning. There are two distinct types of learning. Active learning is interactive and allows the learners to participate in the process of learning. Passive learning requires no conscious effort by the learner, and ideas are fed to the learner without the learner's involvement.

NEUROPLASTICITY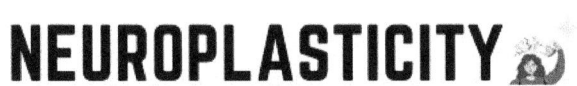

NEUROPLASTICITY IS THE BRAIN'S ABILITY TO CHANGE AND ADAPT DUE TO EXPERIENCE. NEUROPLASTICITY IS AN UMBRELLA TERM REFERRING TO THE BRAIN'S ABILITY TO CHANGE, REORGANIZE, OR GROW NEURAL NETWORKS.

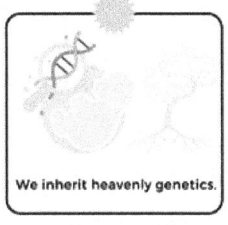

We inherit heavenly genetics.

We are born again. The rewiring of the brain through genetics.

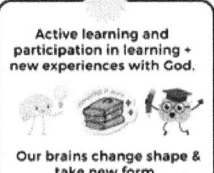

Active learning and participation in learning + new experiences with God.

Our brains change shape & take new form.

We learn new things. The rewiring of the brain through learning.

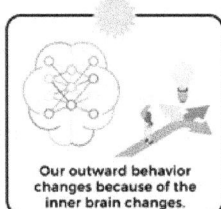

Our outward behavior changes because of the inner brain changes.

As a man thinks so is he. Proverbs 23

In passive learning scenarios, learners merely recite information, and they memorize facts. Conversely, in active learning scenarios, learners engage with their teacher and participate in solving problems. Passive learners may have information, but they don't have applied knowledge.

Studies have shown active learners use and change more of their brains than passive learners. Active learners build and transform the neural pathways and structures in the brain, because they have involved themselves in the learning process. Applied learning through a personal relationship with Jesus Christ and the scriptures changes the structures of our brains. Applied learning allows the brain to undergo deeper psychological transformation. When we are engaged and eager to spend time with God and to learn the ways of God, we will change and rewire the structures of our brains.

Experiencing a relationship with Christ is far more transformative than merely acquiring knowledge about Him or studying the scriptures. There exists a significant distinction between truly knowing Jesus and simply being informed about Him. Our relationship with Jesus and the level of trust we place in Him significantly influence both the depth and speed of our learning. We have the opportunity to draw nearer to God, much like individuals in the Bible who sought to be close to Jesus, in contrast to those who merely observed Him from a distance.

The differing choices of these two groups resulted in varying experiences and insights, highlighting the importance of our chosen proximity to God. Submitting to the unrenewed human psyche causes us to be overcome by our surroundings and our environment when we were designed to dominate and subdue them. The unrenewed brain will be overcome by doubt in situations of trial or testing, because it has not been adequately prepared with the appropriate brain pathways and changes it needs to pass the test.

From a developmental perspective, our brains may operate at a first-grade level, when they should be operating on a much higher developmental level in the spirit realm. A first-grade level brain cannot solve trigonometry, even if it tries, because it is not developmentally and academically prepared to do so.

When walk with Christ, and we learn the lessons that He gives us, we will experience and learn spiritual lessons, and these experiences and lessons will strengthen and form our brain. A mind that has been renewed and transformed by God's word and their experiences with God, will not process our external situations in the same way. Our brain, once renewed, is fundamentally different. A renewed brain is a brain that has been transformed to be spiritually dominated as opposed to physically dominated.

A spiritual mind, given to us by God, as opposed to a carnal one, given to us by our human nature, is the only thing that can overcome the devil, the flesh nature, and the world. A renewed mind produces power and perspective over the spirit of fear.

When we spend time with God learning the Bible, we are endowed with the spirit of faith. The encounter with the spirit of faith then produces positive changes in our brains through our learning experiences. The spirit of faith opposes fear. The spirit of faith encourages, motivates, and frees us from the thoughts, beliefs, and actions of carnal men. Romans 8:15 teaches us, "For you did not receive the spirit of slavery to fall back into fear, but you have received the Spirit of adoption as sons, by whom we cry, 'Abba! Father!'"

A renewed mind is a mind that operates like God's mind. Without the renewing of the mind, our thoughts are not like God's thoughts. Isaiah 55:8 declares, "'For My thoughts are not your thoughts, Nor are your ways My ways,' declares the LORD."

It is no wonder that people struggle through life as unbelievers or carnal-minded Christians. When we do not renew our minds with God's Word, we are led by our human mind working in opposition to the ways of God. When our brain has been trained in God's word, it takes on the shape of God's truth. Only then will our brains influence our outward behavior and actions through a God-ordained lens.

Scientific research has shown genetics also play a role in the shape of our brain. Through our new birth with Christ, we become new creatures, and we get spiritual DNA. We are adopted and changed through our experiences and relationship with our new family.

Our DNA, thoughts, and our behaviors were changed when Adam and Eve sinned against God. Humans, once made in God's image, became sinners, and their God-given nature and psychological perspective was altered, perverted, and polluted. To transform out of the sin nature into the divine nature requires a person to experience the new birth through Jesus. This new birth is the only way to reactivate the God-given nature within the man or woman.

Christians often miss out on God's best on the earth, because they are relating to God in a relationally and emotionally unhealthy way.

By relating with God through the human sin nature, and an unrenewed mind as opposed to the God-divine nature with a renewed mind, humans miss God's plan for perfection and union with Him. Becoming a healthy person takes discipline, work, and effort. God expects us to conform to Him and to put in effort to become the person we are created to be. Romans 12:2 says, "Do not conform to the pattern of this world but be transformed by the renewing of your mind. Then you will be able to test and approve what God's will is—His good and perfect will."

Children who grow up in dysfunctional families can transform into healthy adults and members of society. People who were trained and accustomed to being unhealthy can consciously decide to replace bad habits, thoughts, and traits with healthy ones through deliberate learning and effort.

Likewise, Christians who want to learn to be healthy, and to stop being ruled by wrong thinking and behaving, as the result of the Adam family of origin, must deliberately replace their unhealthy sin nature with a healthy new Christ divine nature. They must learn how to relate to God and to the world in a healthy way, based on the rules and norms of their new family, through the deliberate learning of new ways of thinking, behaving, and acting.

Without the renewing of the mind, a person is unable to consistently progress in the kingdom. God gives humanity seed, and He expects people to plant it appropriately so they can be given more. Second Thessalonians 3:10 teaches, "For while we were yet with you, we gave you this rule and charge: If anyone will not work, neither let him eat."

A man or a woman who is given seed or the wisdom of God and refuses to work to plant the seed will not be given more seed or anything else to eat. God doesn't reward laziness. Proverbs 19:15 declares, "Slothfulness casts one into a deep sleep, and the idle person shall suffer hunger."

If humans want to be healthy, they must work. This is true for physical, spiritual, or emotional health. If you want to be healthy, then you must pursue well being, work on it, and go after it every day. Consistency is key in achieving health goals. Working out at the gym once a month will not produce the desired results for physical health.

To see true lasting physical change, we must go to the gym regularly and consistently. We must watch our nutrition, our calorie intake, and our time spent in the workout regimen. To understand God and achieve the totality of our spiritual health, we must put forth steady effort and spend time with God in His word. We must regularly be eating the words of God and being refreshed by the water of the Holy Spirit. Commitment and consistent effort are crucial components of health. Matthew 5:6 teaches, "'Blessed [joyful, nourished by God's goodness] are those who hunger and thirst for righteousness [those who actively seek right standing with God], for they will be [completely] satisfied."

I lived many years being tossed around by the waves of life and being overly ruled by my emotions. For a few years I was saved, but I still felt like I was drowning emotionally. Like the disciples, my mind was not fully psychologically renewed. Even though I loved Jesus, my state of mind, contributed to my not fully relying on God and His love and protection. My ignorance enabled me to be dominated by the spirit of fear instead of the spirit of faith.

After years of renewing my mind, I can finally see clearly and properly in the Spirit. Changing the brain takes time. When we are new creatures in Christ, we receive a new identity, but to rewire and reroute the pathways of wrong thinking, believing, and behaving, we must continually sow God's word, experience Christ, and create positive brain changes.

When Mary was informed about baby Jesus in her womb, she was unaware of the particulars of her future life. Mary couldn't have reasoned the conception or the birth of Jesus with her psychological mind. Mary received the angel's message from God in faith, not in fear.

Luke 1:30–35 says, "Then the angel said to her, 'Do not be afraid, Mary, for you have found favor with God. And behold, you will conceive in your womb and bring forth a Son and shall call His name Jesus. He will be great and will be called the Son of the Highest; and the Lord God will give Him the throne of His father David. And He will reign over the house of Jacob forever, and of His kingdom there will be no end.' Then Mary said to the angel, 'How can this be, since I do not know a man?' And the angel answered and said to her, 'The Holy Spirit will come upon you, and the power of the Highest will overshadow you; therefore, also, that Holy One who is to be born will be called the Son of God.'"

From the first temptation, Satan gained entrance into the human psychological state of mind, by having humans question God and His word. Satan tempted the woman and the man to trust in their own senses. Satan has historically influenced the human mind and perception through deception. When people live through the lens of the five senses of sight, sound, touch, smell, and taste, they limit God's power and keep themselves from their full spiritual experience.

Thankfully, whenever we struggle with unbelief and a lack of faith in God's Word, we can ask God for help humbly from within our human weakness, and He will help to strengthen our faith. Mark 9:23–24 tells us, "[You say to Me,] 'If you can?' All things are possible for the one who believes and trusts [in Me]!" Immediately, the father of the boy cried out [with a desperate, piercing cry], saying, 'I do believe; help [me overcome] my unbelief."

Walking in the truths of God means discarding the lies of the world, the human mind, emotions of the flesh, and the temptations of the devil. We make a conscious decision to walk in faith and not by sight. God's truths must be brought into a first-place position to manifest God's perfect will into our lives. Our personal preferences, thoughts, emotions, and concerns become secondary to God's truth. When God's truth becomes first, and we become second, God's Spirit and God's truth reigns over the circumstances of our lives.

Submitting our lives to God entails yielding and accepting God's authority. To submit to God, we must let go of the desire to steer our own ship, make our own rules, and come up with our own theology about life. We must believe God knows what is best for us, so we can trust Him with our life's outcomes. We don't need to try to go our own way without God's help, because we know our own way leads to problems and God's way never does. The harder we press into God's teachings and into Jesus' love, the quicker we will develop into the best version of ourselves.

The Bible contains systems of thought unlike anything the world has ever known, seen, or heard of before. First Corinthians 2:9 explains, "But just as it is written [in Scripture], 'Things which the eye has not seen and the ear has not heard, and which have not entered the heart of man, all that God has prepared for those who love Him [who hold Him in affectionate reverence, who obey Him, and who gratefully recognize the benefits that He has bestowed].'"

The Bible shows the corruption of humanity and the evil within the world and the world's systems, but it also shows a way out of all the chaos, and it provides hope in the face of adversity. The Bible provides a positive expectation of things to come. The positive hope and the escape from corruption seems too good to be true, because the gospel is a supernatural phenomenon that makes no sense to the unrenewed human psyche.

A biblical worldview is contrary to a humanistic one. Born-again believers take steps and intentional effort through a concentrated vetting process to replace unhealthy and distorted views buried within the soul and mind. Through our belief in the inherency of scripture, God allows for weeds, roots, and faulty soil to be dug up. He gives us brand new soil and brand-new seeds to plant. Sanctification, the process of being perfected through Christ Jesus, is a systematic processes helping us plant a beautiful garden through a collaborative work with God. God wants to help us eliminate unhealthy beliefs, and He wants to give us beneficial new ones.

Before I was born again, I was a skeptical, outspoken, conspiracy theorist basing my beliefs solely on observation and doubt of the goodness of people and society. I recognized things weren't as they appeared, but I didn't have any proof. With no evidence to back up my beliefs, I had no strategy on how to resist or fight corruption in the world. It didn't seem possible to change my own life, much less change anything in the lives of others. The feelings of imprisonment, victimization and marginalization, and a broken world often left me feeling empty of joy, peace, or hope.

The Bible has provided me with so many answers about life. It has provided me with assurance, trust, and security, and these were things I didn't have before my salvation. First John 4:18 tells us, "In love there is no fear; indeed, perfect love casts out fear, because fear has to do with punishment, and whoever fears has not yet achieved perfection in love."

Knowing the truth about God's love and redemption plan for humanity has driven fear out of my life. Faith has provided me with hope and the possibility to change my life, the lives of others, and society.

It is impossible for us to understand and overcome unbelief and fear if we have not become planted in God's house and garden. God's house is rooted in His love. Without a revelation of God's love and protection, all people have a hard time not being afraid. In the fallen world, there are many things to fear. Yet, the hearing and the receiving of the Bible's promises is encouraging and inspiring, because God's message of transformation brings hope and healing to humanity when we desperately need it.

Spending time renewing our mind is worth every bit of the effort we put in. Without God's healing, and God's love, life on earth would be very difficult, but with God's healing and His help it is meaningful and enjoyable. Psalm 25:12 informs us that God will instruct us into proper thinking and behaving when we fear Him. "Who is the man who fears the Lord? He will be instructed in the way that he should choose."

Fearing God means submitting to God. Peter exemplified unbelief because he submitted to the spirit of fear. In the same way we can submit to fear, and to unbelief, we can submit to God, and the spirit of faith. First Corinthians 10:13 teaches, "No temptation [regardless of its source] has overtaken or enticed you that is not common to human experience [nor is any temptation unusual or beyond human resistance]; but God is faithful [to His word- He is compassionate and trustworthy], and He will not let you be tempted beyond your ability [to resist], but along with the temptation He [has in the past and is now and] will [always] provide the way out as well, so that you will be able to endure it [without yielding, and will overcome temptation with joy]."

God provides born again believers with a new identity. The devil's deception of man thousands of years ago gave humans an identity separate from God's original design. The corrupted identity is reproduced in humanity because the prototype human seed was corrupted. To receive the inheritance and the blessings of God, we must be born again. We must receive the uncorruptible seed of God. First Peter 1:23 tells us, "For you have been born again [that is, reborn from above—spiritually transformed, renewed, and set apart for His purpose] not of seed which is perishable but [from that which is] imperishable and immortal, that is, through the living and everlasting word of God."

The old identity dies when we are reborn. We are removed from our corrupted heritage, and we are joined into a new family as an adopted child of God. Romans 6:3–7 tells us, "Or are you ignorant of the fact that all of us who have been baptized into Christ Jesus were baptized into His death? We have therefore been buried with Him through baptism into death, so that just as Christ was raised from the dead through the glory and power of the Father, we too might walk habitually in newness of life [abandoning our old ways]. For if we have become one with Him [permanently united] in the likeness of His death, we will also certainly be [one with Him and share fully] in the likeness of His resurrection. We know that our old self [our human nature without the Holy Spirit] was nailed to the cross with Him, in order that our body of sin might be done away with, so that we would no longer be slaves to sin. For the person who has died [with Christ] has been freed from [the power of] sin."

The identity we received from Adam and our unhealthy family of origin produces doubt, sin, cursing, sickness, disease, lack, and death. The identity we receive in Christ and our adopted healthy family is the direct opposite. God's new identity for us contains faith, holiness, blessing, health, wellness, provision, and life.

God heals, restores, and helps all who want to escape the torment of the Adam family tree. When we are born again, we are transferred out of our unhealthy dysfunctional family or origin, and positioned into a healthy, conjugal family. John 3:6 says, "That which is born of the flesh is flesh, and that which is born of the Spirit is spirit."

Without a born-again nature, and the inner dwelling of the Holy Spirit, people are subject to experience the devil's torment. Mark 5:4–9 talks about a man who was suffering from demonic possession. "For he had often been bound with shackles [for the feet] and with chains, and he tore apart the chains and broke the shackles into pieces, and no one was strong enough to subdue and tame him. Night and day he was constantly screaming and shrieking among the tombs and on the mountains, and cutting himself with [sharp] stones. Seeing Jesus from a distance, he ran up and bowed down before Him [in homage]; and screaming with a loud voice, he said, 'What business do we have in common with each other, Jesus, Son of the Most High God? I implore you by God [swear to me], do not torment me!' For Jesus had been saying to him, 'Come out of the man, you unclean spirit!' He was asking him, 'What is your name?' And he replied, 'My name is Legion; for we are many.'"

A modern humanistic perspective lacking a spiritual lens would assume this man is suffering from a mental health condition. Without a spiritual examination, a man in these conditions would be treated by doctors or other medical professionals through medicines, confinement, surgeries, talk therapy, or other interventions.

Many people with mental health diagnoses are confined and separated from society like this man was in the Bible. They are treated for suicidal tendencies and self-harm. Modern medicine tells us they are presumed to be unwell, but they are not properly diagnosed if the diagnosis does not consider the supernatural influences contributing to the symptoms of the disease.

Some medical situations and problems are the direct work of the devil. The devil gains access to people's lives at varying levels. This man was invaded by thousands of demons as indicated in scripture. Scripture tells us there are altitudes and degrees of demonic influence or possession.

The sea is darker at the bottom than it is at the top. To get to the bottom of the ocean, a person would have to sink lower and lower, changing altitudes. Science tells us that vessels implode at a certain point. Throughout scripture, humanity is illustrated as vessels of good or of evil. When people sink into demonic depths and influence, they wade deeper and deeper into the darkness, and at some point, they will implode.

Jonah was able to escape the deep waters of the sea, because he called out to God and God rescued him as he was sinking. Jonah knew he could not survive the sea and the monsters of the sea without God's help. Individuals who open themselves to the devil and the devil's agenda live in a state of darkness, sinking lower and lower into the depths of Satan. People do not suddenly begin living incredibility wicked behaviors, thoughts, and lifestyles. Those who sink to the bottom of the sea first intentionally ignore the danger signs in their lives. Revelation 2:24–29 tells us, "But to the rest of you in Thyatira, who do not hold this teaching, who have not explored and known the depths of Satan, as they say—I tell you that I do not lay upon you any other [fresh] burden."

Explorers are known to operate in different capacities. Some explorers venture far beyond normal places, and they go into places people are not meant to be. Others venture out a little and then turn around when they note obvious signs of danger or problems.

The Bible tells us that Satan has depth, and his territory can be explored by humanity. When a human vessel explores the darkness and doesn't turn back at signs of problems, that person will sink lower and lower into the depths of Satan. The darker the water comes, and the lower the vessel sinks, the harder it is to survive without full implosion.

Capacity is the ability to hold, contain, perform, or withstand. Some vessels are built in different proportions than others, and God creates people with various levels of capacity. God will not take us to altitudes or depths in the spirit too quickly because He knows it would cause an implosion. God helps us to understand and to grow in His ways and His thoughts little by little, and He elevates us in the same way Satan drowns us.

We learn and we explore the depths, the heights, and the elevations of God. We venture into the light, exploring the holy and consecrated places with supernatural assistance. First Corinthians 2:10 tells us, "For God has unveiled them and revealed them to us through the [Holy] Spirit; for the Spirit searches all things [diligently], even [sounding and measuring] the [profound] depths of God [the divine counsels and things far beyond human understanding]."

People who explore and sink into the depths of Satan have supernatural assistance. Demons and the devil lure the individual deeper into the darkness and into the waters that will eventually kill the person if he or she doesn't turn around. People learn the thoughts and ways of Satan, and they venture into darkness.

Demons cause various degrees of physical and mental problems in the lives of people. The man who had a legion of demons was close to full implosion as the result of his yielding to Satan. When Jesus cast the demons out of him, the demons went back into the sea because the pig's capacity to handle the demons was less than the man's capacity to hold the demons. Matthew 8: 31–32 says, "And the demons begged Him, saying, 'If You are going to cast us out, send us into the herd of pigs.' And He said to them, 'Go!' And they came out and went into the pigs; and behold, the whole herd rushed down the steep bank into the sea and drowned in the waters."

People who have yielded themselves to the devil and to demons cannot be helped, limited, or treated without turning around and submitting to God. Mark 5:26 explains, "She had suffered a great deal under the care of many doctors and physicians and she spent all the money that she had, yet instead of getting better she grew worse."

Some people will go to doctors and will spend their time and money trying to get well. The doctors and the medical treatment will be unable to heal them, and they will get worse instead of better because they are yielding to demon spirits.

Mark 5:2–4 shows us, "When Jesus got out of the boat, immediately a man from the tombs with an unclean spirit met Him, and the man lived in the tombs, and no one could bind him anymore, not even with chains. For he had often been bound with shackles [for the feet] and with chains, and he tore apart the chains and broke the shackles into pieces, and no one was strong enough to subdue and tame him."

Society attempted to restrain and control the man's mental illness in the best way they knew how. At the time, if there had been antidepressants and other mental health drugs, I am sure this man would have been on them. Yet, despite society's best effort to contain, control, and stop the mental instability and sickness in this man, the efforts were unsuccessful, and he was still continuously in torment. Human intervention alone cannot stop demons.

Many people all over the world live in a state of mental torment as the result of demons. The devil is behind the mental health issues and concerns of society today, just as he was in the days of Jesus. A mind that is not submitted to the authority of Christ and is not renewed will be subject to demonic thought and coinciding demonic behavior.

Many doctors want to help alleviate the problems and try to solve them in a humanistic manner. Yet, without the presence of Jesus and the supernatural power of the spirit, these problems cannot be resolved and will become worse as the individual sinks deeper into darkness. Psalm 108:12 teaches, "Oh give us help against the adversary, for deliverance by man is in vain."

Jesus healed the sick, and cast out devils, to free people from the bondage they were living in. Jesus freed people from the depths of Satan, through His supernatural healing ministry of authority and power. One interaction with Jesus pushed thousands of demons back into the sea. One meeting with Jesus reversed years of mental health disease and torment.

Today, God restores mental suffering and torment in an instance, and He pulls people out of the sea and places them back on solid ground when they call out to Him. Demons, regardless of the degree, must flee and obey the commands of Christ. Psalm 72:4 says, "May He vindicate the afflicted of the people, save the children of the needy and crush the oppressor."

Jesus came to set captives free. He came to save, heal, and deliver people from their diseases and infirmities. Jesus came to conquer the works of the devil and to restore anyone who calls on His name. Matthew 12:15 teaches, "Many followed Him, and He healed all who were ill."

The religious leaders and the rulers of society tried to keep Jesus from healing people who wanted to be healed. This same spirit of the Antichrist is alive and active today. The devil uses people living on the earth to try to stop others from being delivered and healed by God. Sometimes, the resistance is from within the Church, as it was in the days of Jesus's ministry. At other times the resistance comes from governmental leaders, medical professionals, or any other individuals who have not fully yielded themselves to God's Spirit.

The devil will teach anyone who is willing to oppose the works of God. Satan's main objective is to stop God's divine healing and deliverance. Satan hates anyone who operates in the gifts of healing, because healing stops him from dominating and taking people deep into the sea. The supernatural ministry of deliverance and healing is the only thing that stops Satan from destroying people's lives.

Today there are those in our society who condemn, critique, and oppose deliverance and healing ministries. Ministries that affirm the words of Christ, and do the work of the ministry, will face persecution and opposition. Matthew 10:22 tells us, "And you will be hated by everyone because of [your association with] My name, but it is the one who has patiently persevered and endured to the end who will be saved."

Those of us who have been called to heal, deliver, and set free, through Christ's authority and power, know persecution will come, but we don't slow down or stop our ordained work because we are persecuted. When Jesus faced persecution for His ministry of healing the sick and setting the captives free from demonic forces, He continued His work. The devil consistently persecuted Jesus by using other "religious" human beings to attempt to defeat Jesus. As Jesus's deliverance and healings increased, so did the devil's desire to stop Jesus Christ's ministry.

Matthew 12:9–14 explains, "Leaving there, He went into their synagogue. A man was there whose hand was withered. And they asked Jesus, 'Is it lawful and permissible to heal on the Sabbath?'—they asked this so that they might accuse Him and bring charges into court. But He said to them, 'What man is there among you who, if he has only one sheep and it falls into a pit on the Sabbath, will not take hold of it and lift it out? How much more valuable than is a man than a sheep! So, it is lawful and permissible to do good on the Sabbath.' Then He said to the man, 'Reach out your hand!' The man reached out and it was restored, as normal and healthy as the other. But the Pharisees went out and conspired against Him, discussing how they could destroy Him."

Jesus performed the will of the God the Father perfectly. Jesus did exactly what God sent Him to do. John 6:38 says, "For I have come down from heaven, not to do My own will, but to do the will of Him who sent me."

A believer who is anointed and performing the healing work of ministry will offend both religious and wicked secular people alike. These believers will have those who are inspired by Satan try to stop their ministry. However, regardless of man's opinion of us, we are called to do the work of God, helping people and delivering them from all manner of infliction and disease. We are called to bind, cast out and to take authority over demons and demonic forces.

Mark 6:7–13 tells us, "And He called the twelve [disciples] and began to send them out [as His special messengers] two by two and gave them authority and power over the unclean spirits. He told them to take nothing for the journey except a mere walking stick—no bread, no [traveler's] bag, no money in their belts— but to wear sandals; and [He told them] not to wear two tunics. And He told them, 'Wherever you go into a house, stay there until you leave that town. Any place that does not welcome you or listen to you, when you leave there, shake the dust off the soles of your feet as a testimony against them [breaking all ties with them because they rejected My message].' So, they went out and preached that men should repent [that is, think differently, recognize sin, turn away from it, and live changed lives]. And they were casting out many demons and were anointing with oil many who were sick and healing them."

We are called to proclaim and teach the message of Jesus, providing individuals with the opportunity to attain salvation. If someone chooses to reject this message and persists in living in darkness or exploring the ways of Satan's kingdom, Jesus instructed us to allow them to remain in their current state. Nonetheless, we can be confident that when we share the message of salvation and individuals encounter and accept Christ, they will receive a new identity and begin to experience a transformation of their minds.

Police officers work in authority through their support from the government. Civilians must obey and respond to the authority police officers holds, because they must submit and respond to the governing authorities. Without the support and authority of the governmental system, the criminal would not have to obey a police officer's orders. Likewise, the Church without Christ, has no authority or power to stop evil, but with the support of heaven, we do. Evil must submit to the authority of Christ that lives in us.

The Church has been entrusted with authority and a rightful place and stance over the work of the devil. The Church is backed by the power of God, and the Church of Jesus Christ never operates alone. God is with us, and He has given us the Holy Spirit as our helper, enabling us to fulfill our work. The enemy continues to steal and perpetrate crimes against humanity, but when the Church intervenes, he must stop. The only requirement to begin to move in authority and power is salvation and the baptism and the refilling of the Holy Spirit.

Second Corinthians 4:16 says, "Therefore we do not become discouraged (utterly spiritless, exhausted, and wearied out through fear). Though our outer man is [progressively] decaying *and* wasting away, yet our inner self is being [progressively] renewed day after day." Our belief in Jesus and our renewed mind's assurance of Jesus's help to use us against the forces of darkness are the only requirements to cast out devils, heal the sick, and take authority over any work of the devil. This is primarily why the devil works on the belief and the doubt of humans. As he has done from the beginning, Satan tempts us with fear and conflict in the mind. The enemy knows the deception and manipulation of the human mind is the only chance he has to continue his mission.

6

Demolishing the Spirit of Fear

In the wilderness, the devil tried to tempt Jesus to turn a stone into bread because he saw that Jesus's flesh was in a weakened state from fasting. The enemy also saw Jesus was in a season of change, and He was going to enter full-time ministry. Matthew 4:17 says, "From that time Jesus began to preach and say, "Repent [change your inner self—your old way of thinking, regret past sins, live your life in a way that proves repentance; seek God's purpose for your life], for the kingdom of heaven is at hand."

During pregnancy, a woman's body is in an alternative state from its standard mode of operation. Women's bodies during pregnancies are physically vulnerable. Women are also entering a new season of life and ministry—motherhood. When women become mothers, they become responsible for another person's life and well being. They become leaders, and this new season of ministry provokes the devil.

Every time I found out I was pregnant, I felt strong emotions. I really wanted to be a good mom, and that contributed to my having an intense emotional response. Becoming a mother is so incredibly exciting, but it is an immense responsibility and undertaking. For women who want to be excellent moms, a pressure to perform and succeed is linked with a positive pregnancy test.

There is immense power and influence in the hands of a mother, and the work women perform as mothers is unlike any other. During a woman's pregnancy, Satan attempts to lure women away from God as he attempted to do with Jesus. Satan knows pregnant women have entered a new powerful and fulfilling position in life, and he knows how beautiful being a mother is.

Matthew 4:3 tells us, "And the tempter came and said to Him, "If You are the Son of God, command that these stones become bread." In the first temptation, Satan told Jesus to turn stones into bread. He was speaking to Jesus about physical nourishment and comfort. Satan comes to pregnant women with this same temptation: the temptation of the flesh.

The lust of the flesh manifests during a pregnancy through thoughts such as: "I already have three children. How can I take care of them and another baby? My kids I already have will suffer, and they won't have enough." Satan insinuates that women themselves will have a life of physical hardship or suffering. "You will not have enough for yourself and for your baby" or "you will not be able to continue doing the things that you want to do for yourself."

The lust of the flesh temptation tries to get women focused on themselves alone, so the woman feels the child is an interference to her lifestyle and her well being. Women do have to make some lifestyles changes to accommodate a new baby's arrival, but Satan wants women to feel these changes are to their determent and not their benefit.

The second temptation is the pride of life temptation. Using this temptation, Satan tells women to do foolish things, and he wants them to believe they will be fine in reckless decision-making. For example, the pride of life temptation suggests that if women have an abortion, they will be able to walk away better off without suffering any repercussions. This lie promises women they will not suffer physically or emotionally from an abortion, even when they are having a procedure that is against God and His will. This lie tells women to test God and to do something foolish and hope that God works it out for them.

Matthew 4:5 explains, "Then the devil took Him into the holy city [Jerusalem] and placed Him on the pinnacle (highest point) of the temple. And he said [mockingly] to Him, "If You are the Son of God, throw Yourself down; for it is written, 'He will command His angels concerning You [to serve, care for, protect and watch over You]'"

Women have died from abortions. Women have suffered tremendous health complications such as infertility, uterine perforation, pelvic pain, hemorrhage, infection, and mental instability after abortions. Abortion is not safe. It is dangerous, and it is the temptation of the pride of life.

Pregnant women will experience the pride of life temptation in other ways. For instance, Satan will insinuate that a woman can eat and drink whatever she wants during a pregnancy, and these choices will not affect her baby. These women may believe they are justified to eat ice cream and drink soda during their pregnancy, against good judgment.

God created food to nourish and provide for our needs. But the mainstream food industry, particularly in America, has become largely synthetic and artificial. Many Americans do not know how dangerous the food they eat on a regular basis may be. Satan can use diet to harm a woman and her child by tempting the woman to behave in dangerous ways, and he will promise her that she will be unharmed for doing so.

Matthew 4:8 tells us, "Again, the devil took Him up on a very high mountain and showed Him all the kingdoms of the world and the glory [splendor, magnificence, and excellence] of them; and he said to Him, 'All these things I will give You, if You fall down and worship me.'"

The third temptation, the lust of the eye temptation, offers money, fame, prestige, or other forms of success on the earth. Satan positions women against their babies emotionally or psychologically during or before a pregnancy, suggesting that they will be better off in the world for doing so. This lie tells women to not have children or to abort their child so they can gain success and higher social status.

Many women regularly take hormonal birth control because of the lust of the eye temptation and the pride of life temptation. Although hormonal birth control has been proven to cause reproductive side effects, cancer, mood disorders, cardiovascular issues, weight gain, and more, women believe they will be safe and benefit through restricting a pregnancy with hormonal birth control. Despite the research confirming the dangers of birth control, thousands of women believe they are benefiting themselves because they can achieve social status, education, or other personalized benefits. Satan intends for women to pursue their own visions apart from God and attempt to achieve success, while harming their physical body.

God's wisdom can show us that a woman diagnosed with cancer because of her hormonal birth control will probably never reach her career goals because she will be focusing on restoring her health. Likewise, a woman who is overweight, because of birth control will suffer psychologically, emotionally, and physically due to her extra weight. Being overweight has many proven negative health implications. While these women may not get pregnant, they will poison their bodies, which ultimately limits their possibilities for future success more than any child ever could.

Pregnancy should not be viewed as a curse. Pregnancy is a blessing, and when a woman is married and she is in a relationship with God, a pregnancy will help a woman to become who she is destined to become. Women who are not married, or are not ready to become mothers, should be taught abstinence, and they should not have sex. Self-control and personal responsibility relating to sexuality are vital elements to achieve perfect harmony with our sexual health.

Married women who are not prepared to welcome another baby, need to communicate with their spouse, and come to a mutual agreement about timing, number of pregnancies, and other scenarios for family planning within the healthy marriage relationship.

A pregnancy viewed as a curse creates and contributes to disease in American women, misleading them to believe they will be better off altering their chemistry and their physical, emotional, and spiritual makeup to achieve "something." Ignoring both science and spiritual wisdom, women insert, inject, or ingest chemicals and other toxins regularly. Is birth control through artificial means worth blood clots? Is it worth losing or weakening your body and your life? The real dangers of birth control far outweigh the supposed benefits.

The lust of the flesh, the pride of life, and the lust of the eye are not new temptations. These temptations may present themselves in unique, ambiguous ways, but they are the same lies of the same devil. Doubt and fear come from hearing the enemy's words. Whenever someone senses fear, they can know it is coming from Satan. Satan desires to instill doubt and fear so he can gain control of an individual's decisions. When a person feels scared or intimidated, he or she is easier to control. Fear is the enemy to faith, and it comes from the enemy of our soul.

God wants us to resist doubt and the spirit of fear so we can press into faith. Faith comes from hearing the words of God. The more time a person spends in the God's presence, the more he or she will be encouraged and strengthened from hearing God's words. God's presence is rejuvenating, and God's message to us brings positive expectation of the future to those who believe. Satan may promise a life of success, goodness, and lack of failure or harm, but his track record of lying, stealing, killing, and destroying is enough to cue us into reality. We must make good decisions, and operate out of faith, not fear, if we are going to walk in our divine health.

First Corinthians 10:13 explains, "No temptation [regardless of its source] has overtaken or enticed you that is not common to human experience [nor is any temptation unusual or beyond human resistance]; but God is faithful [to His word—He is compassionate and trustworthy], and He will not let you be tempted beyond your ability [to resist], but along with the temptation He [has in the past and is now and] will [always] provide the way out as well, so that you will be able to endure it [without yielding, and will overcome temptation with joy]."

God led Jesus into the wilderness before the devil came to tempt Him. Jesus was perfectly aligned and in the middle of God's will for His life when He came face to face with Satan. A pregnant woman has been given a gift from God, and the devil wants to steal the gift. Even in circumstances where a woman has heard from God about her life and her choices and has been obedient in God's plan, she may come face to face with her enemy, Satan.

The Bible teaches us to seek God's will and direction in all aspects of our lives. When we do this, we can trust we are safe walking on the road to life. When we stay focused and keep our faith, we will end up at our destination, regardless of the demonic attempt to keep us from getting there. Through consistent focus and consistent, obedient faith, we can make informed, wise decisions aligning with God's will. The voice of God leads into wisdom and perfection, and as we trust His voice, we will reach the quiet and the still waters. Psalm 23:2 declares, "He lets me lie down in green pastures; He leads me beside the still and quiet waters."

Personal decisions shape our lives and influence the outcomes of our lives. We must approach our decision making thoughtfully, considering God in everything, so we can know our decisions please the Lord. By consulting with God for each decision, people ensure that they are making decisions that are safe and aligned with God's plan for their lives. As we consult with God, this silences the lies of the enemy, and it magnifies the voice of God.

Failing to consult with the Lord regarding our decisions is dangerous because this failure gives Satan access into the believer's life. Christians should consult with God for every major and minor decision that they make. Christians need to have God's peace, and His word, to verify that their route is correct. In medical settings, medical professionals may suggest a treatment plan or a medical procedure, and the wise Christian consults with God before beginning a medication or a medical treatment plan. When there is a lack of spiritual peace or a conflict with the Bible, Christians must pause and evaluate before they move forward. Asking God for insight and help safeguards us.

As the creator of the human body, God knows if a person will be helped or harmed through certain procedures, medicines, or other medical interventions. When a medical procedure, treatment plan, or other situation is averse to God's plan or our bodies' God-given makeup, believers will be made aware after they consult with their Father.

Often, patients will seek a second opinion from another professional when they are not pleased with their primary doctor's opinion. Consulting with doctors is not harmful when we are first submitted to Christ and His leading for our health. God is the Great Physician and should be our primary doctor. He knows exactly what our bodies need to thrive and survive. God is protective and preventive, and He keeps future disaster and heartache from our lives. If either the enemy or a failure of human intervention is problematic or dangerous to our lives, bodies, or future, our Great Physician will warn us to keep us safe from harm.

When I found out I was pregnant with my second baby, I was offered a job I knew the Lord didn't want me to take. I perceived in my spirit that I was not supposed to take the job because the thought of taking the job stole my inner peace. I cried for days because I wanted to stay home and raise my two kids, and I didn't have God's peace about working outside of the home. At the time, my husband wanted me to take the job, and the money seemed appealing in our financial situation, as we were expecting another baby.

The devil wanted my husband and me to question God's provision. He wanted us to wonder how we could make it. The devil came to me at a vulnerable time and offered me money, and he offered me a supposed position of power on the earth. I wish I could tell you I stood firm and rebuked the devil. I wish I could say I recognized the lies of the enemy and resisted this temptation.

Unfortunately, I was a new believer, and I trusted in my own human reasoning, and I ignored the Holy Spirit's warning. Today, I am aware that the lack of peace I felt about this decision should have led me to say no to the job offer. If I had not given into the fear of the devil regarding finances, then I would have been ministered too supernaturally from God and His angels. God would have provided a better way for me that didn't involve pain and torment. I know God would have given me something better than what I was offered by Satan. Matthew 4:11 says, "Then the devil left Him; and angels came and ministered to Him [bringing Him food and serving Him]."

A lack of peace is a warning from the Lord. In this period of my life, I was still very much accustomed to walking by sight. Walking by faith was foreign to me, and I did not have a firm revelation on it. I was offered a good job. This job appeared to be a blessing and an answer to my financial problems. However, in the supernatural realm, it was a plot by the enemy to try to destroy my life and get me out of the will of my Father.

My situation got progressively worse as I worked outside of the home during my second pregnancy. My new job was an hour away from my new house. To work outside of the home, I needed childcare arrangements. I also needed a new car because of all the additional driving.

Before I took my job at the school, my car was paid for, and when I bought a new car, I went into debt. We accumulated $18,000 worth of car debt that year. We paid for daycare services, another $13,000. I began eating a fast-food diet during my second pregnancy because I did not have enough time to cook or work out. Without knowing it, I opened the door to the enemy in numerous facets of my life. I brought trouble upon myself by not heeding the warnings of my Father in heaven. What appeared to be good was really a trap and a deception, causing harm and suffering to my physical and emotional health.

As an older and more mature Christian, I know God never intended for me to endure the heartache, suffering, and pain I endured that year of my pregnancy with my daughter. People often say, "You learned something, or God will use it," and while that may be true, the Lord did not plan for me to suffer for a year of my life and miss the time with my son. God didn't plan for me to go deeper into debt and neglect my health.

I caused my own problem by not heading the Holy Spirit. I know I can't go back, and I can only go forward, but I do wish I could go back and make a better decision. I regret not standing firm against the enemy's temptations and not walking in the faith that God wanted me to walk in. I regret having an inferior second pregnancy and an inferior motherhood experience with my firstborn son.

After I got out of my terrible situation, it took me some time to heal, and I became further addicted to the Lord's presence. I was keenly aware of the peace I felt when I was in God's presence, because it is a peace I never feel otherwise. The weight I gained, the emotional turmoil, and the financial setbacks took time to eradicate from my family's life. I remember asking God to please help me know what to do so I could get myself out of the trouble I had brought upon myself. As I was seeking the Lord about renewing my school counselor job contract, He led me to a devotional page that read, "Do not enter into contractual agreements that would be bad."

After the delivery of my daughter, when I got the contract for another year as a public school counselor, I made a different decision than before. When God told me to not sign the contract, I listened. I apologized to God for my lack of faith in the former phase of my life, and I told Him I was going to do my best to never step outside of His will for my life again.

At the time, I didn't know how God would make a way for our family. It appeared risky to walk away from my career as a mom to two children. We had new bills and new responsibilities, and our money was already tight. In addition, the world was going into crisis due to COVID-19, and no one knew what the future would hold. Yet, through it all, I knew what the word of the Lord was for my life. I decided I wouldn't doubt or be afraid of the future this time; instead, I would walk confidently through faith into the new part of my destiny.

Staying home with my children was one of the easiest decisions I have ever made. Although I appeared to walk away from money, prestige, and a profession I had spent six years attending college for, I didn't lose anything. It seemed like I was walking away from a sure thing and walking into an uncertain situation. I appeared to be making a mistake. But I knew I had heard from God, and God's voice caused every bit of fear of the present or the future to flee. For the first time in my life, I knew without a doubt that I was going the way God told me to go, and I knew I would be safe and protected as I went.

My first year as a stay-at-home mom to two kids was supernatural. My husband found a better job, and our finances improved almost immediately. For the first time, we could afford the life of our two incomes through one. Our family had more time together, and I could focus on motherhood, cook, clean, and take care of the house while my husband worked for our family. I was able to support my husband's work because I was home, and our family became stronger than it had ever been. I had discovered joy and happiness. I was finally fulfilled in my *work*.

Facing the spirit of fear and walking in faith for the first time was the best decision I have ever made. I don't want to imagine what would have happened if I hadn't faced fear but had let it control my destiny. To be governed by fear would have changed everything about my life, and I would have gotten myself out of God's will for not just my life, but also the lives of my children.

Going the way of the flesh or the way of Satan causes severe problems and implications, even if it appears to be harmless. I am so thankful I chose to seek God, listen to God, and walk the way of the Lord. He has provided a superior way for my family, and I am forever thankful to Him for what He alone has done. Proverbs 4:18 says, "But the path of the just (righteous) is like the light of dawn, That shines brighter and brighter until [it reaches its full strength and glory in] the perfect day."

Many times, in my walk with Christ, I have heard the enemy's voice, taunts, and lies.. He says things like, "You can't do it," and "What makes you think you are capable or called." Satan loves to get us focused on ourselves and our own needs, abilities, or capabilities, as opposed to those of God. He loves to trick humanity into thinking their God is smaller than He is. The truth is, I am not sure how God has done the things He has done for my family. He gets all the glory, but I know God is with me, and I know He is pleased with me, and there is visible fruit our families' life.

In my own strength, I am not capable of the things I have done. I am often in awe of the things God does for me and through me. I have so many testimonies and stories telling of the Lord's supernatural goodness and provisions, and I know because of Him I am successful. My strength and my reasoning will never be enough. Yet, because I walk with God, and I talk with God, I am victorious. Moses didn't open the sea with his personal determination and strength. He opened the sea through the power of God in his life and on his hand.

Both of my c-sections were fear-based decisions, influenced by the enemy. I didn't recognize these medical decisions were an attack, because I was looking at things in a natural, humanistic way. My blind decision to trust the doctors without question opened the door to the devil and his influence over the trajectory of my first and second birthing experiences.

The Lord prompted me to resist, and He warned me both times I had cesarean births through the anguish and lack of peace within my spirit I felt regarding these decisions. My uneasiness should have inspired me to question the medical decisions being made for my children, and me and I should have fought for my health and the health of my kids.

During my first birth, I was denied a chance to go into labor and trust God's perfect timing. I was intimidated through fear. The fear of not being able to safely deliver my son surrounded me, and as a new mother, *I didn't know enough* about God, the Holy Spirit, human physiology, childbirth, or parenting, to rebuke my doctor's claims.

When I doubted that I was hearing the voice of God, and I ignored the spiritual component, I became prey to carnal reasoning, and the overreliance on the understanding of a human. The fear and uncertainty of a hypothetical problem regarding a dangerous birth pushed me into the devil's territory. Fear and uncertainty influenced my decision because I heard the words of the enemy, and I believed them instead of rebuking them.

The night before my first c-section, I asked God if I was supposed to have my baby naturally, because I felt in my spirit I was supposed to. But the guidance of the healthcare system contrasted with my feelings of spiritual discernment. My doctor's recommendation was to have a c-section for my birth. I heard two very different voices, and I was presented with two very different paths.

My first cesarean birth was done against my will, even though I consented to it. I knew what to do, but I didn't do it, because I was afraid of potential harm to my life or my baby's life, and my lack of knowledge led me to reluctantly consent. Fear controlled my decision, but I know if I had just trusted in God's perfect plan and His protection, God would have provided for me and for my son without the need for medical surgery.

No peace, or a lack of complete peace, is a sign to the believer to slow down, pray, and wait. When believers feel uneasy in their spirit about a choice, they shouldn't go forward until they have peace. The enemy attempts to push us into situations out of fear. God will not push His people into decisions with negative or harsh consequences, and He won't have us make fear-based decisions. God always instructs His people, and He gives His people peace. Being confined, insecure, uncomfortable, and uneasy cues us in to perceive the hand of the enemy, not the hand of God.

I chose a different doctor for my second baby, because I knew the first time I had been coaxed into a cesarean birth unnecessarily. When a new doctor learns about your previous pregnancies, he or she begins mapping out plans for your next birth. The new doctor knew I had just had a cesarean birth, and even though she acted as if she supported my decision for a v-bac/vaginal birth after cesarean, she did not. When I got to 38 weeks, my doctor told me I should have a c-section because "I had one before, and I could get it done, and it would be safest and easiest." She waited until I was vulnerable and in the final days of my pregnancy to change my birth plan.

When my daughter was about to be born in March of 2020, COVID-19 was a new pandemic. The public panic combined with my doctor's advice that, "I needed to have my baby through cesarean immediately to protect our health" intimidated me. My doctor also informed me that my husband and son would not be allowed to witness my daughter's birth or to visit us in the hospital after she was born unless I had my baby that day. My doctor also shared with me the "possible dangers" of vaginal birth after a cesarean, as she attempted to have me sign for my cesarean birth. Both the fear of the unknown, fear of complications during birth, and the fear that I was going to be alone during my labor, my delivery, and throughout my first few days of recovery bothered me.

My doctor and others in the hospital assured me that I was making the right decision to have a cesarean birth, because I could "get in and out quickly" before more people came into the hospital with COVID-19. They told me it was convenient because my husband would be in attendance, and if I waited for organic labor, they might shut down hospital visitors. Two separate doctors, at two different hospitals, during two separate pregnancies, advised me to give birth medically instead of physiologically. Both doctors used fear and allopathic "medical science" to coax me to comply with their recommendations, against my own spiritual discernment.

During my first and second pregnancies, in the days leading to labor, I was scared and was told all the reasons I was unable to give birth to my baby without the medical establishment's intervention. This sudden change in my birth plan was brought to me quickly. Throughout both of my first pregnancies, I was told I was healthy and capable of having a healthy baby, and I was told there was no reason to suppose I was unfit or incapable of a natural vaginal birth. It wasn't until the end of my pregnancies, in an abrupt manner, I was instructed to change my birth plan and have cesarean births.

The fear, heightened by my doctor's advice, contributed to my forfeiting my rights. Various scriptures in the Bible tell us not to worry or fear. The enemy's tactics are always similar, but they come in different formats and circumstances. The enemy speaks to us, claiming there will be problems and we are unsafe. The enemy speaks fear for our life and fear our future, and he wants us to feel we are hopeless and helpless. More than anything, the devil wants people to rely on anyone or anything other than Jesus Christ. He wants us to be vulnerable and weak, lacking strength, so we can be preyed on and controlled.

The enemy spoke to me about my future and my delivery through a person. Throughout scripture, the devil used people to perpetuate his plans and thoughts. There are evil prophets and prophetesses who consistently speak the lies of Satan, and sometimes, even well meaning Christians can be used as tools for the enemy's agenda when they speak against God's will. Matthew 16:23 tells us, "But Jesus turned and said to Peter, 'Get behind Me, Satan! You are a stumbling block to Me; for you are not setting your mind on things of God, but on things of man.'"

Jesus does not want believers to be stumbling blocks for other believers in their words or actions. A stumbling block delays or stops the will of God from coming to pass in a person's life. When Peter tried to stop Jesus from doing the will of God, he was wrong, even though he was well intended and loved Jesus. Even good, God-fearing people may at times need to be rebuked. All words and thoughts opposed to God's plan can still be a stumbling block in our lives if they are not properly recognized and rebuked.

Stumbling blocks are not the same as acts and words of manipulation. Manipulation involves intentional planning of evil and harm. Manipulation involves a scheme to harm others. Manipulative people target others, and they perpetuate evil against their victims deliberately and with precision. More than carnal thinking, manipulative deeds and words are sent to cause destruction in the hearer or receiver.

Manipulative people are proud of their cunning and evil behavior because they are arrogant, proud, and vain. Manipulative people must be stopped and rebuked quickly. Tolerance of a manipulative person's plans, words, or actions towards us as believers allows manipulative individuals to gain control over our lives.

Some medical professionals are stumbling blocks in believers' lives, while others are manipulative and intentionally vile. A person needs to use keep observation through the help of the Holy Spirit to discern when a provider is well intended and simply off course and when a provider is manipulative and vile. Whether the behavior is malicious or unintentional, believers must be firm and rebuke the enemy in their lives. If we blindly trust and lack a testing or discerning of spirits, there is potential for danger ahead for the believer. In the world, some people are opposed to God intentionally and unintentionally, and our responsibility is to pay attention and rebuke individuals and groups that set themselves against God's purposes in our lives.

Busyness can also be a barrier in our lives causing us to stumble. My busy schedule limited my time to be refreshed and properly directed by Jesus. I was working full time, and I was a pregnant mom of a one-year-old boy. We were in the process of moving and buying a new house, so a lot of our time was spent moving things, organizing things, buying appliances, setting up the internet, and trying to coordinate everything. Women can be busy doing things that are not to their benefit. Busyness does not necessarily mean being productive or fruitful in the kingdom.

Some things may not be bad to do, but if they are done outside of your God-given position and domain, they are bad for you to do. Working outside of the home may be acceptable for some women during certain seasons of their life, but working outside of the home was not my portion during this season of my life. I went outside of God's perfect plan on my own accord and suffered physically, emotionally, and spiritually as a result.

Martha was a woman in the Bible who was busy working. She was diligent and was trying to do the right thing by serving people in her house. She was working hard, and she appeared to be doing something helpful and harmless. Yet, she was anxious and bothered by many things because she did not make arrangements to spend time with Jesus.

Luke 10:38–42 explains, "Now while they were on their way, Jesus entered a village [called Bethany], and a woman named Martha welcomed Him into her home. She had a sister named Mary, who seated herself at the Lord's feet and was continually listening to His teaching. But Martha was very busy and distracted with all of her serving responsibilities; and she approached Him and said, 'Lord, is it of no concern to You that my sister has left me to do the serving alone? Tell her to help me and do her part.' But the Lord replied to her, 'Martha, Martha, you are worried and bothered and anxious about so many things; but only one thing is necessary, for Mary has chosen the good part [that which is to her advantage], which will not be taken away from her.'"

God wants us to spend time with Him especially in times where we feel weak or vulnerable. Feeling weak or vulnerable is not a sin. Second Corinthians 12:9 says, "And He has said to me, 'My grace is sufficient for you, for power is perfected in weakness.' Most gladly, therefore, I will rather boast about my weakness, so that the power of Christ may dwell in me."

Presenting our requests to the Lord in our moments of weakness enables God to come into the intimate moments of our lives. God adores when we are open, honest, and vulnerable with Him through acknowledging our inability to be self-sufficient and well without Him. Through our openness and vulnerability, we can partner with God and receive His help and guidance. To receive from God, we must realize that we need Him in our lives.

In the weeks leading to my third birth at home, evil spirits tried their best to scare me into modifying my decision to have Gianni at home. In all three of my pregnancies with my children, the devil came to me at the beginning and at the end to present me with feelings of inferiority.

I felt very vulnerable at the very end of my pregnancy, and it is not a coincidence that was when I had a demonic vision in which I saw myself in an ambulance. In my vision, I watched myself unable to birth my baby safely at home, and I saw my son and myself in danger. No doubt the enemy gave me this vision to induce fear and anxiety and to change my mind about trusting God. After I had silenced the voices of doubt from medical professionals, family members, and others in my circle of influence, Satan used another means to attempt to guide me off course. The vision was given to me because I resisted all other human interference and spoken prophecy.

God previously confirmed my home birth to me in a variety of ways throughout my pregnancy. God instructed me to stay out of the hospital and to have my baby at home under the care of my midwife. I spent enough time with the Lord praying and seeking His will throughout my pregnancy to know I would have my baby safely at home. I fully believed I would be okay during delivery because God promised me that He would take care of me.

Once again, I was presented with two distinct choices at the end of my pregnancy. One route was a road of fear, anxiety, worry, and doubt. In this road I needed people's help, and I was weak and vulnerable. The other was a route of peace, comfort, protection, and rest. I was strong and capable to have Gianni, with or without help from humans, because Jesus Christ was my Great Physician, and He was going to take care of us, because He loves us.

The time I dedicated to consulting with God as my Physician during my pregnancy instilled in me a confidence in my birth plan. During my first and second pregnancies, I was fooled and manipulated by the spirit of fear weeks before giving birth. Yet, during my third, I knew I was going to have Gianni at home, and I knew God would not instruct me to have a midwife and a home birth and at the last-minute scare me into doing something else.

A few people in my life with good intentions could have become stumbling blocks for my faith if I had heeded their words. The devil wanted to use well-intended people to speak fear and apprehension through their opinions and words, just as he did in the life of Peter. Some people in my life expressed their concern about my choice to give birth to my baby at home, but I remained steadfast in God's word and promise for me and for Gianni, because I knew what I had heard God say regarding my health and my birth.

I could have had my first and second children naturally without the doctor's intervention and medical surgery. The only difference between my third birth and my first two births was the faith I had in God's plan and His protection for my life and my baby. I had the privilege of spending time in reflection with Jesus throughout my third pregnancy. As Mary did, I gleaned wisdom from Him and became aware of His divine plan for my delivery. I embraced the assurance of God's love for both myself and my son, and I had confidence in the promises, particularly regarding protection during Gianni's birth, refusing to entertain any terms set forth by the enemy.

If there is spiritual vulnerability, there is also a decrease in confidence. True confidence comes from an understanding of God's love and protection. Perfect love casts out fear, and when our revelation of

God's love is in full display, a confidence follows. A confident person will stand against the crowd unashamed. A confident person refuses to be pushed around by anyone trying to stop his or her advancement. But, if we want to be confident people, we must first be assured God loves us, and He is with us in our decisions.

Lack of confidence leads people to consult the wisdom and guidance of humans instead of the wisdom and guidance of God. A lack of God-given confidence in right and wrong choices opens a demonic doorway. The devil looks for people who are indecisive or double-minded and open to suggestions, because then he can infiltrate their thoughts and plans. Any uncertainty in the way we should go should lead us directly to prayer. If we are going to make God-given decisions, then we must take time to consult with God, believing God will reveal the path of life.

Scholars believe Mary was around the age of 14 when she learned she was going to be a mother to baby Jesus. I imagine Mary was overwhelmed with many feelings when she discovered she was going to have a child even though she was not yet married. Fear of her soon-to-be husband's response would have been enough to consume some women. Notably, the Bible says that the angel looked at Mary and told her to not be afraid. Luke 1:30 says, "And the angel said to her, 'Do not be afraid, Mary, for you have found grace (free, spontaneous, absolutely favor and loving-kindness) with God.'" God immediately comforted Mary, knowing she would face fear. God instructed Mary not to yield to the spirit of fear, but instead to rest in His plan.

All of us on the earth will encounter the devil and his demonic forces. In these encounters, God gives us assurance of our safety when we spend time in His presence. Obstetricians and pediatricians often present women with fear so women will agree to their treatment plans. Phrases such as, "what if, just to be sure, out of caution," all have their roots in fear. Fear is not from God, and we should avoid fear at all costs. A fear-based decision is a Satan-inspired decision, and Satan-influenced decisions steal, kill, and destroy our bodies, minds, and spirits.

Hebrews 2:14–15 says, "Therefore, since [these His] children share in flesh and blood [the physical nature of mankind], He Himself in a similar manner also shared in the same [physical nature, but without sin], so that through [experiencing] death He might make powerless (ineffective, impotent) him who had the power of death—that is, the devil— and [that He] might free all those who through [the haunting] fear of death were held in slavery throughout their lives."

The fear of death is the root of all fear. The Bible tells us we do not have to be afraid of death or anything else on the earth because we have an assurance of our salvation and our future. When we walk with God, we have nothing to fear because the devil cannot do anything to us. We are protected through our faith in God's promises of love and protection.

Unfortunately, many tests, procedures, and words spoken allow the devil to prophecy a future over women and their children. Words spoken hold power, and if words are not resisted and rebuked, those words produce fruit in the lives of both the speakers and the hearers. Some medical professionals unknowingly prophesy for the devil by speaking doom, sickness, problems, and death in their patients' lives. Even within the body of Christ, prophets are to be evaluated and their words should be examined to ensure the words are spoken from God alone. First Corinthians 14:29 says, "Let two or three prophets speak [as inspired by the Holy Spirit], while the rest pay attention and weigh carefully what is said."

Accepting the report and the words of another person without protecting ourselves is hazardous to health. Some words are pleasant and healing to the mind, body and spirit, where others are damaging to the hearer. Proverbs 16:24 tells us, "Pleasant words are like a honeycomb, Sweet and delightful to the soul and healing to the body."

Words can make us well. Words can also make us unwell. To maintain a position of health and well being, we must realize when words are being spoken over our lives to cause us problems or harm. At times we must rebuke evil words spoken over us and over our children.

"Fight or flight" has been studied within the psychological world. Many studies have been performed on the fight or flight response in humans. Some people have formed habits of flight or running away from people, words, or situations they are afraid of. However, the more we run from fear, the more the devil gains access and control, and the worse things become, because God commands us to stand firm and to fight the good fight of faith. If we stand in faith and challenge the devil, the devil will flee. Proverbs 28:1 explains, "The wicked flee when no one pursues, but the righteous are as bold as a lion."

A fight must take place to overcome the devil, and his attack through the spirit of fear. Like with any war or battle, before people are ready to fight, they must first put on their armor. The armor of God will make the devil flee from our lives and is successful every single time against our defeated enemy. Ephesians 6:11 says, "Put on the full armor of God [for His precepts are like the splendid armor of a heavily armed soldier], so that you may be able to [successfully] stand up against all the schemes and the strategies and the deceits of the devil."

Fighting and putting on our armor requires action. For instance, putting on the shield of faith requires us to know and believe God and His word and to put it to work through engaging our faith. To engage means to become involved in something. To engage our faith, we must lift up God's word and tear down the enemy's words. Ephesians 6:16 instructs, "Above all, lift up, the [protective] shield of faith with which you can extinguish all the flaming arrows of the evil one. And take the helmet of salvation, and the sword of the Spirit, which is the Word of God."

The helmet of salvation requires us to be saved and sanctified through the blood of Jesus. To have the helmet, we must believe and confess Jesus is the Son of God, and Jesus died for our sins to be forgiven. Without our salvation on our head, our thoughts are uncovered and are subject to carnal beliefs and demonic suggestions.

The breastplate of righteousness calls us to live holy, and we must choose not to participate in the works of darkness. By living pure and honest lives, we limit Satan's ability to influence us. We saw this principle in the life of Daniel, when wicked men created a law to try to trap Daniel, because he was living a pure and honest life, and they had no other way to destroy him.

The more pieces of armor a believer has on, the safer he or she is from the attacks of the evil one. The helmet of salvation combined with the shield of faith is stronger than one without the other. For this reason, we are instructed to put on the full armor and to not leave any part of our being uncovered and vulnerable to Satan. When a believer has all his or her armor, the devil can't penetrate or perpetuate his plans against that Christian. A Christian who is armed for battle takes ground for the kingdom and becomes an offense-ready warrior as opposed to a defense-positioned victim. We stand boldly like a lion confident in our beliefs, and we do not shy away in fear, because we are assured that our God walks alongside us.

7

Prophecy and Prayers of Protection

Jochebed, the mother of Moses, loved God and trusted Him with her life and the lives of her children. When pharaoh ordered that all the Hebrew baby boys should be killed, Jochebed wouldn't comply. She concealed and protected her Moses against pharaoh's orders. Jochebed was determined to protect Moses at all costs. She knew the Lord had a plan for her son.

Pharaoh instructed the midwives, "When you help the Hebrew women in childbirth, look at the child when you deliver it. If it is a boy, kill it, but if it is a girl, let it live." (Exodus 1: 16)

If Jochebed had been discovered, her punishment would likely have been the death of her entire household, including her other child, Miriam, but Jochebed was not intimidated by her enemies. She understood God would protect her entire family, and understanding God's power and love made her fearless. Jochebed and her husband's decision to keep and raise Moses for three months was heroic. Hebrews 11:23 declares, "Moses' parents had faith. So, they hid him for three months after he was born. They saw he was a special child. They were not afraid of the king's command."

Jochebed could not continue hiding Moses in her home. When she needed it, Jochebed received instruction from God. Jochebed's spiritual insight influenced her outward actions as a mom. It is abnormal to protect a child out of love and then release the child into the river as an infant without a justified reason to do so. But Exodus 2: 2–4 tells us, "But when she could hide him no longer, she got a papyrus basket for him and coated it with tar and pitch. Then she placed the child in it and put it among the reeds along the bank of the Nile. His sister stood at a distance to see what would happen to him."

God orchestrated for the princess, pharaoh's daughter, to be at the river when baby Moses was released. God ensured His daughter, Jochebed, heard the instructions for the protection of Moses, at the exact time she needed to receive them. We know Jochebed heard from God that her son Moses would be safe, because of her level of assurance. Her guarantee in her family's safety was the key, enabling her to act in the way that she did. Without confidence from God, Jochebed would not have been able to place her son in a basket, and she would have been afraid for Moses's future.

God has a history of providing His people insight of the future. He gives us information ahead of time, so we are never caught off guard and harmed by our enemies. Through providing Jochebed with foreknowledge and a vision of the future, God safeguarded Jochebed and her family. God spoke specifically to Jochebed about her son Moses, and she received an intimate and private message. Some situations, like the situation with Moses and his mother, require unique and specified instructions.

God continues to speak to us directly. God delivers personal mail to us. These messages are distinctive to the individual receiving the message. God speaks to us intimately, and He provides us with information exclusive to us alone. God does not instruct all mothers to place their children in a basket and float them down a river. God spoke that personal and intimate message to Jochebed because she uniquely needed the instruction to keep Moses safe.

God is not limited in how He speaks to us. Even if we do not know precisely how Jochebed received revelation from God, we know she did. As believers walk with God, they will continuously receive divine messages and instructions. These instructions and messages can come in a variety of ways. Sometimes the Lord speaks to His people through dreams, visions, angelic visitations, or through written or spoken prophecy. God confirms His message to us in a multitude of ways, and God will provide us with an assurance of the message sent.

Jochebed's son Moses was the first person to write down God's word. Until Moses recorded the Ten Commandments, humans did not hold the written word of God. Before the Ten Commandments were documented there was only spoken word. Genesis 12:7 tells us, "Then the Lord appeared to Abram and said, 'To your descendants I will give this land.'"

God's people have always verbally communicated God's message to others, but without the written word, a verbal form of communication was the primary way the Lord interacted with His people.

Today, when a spoken word is from the Lord, it always testifies to the validity of scripture. God is not a liar, and as He speaks to us personally, He will confirm what the Scriptures already say. Everything God uses for communication will always endorse the truths of the Bible, because the Bible was written by people who knew and heard the instructions of God. We should never receive a word from a person, a dream, a vision, or an angel or demon that contradicts the Scriptures. Galatians 1:8 says, "But even if we, or an angel from heaven, should preach to you a gospel contrary to that which we [originally] preached to you, let him be condemned to destruction!"

The messages and the guidance given to Jochebed were not in opposition to God's former word spoken through the former prophets. In fact, they fulfilled them. God's spoken word to Jochebed perfectly corresponded with the earlier prophets' predictions. The former prophets foretold of delivery of Egyptian bondage. They saw and spoke to others of God's people being freed in the future.

Jochebed responded to God's prophecy of deliverance for her people at large, and she responded to a personalized spoken prophecy for her and her family. Jochebed believed in the predicted prophecy for the Israelites as a group, but she also believed God's prophetic prophecy for her son Moses.

Today, the Church receives God's word through a combination of written word and spoken word. We believe the messages of the former prophets, who recorded through writing the words of God, but we also receive personal communication from the Lord.

As those created in the image of God, we have the capability to deliver a message written on paper, and we also have the capability to speak messages from our mouths. We can speak verbally or in a written format. We can communicate messages to large groups of people, but we can also privately communicate messages in an intimate and personal manner.

God speaks to His people through written word and spoken word. He speaks to groups, and He speaks to individuals. A failure to understand and communicate with God through both the written word and the spoken word, publicly and privately, is a failure to properly connect and communicate with God.

Prophecies frequently relate to individuals and groups of people simultaneously. In the book of Daniel, an angel gave a prophetic message to Daniel personally, but the message also applied to his people at large. Daniel 10:11–14 says, "He said, 'Daniel, you who are highly esteemed, consider carefully the words I am about to speak to you, and stand up, for I have now been sent to you.' And when he said this to me, I stood up trembling. Then he continued, 'Do not be afraid, Daniel. Since the first day that you set your mind to gain understanding and to humble yourself before your God, your words were heard, and I have come in response to them. But the prince of the Persian kingdom resisted me twenty-one days. Then Michael, one of the chief princes, came to help me, because I was detained there with the king of Persia. Now I have come to explain to you what will happen to your people in the future, for the vision concerns a time yet to come.'"

Prophecy is a supernatural phenomenon. To believe in prophecy, a person must believe in an all-powerful and all-knowing God. Humans often question the events and circumstances of their life, because they do not know the outcome of their lives. Life without God's assured hope and plan is scary, because people do not inherently know the future. This truth is the reason why Christians have hope and promise of a future. Christians put their hope and trust in the Lord, and the Lord tells us our glorious future.

A prophecy can be experienced in the present tense, where the things that are happening now have been prophesied in years past. Prophecy can also be past tense, as some prophecies in the Bible have already been fulfilled. Prophecy is also foretelling for the future, and this definition is the one that most people use when they are referring to prophecy. But in all three definitions, prophecy is supernatural, because God who knows everything, has chosen to share pieces of the future with human beings.

In the book *The Gifts and Ministries of the Holy Spirit*, Lester Sumrall writes, "In the Old Testament, the position of a prophet was one of divine guide. He was sent by God to lead the people of Israel. The prophet at that time was also called a seer. First Samuel 9:9 says, 'Beforetime in Israel, when a man went to inquire of God, thus he spoke, Come, and let us go to the seer: for he that is now called a Prophet was before time called a Seer.' The Hebrew word *ra'ah*—to see or to perceive—tells us what the ministry of the prophet is all about. Also, the word *chozeh*—beholder of visions—is used of a seer or a prophet. So, prophets are not new, and they are dramatic in their foretelling of what will come to pass. They have no earthly means of knowing what they foretell. Enoch made no calculations by the moon or the stars or with the soothsayers. Only God told him."

Throughout scripture, God used prophets, male and female, to speak the truth. God uses prophets to instruct and tell the future of things before they happen. Moses was a prophet who prophesied about the coming birth and ministry of Jesus years before Jesus was born. Acts 3:22 explains, "Moses said 'The Lord your God will raise up for you a Prophet like me from among your brothers. You must listen to everything He tells you.'"

The Lord used the prophet Micah to prophesy about Jesus's birthplace. Micah prophesied approximately 700 years before Jesus's birth happened, and he told about the future because God told him. Micah 5:2 tells us, "But you, Bethlehem Ephrathah, though you are small among the clans of Judah, out of you will come for me one who will be ruler over Israel, whose origins are from of old, from ancient times."

At the core of prophecy and a prophet's ministry and mission is the preparation of God's plans and pursuits on the earth. God gives prophets a knowledge of Him and His ways, so they can prepare a way for His plans to come to pass. When God's people receive prophecy, they are strengthened and encouraged, knowing God will fulfill what He says He will fulfill.

God appoints prophets, and He gives them the ability to hear and to see in the spirit. To be a prophet, a person must hear and see in the realm of the spirit. Hearing and seeing requires listening, watching, and responding to the supernatural realm. Luke 1:76 says of John, "And you, child, will be called the prophet of the Highest; For you will go before the face of the Lord to prepare His ways, To give knowledge of salvation to His people by the remission of their sins, through the tender mercy of our God."

God uses the voices of His prophets to prove He is the one true God. Prophecy magnifies God and shows He is all knowing and all-powerful. Prophecy proves God knows the beginning from the end.

Like many of the gifts of God, the gift of prophecy has been counterfeited by Satan. Many people attempt to receive insight, instruction, and divine guidance from sources such as psychics and fortunetellers, not knowing they are being deceived. Psychics and witches can give people half-truths and a fraction of supernatural insight. Satan can give people information, but because he is a liar, the information he gives cannot be trusted. John 8:44 teaches, "For you are the children of your father the devil, and you love to do the evil things he does. He was a murderer from the beginning. He has always hated the truth, because there is no truth in him. When he lies, it is consistent with his character; for he is a liar and the father of lies."

Through all generations, Satan has used people to speak for him. Satan has chosen people to be his prophets speaking about future things to come. These individuals are dishonest and deceitful, and their words are not trustworthy.

Trust is defined as a firm belief in the reliability, truth, or ability, and strength of someone or something. Trust is established from a relationship of continual truth. Honesty and integrity are core components in building and maintaining trust in a relationship, but when people believe the prophecies of Satan, they are deceived into thinking they are hearing things that are true about them or those around them, when in fact they are not.

When an individual is deceived by someone they once trusted, it reflects a betrayal of trust placed in that person, ultimately leading to the painful realization of having been misled. Satan and his prophets interact with humanity in this fashion. Even in situations where there is partial honesty or honesty for a period within a relationship, there comes a time when the truth is discovered, and the lies are unveiled. Satan will trick people by telling them things that are partially true or appear to be true, but are not. Satan is the master at deceiving, lying, and twisting the truth.

All witches and psychics have been given half-truths by Satan. The information Satan shares with humanity is often enough to fool them into thinking they are in a trustworthy, supernatural companionship. Matthew 24:24 says, "For false messiahs and false prophets will appear and perform great signs and wonders to deceive, if possible, even the elect."

The devil uses many forms of witchcraft and fraud to fool people into believing they are gaining authentic supernatural insight and wisdom. If human beings can fool, trick and manipulate other human beings through lying and deceit, imagine how much more Satan, the master and father of lies, can deceive through his supernatural sorcery.

Scripture identifies two groups of deceived prophets. In 1 Kings, the prophets of Baal, and the prophets of Asherah were two distinct groups of prophets who served the devil through the worship of false gods. These prophets believed they were serving the most powerful god or gods, or they wouldn't have agreed to go against Elijah in a "competition of the gods." The Bible says these two groups of false prophets joined alliances and both "ate at Jezebel's table." The table of Jezebel was a table of hatred and murder towards God's Word and God's people who proclaim it.

The table of Jezebel was ultimately overtaken and destroyed, and God proved through His prophet Elijah that He was far superior to the people's false gods. Elijah spoke on God's behalf saying, "I have not troubled Israel, but you and your father's house have, in that you have forsaken the commandments of the Lord and have followed the Baals. Now therefore, send and gather all Israel to me on Mount Carmel, the four hundred and fifty prophets of Baal, and the four hundred prophets of Asherah, who eat at Jezebel's table" (1 Kings 18:18–19).

The devil has power, but he does not have *the* power. Satan is weak when he is against Jehovah. Jezebel's mission was to eradicate Israel's love and commitment to their God. To eliminate God's platform before the people, she introduced pagan worship and pagan gods, and she got rid of the true prophets. Getting rid of the prophets was necessary, because the prophets of God would testify of God and His power and authority on the earth. Jezebel needed to silence the prophets if she wanted to deceive the people to serve false gods and to receive false information. Without eradicating the prophets of God, the prophets of Satan could not overtake the platform. First Kings

18:4 declares, "For so it was, while Jezebel massacred the prophets of the Lord, that Obadiah had taken one hundred prophets and hidden them, fifty to a cave, and had fed them with bread and water."

The devil has always attempted to destroy God's word and God's people that proclaim it. But there has always been a remnant of people chosen by God, who survived and thrived in the face of adversity to oppose the works of the devil. In every generation, God has always kept people alive to continue in His work. Satan will never win in the battle against the Lord. Revelation 20:10 prophecies, "Then the devil who had led them astray [deceiving and seducing them] was hurled into the fiery lake of burning brimstone, where the beast and false prophet were; and they will be tormented day and night forever and ever (through the ages of the ages)."

When the Church exits as the result of the rapture, we will leave the authority of the earth in the hands of Satan, the Antichrist, and the False Prophet. The most powerful false prophet to ever exist is yet to come and will be empowered by Satan. The false prophet will speak lies against God, through the Antichrist spirit's power, granted to him by Satan, as the Church speaks truth about God, under Jesus' Spirit's power, granted to us by God.

During the reign of the unholy trinity, the evil authority and dominion will plunge the world into complete chaos and darkness. The False Prophet and the Antichrist will perform mighty supernatural things on earth and will deceive many into following Satan.

Revelation 13:2–6 prophesies, "And the beast that I saw resembled a leopard, but his feet were like those of a bear and his mouth was like that of a lion. And to him the dragon gave his [own] might and power and his [own] throne and great dominion. And one of his heads seemed to have a deadly wound. But his death stroke was healed; and the whole earth went after the beast in amazement and admiration. They fell down and paid homage to the dragon, because he had bestowed on the beast all his dominion and authority; they also praised and worshiped the beast, exclaiming, Who is a match for the beast, and, Who can make war against him? And the beast was given the power of speech, uttering boastful and blasphemous words, and he was given freedom to exert his authority and to exercise his will during forty-two months (three and a half years). And he opened his mouth to speak slanders against God, blaspheming His name and His abode, [even vilifying] those who live in heaven."

God protected Moses from infancy because his parents believed in God's prophecies and plans. The devil wanted to stop the Church's advancement by killing the baby boys. Satan was unsuccessful, because God showed His people how to survive against their adversary. God's power is unmistakable, and God's plan will always succeed over the devil's plans. God caused pharaoh to be responsible for Moses' upbringing. God provided for Moses using the enemies' financial resources, not the other way around.

Believers and their children are supernaturally preserved from the forces of darkness. We are given insightful revelation for our protection ahead of time, so we can remain free from harm. The devil tries to create plans to do away with us, but he cannot carry out his plans, because God goes before us making a way for us to prevail. God will bless us, and He will make the enemy pay for it.

Moses and Aaron permitted the Egyptian magicians to boast in their magic before they embarrassed the magicians. The magicians were able to perform miracles and wonders, but they couldn't do everything God's people could do. The demonic magicians had *enough* power to replicate supernatural miracles such as water turning into blood, but they could not replicate miracles such as summoning mosquitoes or turning the sky dark. Demonic magic allowed the magicians to harness a degree of wicked power, but no matter how hard they tried their power could not match God's power.

Exodus 7:20–22 tells us, "Moses and Aaron did just as the Lord had commanded. He raised his staff in the presence of the pharaoh and his officials struck the water of the Nile, and all the water was changed into blood. The fish in the Nile died, and the river smelled so bad that the Egyptians could not drink its water. Blood was everywhere in Egypt. But the Egyptians magicians did the same things by their secret arts, and the Pharaoh's heart became hard; he would not listen to Moses and Aaron, just as the Lord had said."

God instructed Moses to speak on His behalf before the Pharaoh and the other Egyptians. God made Moses "like God to pharaoh." God gave Moses full power over darkness, and in advance, He explained to Moses precisely what would happen. Moses was not surprised or intimidated by the evil before him because he knew what the outcome would be before he ever entered the situation. Moses knew God was with him, and Moses knew the future of his life and the lives of those surrounding him.

Exodus 7:1–5 explains, "Then the Lord said to Moses, 'See I have made you like God to Pharaoh, and your brother Aaron will be your prophet. You are to say everything that I command you, and your brother is to tell Pharaoh to let the Israelites go out of his country. But I will harden Pharaoh's heart, and though I multiply my signs and wonders in Egypt, he will not listen to you. Then I will lay my hand on Egypt and with mighty acts of judgment I will bring out my divisions, my people the Israelites. And the Egyptians will know that I am the Lord when I stretch out my hand against Egypt and bring the Israelites out of it.'"

Demonic power has been, and will always be, inferior to God's power. When Joseph was in Egypt, he became a ruler when the magicians could not interpret the Pharaoh's dream but Joseph could. The intensity of miracles and power that God holds and will demonstrate through His people, is vastly different, apparent, and recognizable to all—even to those who hold wicked power. There is not a power struggle between God and Satan. God is the highest power.

Exodus 8:16 declares, "Then the Lord said to Moses, 'Tell Aaron, "Stretch out your staff and strike the dust of the ground," and throughout the land of Egypt the dust will become gnats.' They did this, and when Aaron stretched out his hand with the staff and struck the dust of the ground, gnats came on people and animals. And the dust throughout the land of Egypt became gnats. But when the magicians tried to produce gnats by their secret arts, they could not. Since the gnats were on the people and animals everywhere, the magicians said to pharaoh, 'This is the finger of God.'"

Throughout time and without error, God has proved himself to be truthful and reliable. When God speaks, His words always come to pass. The Bible has prophesied the future through the ages and some prophecies have yet to be fulfilled, but we know they will be fulfilled. Second Peter 3:9 tells us, "The Lord is not slow to fulfill His promise as some count slowness, but He is patient towards you, not wishing that any should perish, but that all should reach repentance."

God wants to work and to demonstrate His power on the earth. God wants to fulfill His word. Jeremiah 1:12 teaches, "Then said the Lord to me, 'You have seen well, for I am alert and active, watching over My word to perform it.'" God is observing us to see if we will partner with Him to bring His plans to pass on the earth. When we partner with God, we align ourselves with His word, and we become active participants in the fulfillment of prophecy.

Jochebed was a woman whom God used to bring His plan to the earth. If Jochebed had operated in unbelief, and if she had refused to use her faith and protect her baby, then God would have instructed another willing and obedient woman to fulfill His prophecy of deliverance for His people. But because God sees the future, God knew Jochebed would partner with Him to bring His plans to pass. He knew from the beginning that Jochebed, and her son Moses would be the fulfillment of His written and spoken prophecies.

All over the world, there are God's prophets, and the devil's prophets. God gave humanity the choice to serve Him or the devil. Prophets determine whom they speak for. God already knows who will speak for Him. He knows the beginning from the end, and He is never surprised by what the devil is doing. If we listen to our Father, we won't be taken by surprise either!

When we are committed and loyal to God, we will only testify God's truth, even when humans or devils don't like it. True prophets speak only for the Lord.

2 Chronicles 18:6–13 tells us, "But Jehoshaphat said, 'Is there not another prophet of the Lord here by whom we may inquire?' King [Ahab] of Israel said to Jehoshaphat, 'There is another man, Micaiah son of Imla, by whom we may inquire of the Lord, but I hate him, for he never has prophesied good for me, but always evil.' And Jehoshaphat said, 'Let not the king say so.' And King [Ahab] of Israel called for one of his officers and said, 'Bring quickly Micaiah son of Imla.' The king of Israel and Jehoshaphat king of Judah sat each on his throne, arrayed in their robes; they were sitting in an open place [at the threshing floor] at the entrance of the gate of Samaria; all the prophets were prophesying before them. And Zedekiah, son of Chenaanah had made himself horns of iron, and said, 'Thus says the Lord: With these you shall push the Syrians until they are destroyed.' All the prophets prophesied so, saying, 'Go up to Ramoth-gilead and prosper; the Lord will deliver it into the king's hand.' The messenger who went to call Micaiah said to him, 'Behold, the words of the prophets foretell good to the king with one accord. So let your word be like one of them, and speak favorably.' But Micaiah said, 'As the Lord lives, what my God says, that will I speak.'"

God gives prophets divine wisdom and insight into the future. Prophets of God do not guess when they prophesy. It is wise to hear the word of a trusted prophet, because of the power in a prophet's prophecy. All believers have a duty to determine if a prophet's spoken prophecy is trustworthy and accurate. Believers are specifically instructed in scripture to test the prophecies spoken, to determine the origins of the prophecies. First Thessalonians 5:20–21 "Do not spurn the gifts and utterances of the prophets [do not depreciate prophetic revelations nor despise inspired instruction or exhortation or warning]. But test and prove all things [until you can recognize] what is good; [to that] hold fast."

Hearing and receiving the word of the Lord is the first step to planting any words from God within our hearts. Once we hear God's words, whether spoken or written, through God or through His people, the words of God are either rejected or planted into our hearts.

The seeds of God's word can produce and grow when they are given the opportunity to take root within us. If the word is not planted in our hearts, then it will not bear fruit in our lives. Satan wants people to hear and then reject the words of God, so the words never fully take root in the soil of our hearts. Mark 4:15 says, "These [in the first group] are the ones along the road where the word is sown; but when they hear, Satan immediately comes and takes away the word which has been sown in them."

Our hearts are the soil bringing fruit and harvest to our lives. God's word is a seed, and His word produces when it is planted properly in the healthy and receptive soil of the heart. First Peter 1:23 tells us, "You have been regenerated (born again), not from a mortal origin (seed, sperm), but from one that is immortal by the ever living and lasting Word of God."

The word of God changes, transforms, and creates new things when it is given the heart to work and to produce. But like in any relationship between a man and a woman, seed or fruit, two components or parties work together to create and birth life. In humans, the father produces the seed, the sperm, and the mother has the eggs and the womb that nurtures and grows the seed. In plants, the seed needs the soil, or they will not produce.

We are the soil growing the word of God, the seed, when the conditions of our hearts are right. As the bride of Christ, it is presumed we want to use the seed, which is the word of God, to produce spiritual children and a spiritual harvest.

God is a gentleman, and He will never force us to bear spiritual things or to produce when we are not personally invested, interested, and willing to do so. Our relationship with God is one of mutual love and respect. When we join ourselves to Christ, and we desire to bear fruit and to birth life, we will see supernatural fruit and harvest in the spiritual realm of our lives. If we choose to sow into the flesh and reject God's word or seed, we will not be able to produce the same things as someone who is willing to yield himself or herself to God.

Matthew 13:3–9 says, "He told them many things in parables, saying, "Listen carefully: a sower went out to sow [seed in his field];and as he sowed, some seed fell beside the road [between the fields], and the birds came and ate it. Other seed fell on rocky ground, where they did not have much soil; and at once they sprang up because they had no depth of soil. But when the sun rose, they were scorched; and because they had no root, they withered away. Other seed fell among thorns, and thorns came up and choked them out. Other seed fell on good soil and yielded grain, some a hundred times as much [as was sown], some sixty [times as much], and some thirty."

The believer who sows the word of God in his or her heart will begin to store up goodness within the heart. Over time, the heart is full of God and His word, and it begins to bear fruit supernaturally. All seeds take time to grow, but in the same way that we cannot explain how a seed can produce a harvest of fruit, or a sperm can produce a newborn baby, we cannot explain the supernatural phenomenon of God's word producing a supernatural harvest. But, if we keep the seed planted in our hearts, and we continue to plant more seeds, we know we will have an abundant harvest, and it will be bountiful.

Luke 6:45 tells us, "A good man brings good things out of the good stored up in his heart, and an evil man brings evil things out of the evil stored up in his heart. For the mouth speaks what the heart is full of."

We bring forth or birth into existence the things stored up in our hearts by confession and speaking. Confession is the birthing process of things that have been conceived. When we confess, we birth the thoughts, ideas, and the beliefs we have allowed into our minds and our hearts. Confession comes after hearing and planting the words of

God or the words of the enemy within our hearts, as birth follows the conception and the nurturing of a baby in the womb.

Our confession and words we speak are the tangible fruit of the things already planted within the heart. They are the babies in our life of the things that we have created through our choices to either protect or to neglect what enters the heart. Proverbs 4:23 says, "Watch over your heart with all diligence, For from it flow the springs of life."

Hearing the word of God instills faith into our hearts. The more we hear, believe, and receive God's word, the more we will store these words in our hearts. The storing up in the heart helps bring forth the confession and the activation of God's promises. Confession without heart implantation will not produce, just like planting seed without soil, or sperm without a womb implantation, will not produce.

Often, people want to recite or memorize scripture alone, and although this can be beneficial, it is not enough to produce a harvest in a person's life. The harvest can only be accessed through the implantation process of the heart. Without the seed going into the heart and implanting, there will be no harvest. Recitation without understanding is insufficient for proper growth. We must confess God's word because we understand it and we believe it to be true if we are going to see it produce in our lives.

Memorization is consistently shown to be the lowest form of learning. Research shows us that people often memorize without understanding. For all forms of learning, we know memorizing and speaking alone can't bring forth the same things as applied learning and progress. Unless there is first a decoding of the information, followed by a storing of the information, progress and growth will be limited. If we are going to learn and grow and to produce for the kingdom of God, we must first learn and understand through planting the seed in our hearts, and then we will speak or birth the things that have been planted.

Second Peter 1:21 teaches, "For no prophecy was ever produced by the will of man, but men spoke from God as they were carried along by the Holy Spirit." When the Holy Spirit says something to us personally, it gives us confidence. Through our experiences and encounters with God and His Spirit, we gain assurance regarding the direction of our lives. By engaging in active learning, as opposed to mere memorization and passive absorption, our minds become properly molded to remain focused on God's purposes rather than our own.

I regularly hear and see personal revelation and truth directly from the Holy Spirit. When God speaks to me, I am assured in my next decision because I know I have heard directly from my Father, who loves me and protects me. God has also spoken to me on behalf of others, such as my kids, my family members, friends, or others within my community and my country.

Recently I dreamed about a woman from church. This mother was very concerned about the well being of her children. She seemed uncomfortable and distressed. When I woke up the next morning, I felt the Holy Spirit leading me to check on her. I obeyed, and I reached out to her, even though we don't talk frequently. I told her my dream, and shared a scripture God wanted me to share with her.

This woman sent me a picture of a tattoo on her arm of that specific scripture verse. She shared with me that she had been concerned about one of her children, and she was praying for God to help her. God did not share the information with me for me to gossip, judge, or condemn her. Instead he shared it with me so I could encourage her. By revealing a tiny fragment of her situation to me, and by giving me a Bible verse, the Lord reassured her of His love for her and reassured her that He cared about her situation.

My obedience to reach out to this woman and to speak a word from God for her encouraged her, strengthened her, and helped her to know God was aware and watching her situation. It brought her closer to God, and it gave her God's peace, His love, and His assurance about the future of her situation.

Above all else, this is the reason for prophecy! Prophecy shows people God's sovereignty and love. Prophecy brings comfort through the assurance of God's protection and authority over the earth. First Corinthians 14:3 tells us, "But [on the other hand] the one who prophecies speaks to people for edification [to promote their spiritual growth] and [speaks words of] encouragement [to uphold and advise them concerning the matters of God] and [speaks words of] consolation [to compassionately comfort them]."

When God created everything, He spoke. Psalm 33:9 declares, "For He spoke, and it came to be; He commanded, and it appeared at His command." God spoke to the earth and commanded it to appear. God spoke and brought the oceans into existence. The Bible says when the earth began, it was void, yet through God's speaking, the whole world came to be.

Humanity was God's creation that He made in His image. Genesis 1:27 tells us, "So God created mankind in His own image, in the image of God, He created them; male and female he created them." As men and women formed in the image of God, we were designed to speak and create things from nothing. We were made to change situations through our words.

God partners with us to orchestrate His mission on the earth. Declaring and speaking are necessary components in the Christian life. To be saved, a person must first believe, then speak and confess with his or her mouth. All other things within the kingdom work in this way. We must believe first, then we must confess what we believe to be true in our hearts. Romans 10:10 tells us, "For with the heart a person believes [in Christ as Savior] resulting in his justification [that is, being made righteous—being freed of the guilt of sin and made acceptable to God]; and with the mouth he acknowledges and confesses [his faith openly], resulting in and confirming [his] salvation."

As believers, we are God's witnesses. A witness is someone who speaks about the things he or she has seen or heard. Witnesses are supposed to tell others the truth, and their testimony matters in a court of law. A credible witness rightfully testifies about the things he or she has seen so the truth can be uncovered and justice can be served.

As God's witnesses, we see and hear the words and the plans of God. We decipher the truth and the mission of the Lord, and we share this truth with the world, so other people have the chance to see too.

If a person rejects what he or she has been told, then that person alone will be held accountable for his or her sins, but we are responsible to testify to the truth, hoping for all to receive the forgiveness of Christ. Isaiah 43:10 explains, "'You are my witnesses,' declares the Lord, 'and my servant whom I have chosen, that you may know and believe me and understand that I am He. Before me no god was formed, nor shall there be any after me.'"

From the time Jesus was a young boy, He was keenly aware the Father's will for the earth, because He knew God's spoken and written word. Jesus was permitted to speak for His Father, even as a young child, because Jesus spent time in prayer, and He spent time studying the Scriptures. Prayer is talking to God and allowing God to talk to you. When we pray, we should expect God to answer our prayers, because He promised us He will. We may receive a personalized word, or we may receive one that is applicable to the larger society, or other groups of people, but we will receive a word when we ask for one.

If we want to be used mightily of God, we must be willing to do what Jesus did. We must be willing to study and understand scripture, and we must be willing to spend time in God's house, communing with our Father. Matthew 10:24 tells us, "A student is not greater than his teacher. A servant is not above his master."

As children of God and servants to our Lord Jesus Christ, we must submit ourselves to the teaching of the Holy Spirit and to the study of the Holy Scriptures. We must spend time talking to God and letting God talk back to us.

As Jesus spoke or performed any great work on the earth, He confirmed the will the Father. John 5:19–20 says, "So Jesus answered them by saying, 'I assure you and most solemnly say to you, the Son can do nothing of Himself of His own accord, unless it is something He sees the Father doing; for whatever things The Father does, the Son in His turn also does in the same way.'"

As heirs to God's throne, Christians are to hear, know, and perform the will and the plans of God. We are to do the work of God, and we prepare ourselves for work through prayer, and through the knowledge of God's will. We must be God's witnesses to other people, showing them that God is real, active, and alive, through prophecy and the supernatural working of miracles, by the power of the Holy Spirit, and the authority of Jesus Christ.

As you read these prayers today, believe in your heart the Lord is with you and fights for you. Plant God's word within your heart and store up God's truth and provision.

The more we store in our hearts, the more we will produce in our outward life. The kingdom is a seed, so don't grow weary in doing good things, because in due time you will reap a harvest for all seeds that have been sown. Sow and keep on sowing, knowing your seeds are in the ground and are growing! A pregnancy takes nine months, and after a season we meet our precious baby. Birthing spiritual things is a process, but when it is done correctly, the harvest will come through every single time!

Mark 4:26–29 explains, "And He said, 'The kingdom of God is like a man who scatters seed upon the ground, And then continues sleeping and rising night and day while the seed sprouts and grows and increases—he knows not how. The earth produces [acting] by itself—first the blade, then the ear, then the full grain in the ear. But when the grain is ripe and permits, immediately he sends forth [the reapers] and puts in the sickle, because the harvest stands ready.'"

The Church is protected and preserved from the attacks of the devil. We will continue to take ground and to challenge the lies and the taunts of the enemy, because the devil is subordinate to our God. As parents of children, we will stand boldly, believing the words God has spoken about our children. The Holy Spirit is a seal of protection around our lives. The Holy Spirit stands as a helper, working to always defend our families from the attacks of the evil one.

Isaiah 54:15 declares, "'If anyone fiercely attacks you it will not be from Me. Whoever attacks you will fall because of you. Listen carefully, I have created the smith who blows on the fire of coals And who produces a weapon for its purpose; And I have created the destroyer to inflict ruin. No weapon that is formed against you will succeed; *And every tongue that rises against you* in judgment you will condemn. This [peace, righteousness, security, and triumph over opposition] is the heritage of the servants of the Lord, And this is their vindication from Me,' says the Lord."

A Prayer for Moms

Heavenly Father,

Thank you for the victory over my enemies. I take a stand and use my authority now over the devil and all his attacks. I believe You are here with me, fighting on my behalf and on behalf of my children. You have a plan for our lives, and You will fulfill that plan. I trust You with everything, including the lives of my children. As Jochebed released Moses, I release my children into Your loving hands, because I know You have a unique and valuable purpose for their lives. Your word tells me You have a plan to prosper us and to keep us safe. Your word promises me that You will keep me knowledgeable about the way to go before any attack comes. I believe You will speak to me and give me detailed instructions on what to do in every circumstance. I believe and receive Your word.

I assert today that I am protected and my children(names) are protected. I declare (name) will be mighty on the earth. (Name) is a reward and a heritage given to me by You.

Your word says I am blessed because I am a mother. Your word tells me I will not be put to shame, and my children will grow up and call me blessed. We are Your witnesses, and we will testify your power to this generation and the next. In our house, we will talk about miracles, healings, and deliverance. We will walk in Your precepts and only walk on Your path. We will experience You in a supernatural way, whether we are sitting, lying down, or waking up.

We vow from today forward we live an abundant supernatural life with You: A life so incredible everyone will see it. Amen.

"Moses answered the people, 'Do not be afraid. Stand firm and you will see the deliverance the Lord will bring you today. The Egyptians you see today you will never see again. The Lord will fight for you; you need only to be still'" (Exodus 14: 13–14).

8

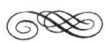

Attachment, Breastfeeding, and Circumcision

God designed the world and everything in it. Within the human design, God authorized free will. God instructed Adam and Eve to refrain from partaking in the knowledge held within the tree to protect humanity from acquiring poisonous information. God instructed Adam and Eve to refrain from possessing the knowledge of evil, because He knew the knowledge of evil and sin would change humanity for the worst. God saw the knowledge of evil would introduce unhealthy mindsets and unhealthy behavior. He understood sin would make humanity unwell.

Learning incorrect things is detrimental. The knowledge of evil has confused, weakened and separated humans from God for thousands of years. Knowledge of evil altered the way people interacted with God and with each other. God didn't change His perspective or behavior towards people, but people changed their perspective and behavior towards God. Genesis 2:9 tells us, "And [in the garden] the Lord God caused to grow from the ground every tree that is desirable and pleasing to sight and good (suitable, pleasant) for food; the tree of life was also in the midst of the garden, and the tree of [experiential] knowledge (reignition) of [the difference between] good and evil."

As God peered into the future, He observed Adam and Eve with the knowledge of good and evil. He saw the elements of the curse coming onto humankind, causing suffering and feelings of inadequacy, insufficiency, and shame. Before sin entered the world, Adam and Eve didn't perceive themselves as weak and imperfect before God. They were able to communicate with Him freely and openly. They came boldly to God as their Father, and they spent time with the Lord without any doubt, fear, or insecurity, because Adam and Eve were fully healthy people.

The knowledge of evil allowed Adam and Eve to become conscious of their failures, and human imperfections before a perfect, and loving God. Adam and Eve sinned and understood their violation of God's law, and as a result, they became sin-conscious, insecure people. Sin consciousness is a state of mind that permits humans to focus on sin's power, magnifying sin instead of God's grace. When we are sin conscious, we pull ourselves away from God, because we feel we are unworthy of His love and affection.

Without sin consciousness, we experience an openness, love, affection, and peace with God. When we are not sin conscious, we know God is not upset with us, and He will respond to us. A sin-conscious mindset impacts the way humans think and behave in their relationships. Romans 3:19–20 says, "For no person will be justified [freed of guilt and declared righteous] in His sight by [trying to do] the works of the Law. For through the Law we become conscious of sin [and the recognition of sin directs us toward repentance, but provides no remedy for sin]."

God's love for humans did not adjust when Adam and Eve sinned. God's love for His children persisted. God is full of grace and love and forgiveness, and God continued to love Adam and Eve. The grace and overwhelming love of God permitted God to have the foresight of humanity's future sin but He still loved and created humanity. Kindness, forgiveness, and gentleness are all characteristics of God. Ephesians 2:8 declares, "For it is by grace [God's remarkable compassion and favor drawing you to Christ] that you have been saved [actually delivered from judgment and given eternal life] through faith. And this [salvation] is not of yourselves [not through your own effort], but it is the [undeserved, gracious] gift of God;"

God should always receive the praise, the glory, and the honor for loving us and creating us, despite our behavior, because He is forgiving, kind, and loving, all by himself. When we try to earn God's love, and we believe we are good or bad worthy or unworthy based on our behavior, we pull ourselves away from God and His grace.

God does not love humanity because of what we do. God loves humanity because of who He is. The knowledge of evil became a barrier between humankind and God, because the knowledge of evil made us sin conscious, insecure, and focused on self. Sin made us feel personally responsible for God's love or lack thereof.

Romans 9:32 teaches, "And why not? Because it was not by faith [that they pursued it], but as though it were by works [relying on the merit of their works instead of their faith]. They stumbled over the stumbling Stone [Jesus Christ]."

Galatians 3:3-5 explains, "Let me ask you this one question: Did you receive the [Holy] Spirit as the result of obeying the Law and doing its works, or was it by hearing [the message of the Gospel] and believing [it]? [Was it from observing a law of rituals or from a message of faith?] Are you so foolish and so senseless and so silly? Having begun [your new life spiritually] with the [Holy] Spirit, are you now reaching perfection [by dependence] on the flesh? Have you suffered so many things and experienced so much all for nothing (to no purpose)—if it really is to no purpose and in vain? Then does He Who supplies you with His marvelous [Holy] Spirit and works powerfully and miraculously among you do so on [the grounds of your doing] what the Law demands, or because of your believing in and adhering to and trusting in and relying on the message that you heard?"

A law violation caused Adam and Eve to realize they were naked. Before sinning, Adam and Eve were naked, but they weren't ashamed. Genesis 2:25 tells us, "Adam and his wife were both naked, and they felt no shame." Adam and Eve were open and intimate with each other and with God. Upon realizing they were naked or insufficient, Adam and Eve tried to cover their sin and nakedness and insufficiency. Covering themselves was an attempt to find meaning apart from God, believing they could do something to fix the problem they created. Genesis 3:7 explains, "Then the eyes of both of them were opened, and they realized they were naked; so they sewed fig leaves together and made coverings for themselves."

To be fulfilled, healthy, and complete, we must find our worth, our help, and our identity in God, not ourselves. Sin introduced self-worth to humanity. Self-worth outside of God is a block between humans and God, because people attempt to find personal meaning and purpose outside of God.

Satan looked at himself before he rebelled against God. Isaiah 14:13 explains, "But you said in your heart, 'I will ascend to heaven; I will raise my throne above the stars of God; I will sit on the mount of assembly in the remote parts of the north.'"

Satan separated himself from God and established a separate identity apart from God. When the human identity and the human self-image is disconnected from God, it is a satanic identity.

The psychological term for withdrawing connection with another is stonewalling. Stonewalling is a negative way of communicating in which one party removes himself or herself from intimate interaction and puts up an emotional wall separating himself or herself from the other person. Adam and Eve's sin caused them to stonewall and reject the love of their Father. The altered perception caused humanity to hold back and not come boldly before the Father who loved and created them for connection. As Adam and Eve judged themselves by their worth. They looked to themselves and their own behavior and blocked God's love and grace, pulling themselves away from their Creator.

Parents experience stonewalling when they attempt to connect with their child after the child has done something wrong and discover a child who is withdrawn and refusing to intimately interact. Healthy children may temporality withdraw from love and affection, if they know they have done something wrong, because they are aware of their sin. Through a healthy parental relationship, these children can learn they are still loved and cared for, even in times of correction and wrong behavior.

However, some children learn to accept a lie through unhealthy parenting or a traumatic event. They feel they must earn a parent's love, or that they are not worthy of love. Sometimes, these children make mistakes and are mistreated for being human, where other times, they are neglected and treated with contempt because of their behavior.

Parents who do not understand that children are as born as sinners and must be reproved and taught the right things to do will punish children too harshly when they make a mistake. They may be cold and distant to withdraw their love from the child, when they need to be connected to the child, even during times of misbehavior, so the child can learn how to relate with others. Some parents abandon, neglect, and harm children for their own issues; children of these types of parents will at times feel they are the cause of the parent's lack of love.

All humans fail and make mistakes. Mistakes are a part of life. Healthy parents will teach children to properly behave through reinforcing consequences for poor behavior, while showing appropriate levels of love and affection. Children who are raised in a stable, consistent environment will learn when they do the wrong thing they will be disciplined, but they are still loved and respected. These children will thrive and will be positioned to understand God and His kingdom appropriately.

To be in right standing with God, a person must acknowledge that they make mistakes, but they are worthy and important to God anyway. We must realize that God made a way for us to be forgiven, but He wants us to be holy and righteous, turning away from our sin. God will always correct us if we sin, and He will show us the way to go to enable us to become successful and healthy people. With His righteousness, we can openly communicate with our Father, and we can defend ourselves from Satan.

Attachment theory focuses on relationships and bonds between people, specifically between a parent and a child. Attachment theory emphasizes that people are born with a desire to have a bond with their caregiver. This theory asserts that the bonds made in the child's life with their primary caregiver, usually the mother, influence how the child views himself or herself and others.

Psychologist Mary Ainsworth expanded on attachment theory as she conducted experiments with children as young as one year old. Ainsworth perceived four attachment styles: ambivalent attachment, disorganized attachment, avoidant attachment, and secure attachment. Out of the four attachment styles, three are unhealthy, and one is perceived as normative.

Attachment styles are established through healthy or unhealthy behavioral interactions. When babies are created, they begin to learn in their mother's womb. They are not inherently secure, avoidant, disorganized, or ambivalent in their attachment towards others. Babies learn healthy or unhealthy attachment through interacting with their parents in the first few years of their lives. God is a perfect parent, who interacts with His children. Adam and Eve were securely attached to God until Satan interfered with the loving bond.

Satan tricked Adam and Eve to feel personally responsible for the love of their Father as a tactic to separate God's children from Him. Sin made Adam and Eve think they needed to earn their God's love, because they were unlovable and unworthy of His love. Satan persists in harming children's attachment to their parents or guardians. Satan inspires sinful family dynamics to train children to feel responsible for earning or losing their parents' love.

Children who are abused, traumatized, and face adversity early in life are more likely to be infiltrated with this lie of the enemy. A child whose parents divorce may feel he or she is responsible for the divorce, even when this isn't the case. Children who see their parents as addicts may wonder why they cannot save their parents, even though the parents are solely responsible for their behavior.

A child's brain is growing, learning, and developing, even within the womb. When a young child experiences the withdrawal of a parent's love, it can create strongholds within the child's brain. These strongholds are Satan's way of sowing tares into the field or mind of the child, to try to prevent the child from proper growth and development. Children with insecure attachments and an unhealthy worldview stemming from their unhealthy family unit need to be loved and taught the truth, so they can heal from their pain and trauma.

Whether children are ambivalent, disorganized, or avoidant, they do not have a secure base or a healthy attachment permitting them to properly explore the world around them. Insecure attachments contribute to difficulties in life because of the origins and deep-rooted maladaptive beliefs about self and others. An adult who has not healed from their childhood trauma will relate to God in an unhealthy way, if he or she relates to God at all, because Satan created a stronghold in his or her mind.

Children with an avoidant attachment style feel their needs, particularly their social and emotional needs are rejected and ignored. Through neglect and rejection, these children believe they are not loved for who they are, and they will translate this into their spiritual journey feeling unworthy of God's love.

When a parent doesn't show the child that he or she is safe, loved, and cared for, the child learns very early in life that he or she must be unlovable. Children with avoidant attachment styles often develop a sense of self-reliance, because they feel they must care for themselves.

These children feel personally responsible to "fix" their problems, as well as others' problems.

Adults with childhood trauma may refuse to go to their Father for comfort, love, and help in times of distress, because they are unsure if He cares about them. If a person has been conditioned to consistently be ignored or abused, he or she questions whether he or she is worthy of love from anyone, including God.

Even Adam and Eve, who were previously attached to God, questioned God's love after they became aware of their sin. Satan plants an attachment stronghold in a child's mind, to try to keep the child from running to the heavenly Father when they need help. Children in this situation may try to "work" to receive others' love, but they will not properly understand God's grace.

To become healthy, a person must create a new attachment to God, and then the person can safely explore and learn new ways of relating to another person within an intimate relationship. Learning how to be loved, what love is, and how to express love to others is often a process that takes time especially when someone has learned unhealthy ways of interacting with others.

God showed us He is committed to loving and caring for humanity because He chose to pursue Adam and Eve. The Bible tells us God's standard of love is longsuffering and holds no records of wrong. God didn't give up on Adam and Eve because they disobeyed Him. Like any loving parent, God forgave His kids, and He tried to talk to them and to teach them, so they would learn right from wrong, and choose to not disobey Him in the future.

Sin has negative personal consequences. Sin gives Satan a "foothold" in our lives. It allows Satan to plant into the fields of our hearts and our minds. When people sin, it doesn't make God stop loving them, but sin steals, kills, and destroys us, because it alienates us from the One who made us.

Unfortunately, the results of poor decision-making and a lifestyle of sin will impact children. Children can be seriously harmed and even destroyed, through a parent's sinful choices. Adam and Eve's sin thousands of years ago still affects mankind today. The sins of the parents are not counted to the child's account, but they do hurt the child and can set the child up to be alienated from the Creator of the universe.

Deuteronomy 30:19 says, "I call heaven and earth as witnesses against you today, that I have set before you life and death, the blessing and the curse; therefore, you shall choose life in order that you may live, you and your descendants."

When there is a separation from God, and an influence of sin and Satan, dysfunction will develop. Dysfunctional families are plagued with divorce, substance abuse, sexual immorality, intense anger, or other demonic strongholds. These families perpetuate sickness and disease in children, because children are not properly attached to their caregivers, and they fail to receive the necessary instruction in the ways of righteousness.

The flu is a disease that can spread through personal contact with another person. Likewise, sin and unhealthy lifestyles of sin can pass from the adult to the child because of close contact. Children watch and model their parents. They imitate and learn unhealthy behaviors and thought processes.

Deuteronomy 4:9–10 tells us, "Only take heed, and guard your life diligently, lest you forget the things which your eyes have seen and lest they depart from your [mind and] heart all the days of your life. Teach them to your children and your children's children—Especially how on the day that you stood before the Lord your God in Horeb, the Lord said to me, Gather the people together to Me and I will make them hear My words, that they may learn [reverently] to fear Me all the days they live upon the earth and that they may teach their children."

Parents are personally responsible to protect their children's lives by instructing their children into righteousness. All parents will give an account of the children they were given before God. God placed children into our care as parents, and He allows us to help them become who He wants them to become. The responsibility to care for and properly provide a life for a child should not be taken lightly. As parents, we can help our children walk into their God-given destiny or we can pull them away from it.

Children from broken or dysfunctional backgrounds can be healed, set free, and born again. They can become whole, healthy adults, but they must be shown Jesus Christ, compassion, and proper guidance. They must be loved and corrected when they are acting unlovable, so they can learn the grace of God. To truly love a child is to correct a child by leading him or her into the paths of righteousness. Proverbs 13:24 tells us, "He who withholds the rod [of discipline] hates his son, But he who loves him disciplines and trains him diligently and appropriately [with wisdom and love]."

Satan targets human minds with the lie that God will never love them because they are unworthy of His love. Rebellion against God caused Satan to be kicked out of heaven, and he wants us to suffer the same fate. Satan wants us to be punished and judged eternally, as he is. He wants God to abandon us, forget us, and write us out of His family.

God's grace allows us to enter God's perfect family, even if we didn't deserve it through our behavior. We are permitted access if we will only believe and receive God's forgiveness. When someone believes he or she must earn God's love by works alone, that person will never enter heaven, because he or she has rejected God's free gift of grace.

When we violate God's law, we realize the need for purity, the need for God. Adam and Eve valued God's love more than ever because they realized the garments they made for themselves were insufficient and did not cover their sin. It is impossible to cover our sin apart from God. God is the only one who can clothe us in His righteousness. Genesis 3:21 explains, "For Adam also and for his wife the Lord God made long coats (tunics) of skins and clothed them."

Genesis 3:9 tells us, "But the Lord God called to the man, 'Where are you?' He answered, 'I heard you in the garden, and I was afraid because I was naked; so I hid.'"

We hide from God. We run away from God, but God never runs away from us. God's relationship with humans is established through His love and His plan to create us in His image. It was never established based on our own work and good deeds. Feelings of inferiority because of sin consciousness should lead us to repentance. We realize we are sinners and unworthy of God's love, but God is so good He loves us anyways, so we thank Him and praise Him for who He is. To know God loves you even though you don't deserve it is the greatest blessing of all.

Psalm 51: 4–6 declares, "Against you, you only, have I sinned and done what is evil in your sight; so you are right in your verdict and justified when you judge. Surely, I was sinful at birth, sinful from the time my mother conceived me. Yet you desired faithfulness even in the womb; you taught me wisdom in that secret place."

Parents know their children will make mistakes and learn to do the right thing through consistent training. Perfect children do not exist. Children learn and develop, and they become who they are to become through proper training, within a healthy relationship with their mom and dad. Parents have children to enjoy them and to love them. They create them for fellowship and relationship. Everything God made, He made for His own enjoyment. He created us to have a relationship with us.

Adam and Eve were not indefinitely cursed and separated from God because of their sin. God restored His relationship with them, and He continued to interact with them. Eve attributed her pregnancy and her fruitfulness to God. She realized God was the source of her life, and He was the one who blessed her with children. Genesis 4:1–2 tells us, "And Adam knew Eve as his wife, and she became pregnant and bore Cain; and she said, 'I have gotten and gained a man with the help of the Lord.' And [next] she gave birth to his brother Abel. Now Abel was a keeper of sheep, but Cain was a tiller of the ground."

Cain and Abel's lives represent two ways to approach sin. Abel realized he needed God. He was willing to obey the Lord and meet the Lord's requirement for his sacrifice. Abel respected God's atonement for his sin, and he obeyed God and met the requirements through his obedience and his faith.

Conversely, Cain tried to work out his own salvation. He wanted God to forgive him and accept him because he felt he had done something worthy of acceptance. He refused to obey God's plan for atonement, and he thought his work was good enough for God.

Being a good person is not sufficient to get to heaven. Trying to obey the law won't atone for sin. Behaviorism, work, and controlling ourselves without an appreciation towards God, is worthless. We cannot work and offer God things instead of our love, honor, and gratitude. We cannot gain heaven apart from repentance and appreciation in God and His grace and His mercy towards us as people. None of us deserve to be loved by God. But because of Jesus, and because of God's mercy, we are loved and welcome to connect to God, even when we don't deserve it.

The Pharisee spirit operating in the world hates God's grace. Pharisees are religious hypocrites who lack mercy, love, grace, and forgiveness towards others. Pharisees believe they are righteous because of their own behavior and religious observances. Pharisees believe they can work their way into heaven because they appear to perform well. The spirit of the Pharisee wants to destroy the Christian witness. It wants to kill and murder a brother, as Cain did to Abel. Pharisees know the law, and they hold people accountable to the law, but they fail to honor God as they perform their religious traditions.

Through the teaching of religious tradition and law, Pharisees turn people away from Christ. The Pharisee spirit teaches people to feel they are worthy only if they perform. This teaching prevents people from coming to Christ to receive forgiveness. When the gospel is presented as a works-based doctrine, it causes humans to run, hide, and turn away from God instead of coming to him, because people feel inadequate and personally responsible to earn God's love and affection.

A refusal to turn to God is suicide, because it results in spiritual death. When a religious person turns someone away from God, it is murder. Pharisees are accountable for their brothers' blood, as Cain was responsible for Abel's. Through teaching others personal responsibility outside of Christ, Pharisees separate people from Christ's atonement plan. They send people to hell and feel justified for doing so. Matthew 23:13 says, "But woe to you, scribes and Pharisees, pretenders (hypocrites)! For you shut the kingdom of heaven in men's faces; for you neither enter yourselves, nor do you allow those who are about to go in to do so."

The book of Hebrews was written to help us understand God's love and grace. Hebrews 4:16 instructs us, "Let us therefore come boldly to the throne of grace, that we may obtain mercy and find grace to help in time of need."

God wants to take away shame, guilt, remorse, and the knowledge of evil and sin consciousness to prevent stonewalling in our relationship with Him. He wants us to know we can come to Him, talk to Him, walk with Him, and receive love from Him because He created us to be in a relationship with Him. All people are born sinners, and all have sinned, but we are all welcome to come to Him and receive forgiveness. We become pure before God if we repent from sin, turn from sin, and accept Jesus Christ as our Savior.

In the old covenant, animals were used to represent atonement for sin. God did not desire the life and the blood of animals. He desired the heart of the people. Animal sacrifices displayed a repentant heart and the need for cleansing from sin. God wanted people to realize their sin was separating them from Him so He could draw near to them again. Only through the realization, the remorse, and the hatred of sin, could a person offer an acceptable sacrifice to the Lord.

Ceremonial rituals and procedures help alter and influence the human mind. Through religious ceremonial rituals, sin consciousness can be removed, and purity can be established. This change in human perception allows people to go confidently before the Lord and talk to him without stonewalling. Religious processes alone do not make us clean; religious ceremonies and rituals simply solidify and express outwardly the inner cleansing of the heart. When a religious ritual or procedure is done from the heart as an outward sign of faith or as an expression of love, then the act helps establish a spiritual truth in our brains. But when a religious ritual, procedure, or ceremony is done simply as a tradition, without heart commitment, it will produce nothing.

Matthew 5:8 says, "Blessed are the pure in heart, for they shall see God." Only when a man or woman's heart is right before God, will the authentic outward behavior follow. The Lord will not accept as an offering the behavior or ritual without the cleansing of the heart first.

Cain made an offering to God, but his heart was not right when he prepared his offering. God knows our hearts, and He knows if we are cleansed from the inside out. Jesus said, "Woe to you, [self-righteous] scribes and Pharisees, hypocrites! For you are like whitewashed tombs which look beautiful on the outside, but inside are full of dead men's bones and everything unclean" (Matthew 23:27).

Abraham did not have to perform an outward religious ceremony for God to accept his sacrifice. God accepted Abraham's sacrifice of his son Isaac because he believed, and God saw the intent of his heart. Genesis 15:6 explains, "Abram believed the Lord, and he credited it to him as righteousness."

When Abraham decided in his heart to offer Isaac to God, in the eyes of God, he committed the act. God counted the sacrifice as complete, because God saw he was willing and obedient within his heart. First Samuel 15:22 declares, "Samuel said, "Has the Lord as great a delight in burnt offerings and sacrifices As in obedience to the voice of the Lord? Behold, to obey is better than sacrifice, And to heed [is better] than the fat of rams."

Obedience and a joyful inner decision to obey is what matters to the Lord. Authentic obedience comes from respect and honor. When children honor and respect their mother and their father, they will obey them because they know they are loved and they know their parents want what is best for them. Without honor and respect, proper behavior is an act and is not genuine. In these situations, even if a child obeys, he or she internally resents his or her parent's instruction.

Abraham was securely attached to the Lord. He knew His father's heart for Him was good and pure. He knew he could trust God to take care of him. Abraham did not doubt, question, or run from God. He ran to God, knowing God would take care of his every need. Hebrews 11:17–19 explains, "By faith Abraham, when God tested him, offered Isaac as a sacrifice. He who had embraced the promises was about to sacrifice his one and only son, even though God had said to him, 'It is through Isaac that your offspring will be reckoned.' Abraham reasoned that God could even raise the dead, and so in a manner of speaking he did receive Isaac back from death."

Throughout scripture, God reveals to us the importance of a clean and pure heart. Ezekiel 36:26 tells us, "I will give you a new heart and put a new spirit in you; I will remove from you your heart of stone and give you a heart of flesh."

Jesus took our sin and gave us His righteousness, so we could become the sons and daughters of God. We did not do anything to become eligible to receive this gift or work out our own salvation. The right to work out our salvation is secondary to God's grace and forgiveness of our sin. We receive opportunities to perform good works because God is gracious, but we did not earn the right to work out our salvation through our own righteousness.

David is called a man after God's own heart because he acknowledged his own shortcomings as he acknowledged the grace of God. David wanted to please God through his behavior, but he admitted he was impure and could not perform good works outside of God's grace. David's heart was pure, and his behavior represented his pure heart. Psalm 51:1–3 declares, "Have mercy on me, O God, according to your unfailing love; according to your great compassion blot out my transgressions. Wash away all my iniquity and cleanse me from my sin. For I know my transgressions and my sin are always before me."

Working out our salvation is our responsibility. After we realize our sin and repent for our sin, we must commit to turn from sin and walk in our covenant with God. God does have a standard for holiness, righteousness, and perfection, but we cannot attain God's standard without the atonement of sin through the blood of Jesus Christ. When Jesus died for us, He permitted us to walk with God consistently, knowing we are sanctified, justified, and renewed before Him in our minds and our hearts. Hebrews 8:10 says, "'For this is the covenant that I will make with the house of Israel after those days,' says the Lord: 'I will imprint My laws upon their minds, even upon their innermost thoughts and understanding, and engrave them upon their hearts; and I will be their God, and they shall be My people.'"

Circumcision is an outward religious ceremony performed as a surgery, meant to aid in the cleansing of the human mind as an expression of faith. Circumcision was needed within the old covenant. However, when God established the new covenant with His people, through Jesus Christ, He annulled the need for the former covenant. We have a new covenant, based on better promises.

The new covenant is imprinted in our minds and our hearts, and we do not need to perform a religious ceremony to cleanse our minds and our hearts or to draw near to the Lord. "When God speaks of a new [covenant or agreement], He makes the first one obsolete (out of use). And what is obsolete (out of use and annulled because of age) is ripe for disappearance and to be dispensed with altogether" (Hebrews 8:13).

During a circumcision, the skin covering the penis, called the foreskin, is removed. In Jewish tradition, circumcision is done on the eighth day after the birth of a male child. In the United States and other developed nations, circumcision usually takes place immediately following the birth of a male child. In the United States, when a circumcision is performed shortly after birth, medical professionals require the child to have a vitamin K injection, because vitamin K is said to aid in healing through impacting the body's blood clotting or blood coagulation.

Modern technology has demonstrated that vitamin K levels are not present in newborn babies. All babies are born with a vitamin K "deficiency." However, vitamin k injections have dangers that far exceed the benefits. The Vitamin K1 injection (Phytonadione Injectable) carries a black box warning and reads, "Severe reactions, including fatalities, have occurred during and immediately after intravenous injection of phytonadione, even when precautions have been taken to dilute the phytonadione."

Christians should wonder why God, as a Creator, would create humans with a "deficiency" leading them to rely on human intervention and help for survival. If this were true, how did thousands of humans survive without the shot or oral injection? Why would God create us without everything we need to survive, and how did humans survive in the past without it? Additionally, a wise parent, should consider if the potential risk of death or other serious reactions are worth the assumed benefit of vitamin K.

When I was praying about circumcision, I wanted to know if I should give my son a vitamin K shot, and if I should circumcise him. God instructed me to do neither, and I was provided with a biblical understanding of the old/new covenant. Before my experience as mother of a male child, I never understood circumcision, blood sacrifice of animals, the old and the new covenant, or any of these similar concepts on a deep, informed level. It is funny how something, like a surgical procedure done to infant boys can teach you so much about the Lord if you are open to learning.

In all medical decisions for our children, we must consult with the Lord to determine if we are making wise decisions. Professionals may or may not have the information we have been given as parents. Procedures and medical recommendations are not always correct.

For instance, female and male babies in the hospital setting have their umbilical cords cut immediately upon the child's birth, unless the mother requests otherwise, even though early cord clamping and cutting prevents babies from receiving a full blood transfer from their mother.

Delayed cord cutting allows blood to continue to flow from the placenta to the newborn baby after delivery. Delayed cord cutting is for the baby's betterment, because it allows the baby to receive blood from the placenta. Delayed umbilical cord clamping, which is defined as cord clamping not done earlier than one minute after birth, is recommended for maternal and infant health. Many medical professionals will tell us we need to do things that we do not need to do, such vitamin K shots and circumcision, while neglecting to do things the babies and the mothers truly benefit from.

Receiving our information from God prevents us from blindly trusting the recommendations of the medical profession and instead, make good, informed sound decisions for our children.

Hebrews 9:11–12 teaches, "But when Christ appeared as a High Priest of the good things to come [that is, true spiritual worship], He entered through the greater and more perfect tabernacle, not made with hands, that is to say, not a part of this [material] creation. he went once for all into the Holy Place [the Holy of Holies of heaven, into the presence of God], and not through the blood of goats and calves, but through His own blood, having obtained and secured eternal redemption [that is, the salvation of all who personally believe in Him as Savior]. For if the sprinkling of [ceremonially] defiled persons with the blood of goats and bulls and the ashes of a [burnt] heifer is sufficient for the cleansing of the body, how much more will the blood of Christ, who through the eternal [Holy] Spirit willingly offered Himself unblemished [that is, without moral or spiritual imperfection as a sacrifice] to God, cleanse your conscience from dead works and lifeless observances to serve the ever living God?"

All rituals and sacrifices were made to cleanse the human conscience. Before Jesus Christ's death and resurrection, without rituals, and sacrifices, people were could not talk to God directly, because a separation blocked them from God. Sin, and the human mind blocked humanity from fully experiencing the love of God. God wanted our consciences cleansed, and our sin to be wiped away so He could communicate with us personally. He wanted His kids to be able to talk to Him confidently in a loving way. When Jesus died on the cross, the veil separating God from humans was torn. This symbolized the separation between God and man being torn down, to be remembered no more.

After the veil was torn, God and man could be reunited. We could personally communicate again. The Church can come boldly to the throne and talk to God directly, as His children. Matthew 27:50–51 tells us, "And Jesus cried out again with a loud voice and yielded His spirit. Then, behold, the veil of the temple was torn in two from top to bottom; and the earth quaked, and the rocks were split, and the graces were opened; and many bodies of the saints who had fallen asleep were raised; and coming out of the graves after His resurrection, they went into the holy city and appeared to many."

Many people view God as an angry, unloving God, who wants to punish and condemn mankind for their sins. But the gospel of grace, and the gospel and the good news of Jesus, frees humans from their sin consciousness and leads people to appreciation and honor. First John 4:19 says, "We love because He first loved us."

God has always showed His love and His plan to be in a relationship with us. God is relational, and He cares intimately about His creation. The insight of God's love, His grace, and His forgiveness leads people deeper into a relationship with their Creator. People are saved because they realize they have a Savior who loved them so much He died for them.

When someone we love does something kind for us, we appreciate that person more. Knowing we don't deserve God's love and can't earn God's love creates an atmosphere of thankfulness and praise. We can go to God knowing He will take care of us, and He will never leave or forsake us. Unlike unholy, imperfect, or sinful parents, God never abandons, neglects, abuses, or forsakes His children He created. He will always answer, always forgive, and always be there for the child who goes to Him for help. *We can securely attach ourselves to Him.*

Circumcision isn't required to cleanse our minds and remind us that our Father loves us. We don't need to perform a religious ceremony of circumcision any more than we need to kill an animal and put it on an altar to prove we are in covenant with God. The new covenant describes rightful circumcision that comes from the heart. Romans 2:28–29 tells us, "For a person is not a Jew who is one outwardly, and true circumcision is not something visible in the flesh. On the contrary, a person is a Jew who is one inwardly, and circumcision is of the heart- by the Spirit, not the letter. That man's praise is not from men but from God."

God didn't create us to abandon us. Isaiah 49:15 says, "Can a mother forget the baby at her breast and have no compassion on the child she has borne? Though she may forget I will not forget you."

God wants to provide everything for us and care for us like tiny babies, dependent totally on their mother. When a woman holds and breastfeeds her child, she looks at her child with tender loving care, and she wants to protect her baby. Through the mother's consistent care and love, the baby will begin to grow. The baby learns to trust and respect the mother, because he or she knows the mother loves him or her deeply and would do anything to keep him or her secure. Similarly, when God's people trust in Him and rely on Him for their nourishment and growth, God will never forget us and let us go.

Mothers help their children feel secure in their love. A mother's unwavering love influences a child's perspective of God, beginning within the breastfeeding relationship. Psalm 22:9 teaches, "Yet you are He who took me from the womb; you made me trust you at my mother's breasts."

Babies who rest in their mother's protection, love, and care learn to trust God as their parent easier than those who have cold and distant mothers. Within the first few years of life, babies can be securely or insecurely attached within interpersonal relationships.

Breastfeeding is usually done between the ages of 0–3, and these three years are exceptionally important for proper child development. Breastfeeding is mentioned frequently in the Bible. Breastfeeding accompanies scriptures on love, strength, blessing, and comfort, where dry breasts or the inability to nurse is portrayed negatively and is associated with cursing. Hosea 9:14 tells us, "Give them, O Lord-what will you give? Give them a miscarrying womb and dry breasts."

God planned for us to recognize the importance of the mother and child relationship and breastfeeding during the formative years of early childhood. God ensured that Moses's mother Jochebed would nurse him, even when he was to be removed from her and placed within the pharaoh's house. Jochebed was granted the first few years with her son, and she was not only able to nurse Moses, but she was paid to nurse him. Exodus 2:9–10 teaches us, "Then Pharaoh's daughter said to her, 'Take this child away and nurse him for me, and I will give you your wages.' So, the woman took the child and nursed him. And the child grew, and she brought him to Pharaoh's daughter, and he became her son. And she named him Moses, and said, 'Because I drew him out of the water.'"

The time Moses spent with Jochebed as a nursing baby influenced him far beyond his formative years. God paints a picture for us, showing us the beauty and the influence of a mother/child relationship in the child's outlook and destiny in life. When Moses left his mother's home and moved into pharaoh's house, full of witchcraft and sin, he refused to *attach* himself to the wicked lifestyle. Moses's mother was a woman from the priestly tribe of Levi, and a woman of great faith. She believed in the destiny of her son, and she imparted to her son spiritual blessings and a spiritual attachment to God. Jochebed formed an attachment within Moses to her God's family.

First Thessalonians 2:7 says, "But we were gentle among you, like a nursing mother taking care of her own children." Breastfeeding a baby requires effort and time. To breastfeed, a woman must be committed to it. The bonding time between a mother and a child is significant. It is a time of deep attachment to one another through personal love and connection. Within the breastfeeding relationship, a baby fully depends on another person, and he or she needs the mother for his or her life to continue.

A newborn baby relies on its mother for both life and comfort. The baby needs the mother and learns if the mother is safe. The baby learns quickly if the mother will provide everything he or she needs. When a mother commits to breastfeeding, she is investing in the child's development, and the connection between the mother and child will provide the baby with strength and security. She is investing in her child's long-term health.

Many children form an unhealthy attachment style due to the unhealthy or healthy/unhealthy mixed message they receive within the feeding or breastfeeding relationship. In America, many women breastfeed for a short time and then stop to return to work or feel it is too challenging to continue.

Some women chose to never breastfeed. In these situations, babies learn that their needs are met by others besides the mother, and they learn to have a disorganized attachment style. In disorganized attachments, caregivers are inconsistent and children become confused, learning their needs are met, but inconsistently. These children will trust others sometimes but at other times, withdrawal.

Life as a mother goes quickly, and even if things are hard to do, it doesn't mean we shouldn't do them. Nothing is more important than caring for the children God gave us. Breastfeeding is often difficult in the first few weeks of a baby's life, but as the relationship is established, it improves. Mothers who push themselves to breastfeed and stick to breastfeeding for the health and safety of their children will be glad they did. The breastfeeding relationship has many benefits for both mother and baby.

Mothers who breastfeed show improved emotional well-being, easier weight management, cost savings, lower risk of cancers, better bone health, faster post-pregnancy recoveries, natural birth spacing, and best of all, better connection to their babies.

Babies who are breastfed receive ideal and whole nutrition enriched with antibodies, and they have lower rates of sickness and disease. Breastfed babies have healthier weights and are less likely to be overweight later in childhood or life. Breastfed babies have higher intelligence, as research consistently shows the long-term brain development differences between breastfed and formula-fed babies.

One of God's names' is El Shaddai. El Shaddai means *mighty in power* and *sufficient in all things*. God's name El Shaddai make evident that God can provide for all the needs of people, like a nursing mother who provides all things for her baby. As mothers nurses their babies, they give their children the same loving care God provides for His children. Mothers who breastfeed are investing in their children's development and growth, even when it requires commitment, effort, and time. They are showing their baby that he or she is worth the time and the effort, and they will do anything to maintain an attachment, even when it isn't easy.

El Shaddai stems from the Hebrew plural word "shad" meaning the breasted one. God believes people are worth His time and His effort. He takes the time to be in relationship with us, and He provides everything we could ever need through that relationship. In any good relationship, spending intimate time together is the glue that helps the relationship remain strong. God is invested in our long-term health and growth.

Breastfeeding is God's ideal method for babies. When God created people, He intended for moms to nurse their children for the first few years of life. Hannah was a mother who took time to focus on her baby. Hannah was devoted to her baby's care, so she placed all other duties aside to ensure her son was properly cared for. Hannah separated from the group that was going to perform the yearly sacrifice to stay home and nurse her baby.

First Samuel teaches, 1:21–23 "Now the man Elkanah and all his house went up to offer to the Lord the yearly sacrifice and his vow. But Hannah did not go up, for she said to her husband, 'Not until the child is weaned; then I will take him, that he may appear before the Lord and remain there forever.' So, Elkanah her husband said to her, 'Do what seems best to you; wait until you have weaned him. Only let the Lord establish His word.' Then the woman stayed and nursed her son until she had weaned him."

A support system is important when it comes to breastfeeding. Hannah's husband, Elkanah, understood and supported Hannah's decision to stay home and nurse Samuel. A woman can breastfeed and be successful without a support system, but breastfeeding consultants, a supportive spouse, and others who support a mom with her decision to breastfeed, will help her form a strong breastfeeding relationship.

Women whose husbands financially provide for the family partner with the mother to enable breastfeeding. By giving the mother the opportunity to stay at home with a baby, the husband partners with the mama's decision to breastfeed. Others outside of the home can also help us achieve our breastfeeding goals. Many groups and resources are devoted solely to helping moms breastfeed their babies.

Gianni was not gaining the recommended weight for a few weeks after he was born, even though it appeared he was nursing. My midwife connected with a speech pathologist, who helped me to remedy the problem quickly without medical intervention or surgery. A recommendation from my encouraging midwife connected me to another support person. After a few exercises with Gianni, moving his tongue in his mouth in specific ways, the speech pathologist improved his latch, and he began nursing without any issue. I am thankful for the women who supported me, helped me, and encouraged me to continue to nurse my son.

My commitment to breastfeeding kept me focused on the goal of finding supportive people who could help me resolve our breastfeeding difficulty. I was one hundred percent committed to breastfeeding all my children. When I encountered a challenge, I refused to stop looking for a solution because I knew breastfeeding was God's ideal nourishment for my son. We are now over a year through breastfeeding, and Gianni is doing fine. I have breastfed all three of my children, and none of them have ever had formula.

Who we have partner with us impacts our journey, but our commitment to finding the people we need to help us is equally important. The speech pathologist was a great breastfeeding consultant! The tongue is a precious muscular organ, and it is directly associated with speech development. Many babies have tongue-ties, lip ties, or other issues of the mouth that can be resolved with the help of a good speech pathologist. The speech pathologist watched my son nurse, and she did a few exercises with his mouth and tongue. She gave me some exercises to do at home, and within a few days our problem was resolved.

Studies have shown a connection between tongue, breastfeeding, and speech development. Our time breastfeeding impacts our children's long-term heath in various ways. Our tongues are vital to our ability to talk and eat. "One of the functions related to brain development is speech ability. Results of a meta-analysis conducted show the effect of breastfeeding on speech development in children. The results of the analysis of cohort studies indicate that breastfeeding increases language development by 1.19 times compared to children who did not receive this type of feeding; the effect observed in cross-sectional studies was 1.54 times greater language development in breastfed children compared to those who did not" (Muro-Valdez, Meza-Rios, Aguilar-

Uscanga, Lopez-Roa, Medina-Diaz, Franco-Torres, & Zepeda-Morales 2023).

As mothers, we set our children up to form healthy lifestyles and patterns of thinking and behaving. We can create strong attachments, and we determine who or what is permitted access into their lives and their early stages of development. An infant's healthy attachment to the mother, who is personally attached to her Father, the Lord, sets the trajectory of success and blessing. A mother attached to God will attach her child into God's family, as Jochebed did for Moses. Moses never lost His attachment to God and the kingdom of God because of his mother's choices. She attached him to the things of God within a few early years of his life, and his tongue was used to speak for God, not the enemy.

Moses experienced many things, and he was exposed to evil, but his attachment to God's will and kingdom never wavered. The family we are attached to early in life impacts us. God wants us to be attached to the kingdom's family. He wants us to learn to connect, love, and respond to others in a kingdom way, and with kingdom wisdom. Kingdom attachment is the only way to truly have a healthy attachment style.

No one is stuck indefinitely in an unhealthy attachment style, despite what "experts" may tell us. With God we can be freed, and we can learn proper healthy ways of interacting with God and the world around us. If we have received an unhealthy mindset as the result of neglect, abuse, abandonment, or other childhood traumas, we can be free. A simple prayer of faith, asking God to help us to be free from the unhealthy patterns formed during our early years of development, will ensure we are set free from all the strongholds of our enemy. God will reprogram our brains. He will create new wave links within the mind as we come to Him for help, instead of running and hiding from Him.

If you have never made Jesus your Lord and Savior you can pray this prayer and have assurance of your salvation.

Dear Heavenly Father,

I come to you in the name of Jesus. Your Word says in John 6:37, "The one who comes to Me I will by no means cast out." Thank you for not casting me out of your family, and instead choosing to take me in. I am calling on Your Name in faith, knowing that you have the power to save me. You said in Your Word, "If you confess with your mouth the Lord Jesus and believe in your heart that God has raised Him from the dead, you will be saved. For with the heart one believes unto righteousness, and with the mouth confession is made unto salvation" (Romans 10:9–10).

I believe in my heart Jesus is the Son of God. I believe He died on the cross and was raised from the dead to pay the penalty for my sins. Although I did not deserve it- I know you have given it freely as a gift because you love me. I confess that Jesus is my Lord. I know I have now become the righteousness of God in Christ (Second Corinthians 5:21). I am now saved and redeemed. I can communicate with you freely from this moment on without fear or shame. I can run to you when I need help and I know you will always help me. Thank you Lord. Amen.

If you prayed this prayer please go to BohannonBoutique.com and find the I just got saved link and fill it out. I would love to send you some more materials to help you grow and develop as believer.

9

The Intentional Birth Plan

All physicians gain credibility through a proven record of successful treatment for their patients. Statistical analysis and testimonial experiences can both be used to determine if a physician can be trusted to provide holistic preventive healthcare and curative healthcare. A good physician instructs patients in healthy lifestyle practices, enabling the patients to prevent sickness and disease within their bodies, while also treating patients if they become ill. A good physician is a healer and a consultant.

The formation of the human body's incredibly complex structure is astonishing. The human body is comprised of trillions of cells. Our anatomy is organized by levels—from cells, to tissues, to organs, and organ systems. As babies form in the womb, the cells, tissues, and organs achieve perfect alignment. Babies by 12 weeks have almost all their organs completely formed, aside from the brain and the spinal cord.

Our advancements in technology have significantly helped us to understand the human body. We understand more about human biology and physiology today than ever before. For instance, ultrasound technology can show us the developing babies within the mother's womb. We can identify the sex of the baby through DNA analysis at 12 weeks, and we can perform complete anatomy scans by 20 weeks.

God created the complex human body. He designed every single part of it. A family who has Jesus as their family's Physician, knows they are safe, because they know they are consistently making wise health decisions. Jesus knows what we need to thrive, and He has a perfect record of healing. Testimony and historical facts alike prove Jesus healed all people of all ages who came to Him for help.

Luke 12:7 tells us, "Indeed the very hairs of your head are all numbered. Do not be afraid; you are far more valuable than many sparrows."

The American medical system was altered for the worst through a series of intentional changes by financially motivated men. Between 1920 and 1935, holistic medicine was intentionally suppressed for the promotion of allopathic medicine. The switch to allopathic medicine was motivated by profit, and the Rockefeller Foundation paid medical schools to change their teaching programs, while eradicating any medical school who didn't align themselves with the new vision.

In *Medical Education in the United States and Canda* by the Carnegie Foundation the author states that suppressing medical educational facilities that "demoralized" the issues in education reform in America was ideal. The authors of this document claimed that any medical education institutions that refused to comply with their updated requirements and standards and beliefs of how medical education and medicine should be, would be stifled and forced to obey, or they would be shut down at a hard deadline.

With a strong plan and a robust financial pull, these men forced their agenda and silenced everyone who disagreed with them. They have successfully impacted the medical education system and the doctors graduating from the system for a hundred years.

To suppress means to forcibly put an end to something. The architects and affiliates of the *Medical Education in the United States and Canada* changed American Medicine and the education system of doctors by force. They proudly gloated that they were going to effectively put an end to all schools and medical institutions disagreeing with them, and they had a plan to carry it out. The motivation of the change was not as it was presented, as the instigators of our current medical system were not changing the system to benefit the public or public health. Instead, the system was changed to become a for-profit organization, benefiting chosen and selected conforming universities, and elite shareholders alike.

The abolition of free inquiry in medical education began when education was strictly regulated. Infiltrated by rich men and women who wanted to control the way information was learned and presented, education became corrupted. These people wanted to control who was allowed entry and access to education, so they eliminated free thought, free study, and open discussion, and they incorporated patented products, strict guidelines, and strict regulations. The agenda was planned, strategic, and comprehensive, so the plan could ensure that they would be permitted to enforce their agenda through the threat of withholding federal funds or credentials.

By dictating which schools and students were accepted and received financial aid, the schools determined who was hired, promoted, or given tenure. The educational system was completely controlled. The financially motivated elite group prepared to rule the entire educational system and ultimately the entire medical system, and they have been successful. They sought to eliminate schools, so they could control medical education and ultimately, medical best practice. Although many medical institutions and schools benefitted their communities and the public's health before the change in policies, because their ways of operating didn't fit the agenda of the elect, they were practically shut out practicing medicine.

When America was founded, it was created to free people from the oppression of governmental forces. America was founded to be a free place to live. Many Americans believed overly regulated, controlled, bureaucratic education was for their good and for their safety. This lie caused the elimination of free-education institutions. It rid the United States from creativity and passion for pure health remedies, and it caused the medical system to be controlled and infiltrated with synthetic medicines and curriculum, so the system and the medicines could be patented and profitable for select men and women.

Synthetic medicines are eligible be "patented" where herbal remedies are not. A patent establishes the right to exclude others from making, using, offering for sale, or selling an invention. The business-minded people who cared about making money found creative ways to produce medicines that could be patented, because patented medicines could make them lots of money. The creators of many of our synthetic medicines today do not care what the additives do to the human body; instead they care about the money they will make by owning and regulating the patented products.

Baby formula is one of the artificial, synthetic, supplements promoted by medical professionals. The U.S. Food and Drug Administration regulates formula, and the FDA determines which infant formulas can be sold to American consumers. According to data compiled by Allied Market Research, four companies—Perrio Company, Nestle USA, Mead Johnson Nutrition, and Abbott Nutrition—control 90 percent of the formula industry. Smaller formula companies have a hard time competing against these large companies due to lack of revenue. It is very expensive to compete against the large established formula companies unless you have a lot of money to invest in your project. The U.S. baby infant formula market size was valued at $3,962.7 million in 2022 and is projected to reach $6.973.7 million by 2032 (Allied Market Research 2021).

Formula is advertised as safe and healthy for newborn children. "However, infant formula is a highly susceptible food product to contamination/adulteration, which hampers the U.S. baby infant formula market growth. In the past, infant formula products were occasionally found to be contaminated with salmonella and E. coli. Although they are uncommon, these events can cause infants to suffer or even die. Some infants may be allergic to the components in baby formulas, such as soy, or cow milk protein. Hives, vomiting, diarrhea, and rashes are some of the symptoms prevalent among infants. Furthermore, certain parents are concerned that formulas do not provide as much nutrition as breast milk or that it may contain nutrient imbalances that are harmful to their child's health. According to several studies, formula fed infants are more likely to acquire health problems such as obesity, diabetes, and allergy as they grow" (Allied Market Research 2021).

After the birth of my first child, I had a hard time breastfeeding in the hospital. The hospital staff threatened me, saying if my son didn't start gaining weight back immediately, they weren't going to let me leave the hospital with him. The nurses entered our hospital room with a formula and said my son needed to be put on formula if I wanted to take him home with me. They were mixing bottles of formula beside my bed as they told me I would not be able to leave with our son if we didn't give him these artificial supplements.

As a mother who wanted to breastfeed, I was devastated. My husband knew how much breastfeeding meant to me, and he stood up for me and for our son. He informed the nurses that we were going to continue to work on breastfeeding. They suggested I pump the milk into bottles to measure how much milk he was receiving. Through my pumping and measuring the breastmilk, we were eventually released from the hospital.

Pumping breastmilk was the way I fed my first child for over a year. I never found a breastfeeding consultant to help me, so I continued feeding my son with pumped bottles of breastmilk, because it was the only method I knew how to do. I wanted to breastfeed him, and I attempted to many times at home, but I never felt confident in my ability to nurse him after my experience at the hospital. I didn't have the information or support, and so I made do with what I had.

A competent hospital staff would have sent a breastfeeding consultant to help me with nursing. Competent caring healthcare professionals would have partnered with me in my desire to breastfeed my son and given me the resources I needed to be successful. I only saw a breastfeeding consultant once in the hospital, and it was shortly after a cesarean birth. As a new mom, with no knowledge of breastfeeding, one breastfeeding consulting session was not sufficient for me to know how to breastfeed. Breastfeeding is an art, and it requires repetitive practice for mom and baby to be successful.

In hindsight, I realize multiple things contributed to my struggle with breastfeeding my first child, and a strong birth plan could have safeguarded me from some of the problems I encountered. For instance, too many visitors in my room impacted my breastfeeding experience, because I felt uncomfortable. Breastfeeding is intimate and personal. A woman must learn positioning, and she must be in an environment where she is comfortable to practice nursing. When family members are around and a woman must reveal her private body parts to nurse, she feels awkward.

If I had limited visitors, I may have been able to continue to practice breastfeeding. By planning to limit visitors, not allow visitors, or curtail visiting times, a woman can exert a level of control within her breastfeeding experience. Women also need to recover and sleep after a delivery of a baby. Women who have had cesarean births have undergone serious surgery, and need even more recovery time. Too many visitors restrict the already interrupted sleep of a new mother and child. Having too many visitors limits proper healing and recovery. If a mom plans to limit her visits, she can control her recovery and her time with her new baby.

I did not have an intentional plan for my first or second babies. As a result, I let medical professionals, breastfeeding consultants, family members, or others dictate my pregnancy, my birth, and my postpartum period. One of the biggest lessons the Lord taught me through home birth under a midwife's care was just how much I had been violated in previous birth experiences and how much control I did not have. In my first and second pregnancies and births, I didn't take proper control, and in return, I was denied the right to decide what I wanted for my pregnancy, birth, and postpartum season.

We often hear women's right advocates and feminists discuss violence against women. However, I was unaware and blindsided about the violations and the violence against women in the field of healthcare relating to pregnancy, birth, and postpartum care. I was very frustrated and felt violated because I didn't stand up for myself. I was angry with other people for violating me, but I didn't take responsibility for my role in allowing the mistreatment.

During my third pregnancy, I realized that I had power. I decided what I wanted for my pregnancy and my birth, and I regained control of my health. I chose to stop being mistreated, and I chose to opt out of being victimized and controlled by others.

In the first and second births, I let the healthcare system turn me into a victim by allowing them to control my life and refusing to take my proper place and responsibility. As the authority over my life and the lives of my children, I get to decide what I allow and what I don't allow. Matthew 18:18 tells us, "I assure you and most solemnly say to you, whatever you bind [forbid, declare to be improper and unlawful] on earth shall have [already] been bound in heaven, and whatever you loose [permit, declare lawful] on earth shall have [already] been loosed in heaven."

Power belongs to us. We decide what we allow and what we permit. We choose what we forbid and what we allow to happen to us and to our kids. I stood as a helpless victim, refusing to take my place of authority, and I assumed that the medical professionals were the best source of guidance for my baby and me. I assumed that they had my well being in mind because I didn't realize the power I had to say no and to make decisions regarding my and my children's health.

The more we spend time in God's presence, the more we will understand the character and nature of Christ, and we will understand who God made us to be. Time spent with Jesus permits us to be comfortable trusting Him for the right thing to do for our own lives and the lives of our kids. It permits us to stand strong when we are violated by someone or something in our lives. I know my kids are safe in

God's loving care, and the wisest decision I ever made was to give God control of my life and my children's lives. Now, I ask God for direction and information. Then I stand strong in the Lord's wisdom, and I refuse to back down or allow anyone to back me off what I know the Lord spoke to me.

After I became born again, I viewed the world differently. I realized the world's system was very different from God's system. Without a firm knowledge of the Bible, at first God primarily used the Spirit to guide me by giving me spiritual intuition. It took time for me to read and understand the Bible, but instantly upon being born again, God helped me by giving me gut spiritual feelings of wrong or right. Many times, early in my walk with Christ, I knew something was wrong, because God warned me in my spirit.

As a naïve, young American woman, I believed the people making decisions about my health were trustworthy because I was taught to love my country. Growing up in America, I assumed our medical system was largely founded upon proper ethics, integrity, and the Bible. America is known as a Christian nation, and Americans are proud of our country. However, many of Americans policies and norms are distorted, and they need to be adjusted to help us succeed as Americans.

An assumption is defined as something accepted as truth without proof. My assumptions about healthcare, God, and America led me to blindly trust things I should have questioned, because our current system regulating American healthcare is not ethical, trustworthy, or founded on integrity and God's Word. The current American healthcare system was founded on elitist greed and control. It was developed through overregulation and infiltration of education, customs, norms, licenses, and requirements to practice medicine, and many other occupations, teaching incorrect practice and simultaneously mandating compliance.

All forms of education should be based on free inquiry, an educational approach allowing learners to construct their own questions, find their own resources, and customize their learning experiences, while allowing for individual summative assessments, demonstrating learning has occurred. Education is important, and all of us should have the right to be educated, but true education is learning and mastering information or a skill. We still have many things to learn about human health, and until we have figured out everything, we should be eager to acquire information through inquiry and questioning the assumptions that have not yet been proven successful or sufficient.

To solve the problem in healthcare, we must first solve the problem in education. Licenses and degrees are not always proof of superior learning acquisition, although they are assumed to be. For instance, many in the holistic healthcare field are very knowledgeable, but they practice holistic healthcare instead of allopathic care, and are assumed to be inferior. As an example, midwives are highly educated and knowledgeable practitioners, but they are often assumed to be less knowledgeable or trustworthy than a physician, even when this is not necessarily the case. My midwife knew more about women's reproductive health than any physician I had ever seen in my 15 years prior!

To question means to investigate or to interrogate, looking deeper into something to separate truth and lies. Learning is always our responsibility. Every believer should be interested in learning and deciphering truth from lies so we can ensure we are not deceived by wicked people and their agendas. Jesus warned us we needed to pay attention, to properly navigate the world with discernment, so we won't become prey. Matthew 10:16 warns us, "Listen carefully: I am sending you out like sheep among wolves; so be wise as serpents, and innocent as doves [have no self-serving agenda]."

Without discernment, even in a "Christian" nation, God's people can become prey to people who want to take advantage of us. Christians are loving, kind, longsuffering, and caring because we share the characteristics of Christ. We want to help others, protect others, and defend others from oppression. However, the unsaved world does not share these characteristics. Many people in the world are malicious, evil, and vile. Others only care about their own interests and those who are in their inner circle.

It is possible for Christians to be deceived. Christians can be weak and vulnerable, even when they are called to be strong and bold. We cannot look to one another to determine right and wrong. We must look to God to for strength and wisdom. We must know what we are called to do, and we must refuse to back down to the enemies that live among us, taunting our God. When David attacked Goliath, he went with God alone. The men who should have been on his side, fighting beside him, were not. Unfortunately, they were afraid, timid, and controlled by enemy forces, but David knew it only takes one man of God to defeat an obnoxious and vile giant.

First Samuel 17:8–11 says, "Goliath stood and shouted to the ranks of Israel, 'Why have you come out to draw up for battle? Am I not a Philistine, and are you not servants of Saul? Choose a man for yourselves and let him come down to me. If he is able to fight with me and kill me, then we will be your servants; but if I prevail against him and kill him, then you shall be our servants and serve us.' And the Philistine said, 'I defy the ranks of Israel this day; give me a man, that we may fight together.' When Saul and all Israel heard those words of the Philistine, they were dismayed and greatly afraid."

The Church must pay attention if we are going to exert dominion in the world. First Thessalonians 5:6 instructs us, "So then let us not sleep as others do but let us be alert and sober." Many world leaders, including American leaders, are demonically inspired. We must recognize we are wrestling against spirits who want to control, not against men and women. Demons need a host to work through, and some individuals partner with the demonic forces deliberately, while others do so blindly.

Many scientific and medical remedies are potions, having their roots in occultic science. Medicines and medical procedures are effective and can produce a level of healing in patients. As it was in the days of Moses, magicians, using magic arts and sorcery exist, and can replicate miracles using supernatural power, but supernatural doesn't always mean holy and godly. Supernatural experiences or healings may appear to be established by God, when they are coming from the kingdom of darkness. The Bible, and our personal relationship with God invoking the indwelling of the Holy Ghost, provides us with the guide we need to walk in wisdom and discernment, identifying the roots of a healing practice.

Psalms 144:1–2 says, "Blessed be the Lord, my rock, who trains my hands for war and my fingers for battle. He is my loving God and my fortress, my stronghold and my deliverer, my shield, in whom I take refuge, who subdues peoples under me."

God will always warn us. He will give us a blueprint to succeed when we want to learn and receive, but we must be willing to fight for ourselves and to stand against evil, as David did. If we run in fear from our giants, they will overtake and dominate us, when we have been granted the authority to dominate them. God's people have a role to play in ensuring that God's will is established and the devil's plan is demolished.

In 2024, the Lord showed me the truth about the devils operating in the medical profession and the medical education system, where I received my bachelor's degree. I received my bachelor's degree in psychology from Virginia Commonwealth University in Richmond Virginia. Virginia Commonwealth University is one of the top accredited medical colleges in the United State, but Virginia Commonwealth University has spiritual ties to the Egyptian practices of witchcraft and sorcery, and they are proud of it.

As a student at Virginia Commonwealth University between 2013–2015, I was unaware of the school's background or its alignment with these spiritual forces. I wanted to help people and understand human behavior, so I went to an accredited school near my hometown. To my knowledge, the school never mentioned the origins of the university, and I never considered looking it up. As an unbeliever, I didn't have the spiritual understanding to see it or understand it. Second

Corinthians 4:4 tells us, "Among them the god of this world [Satan] has blinded the minds of the unbelieving to prevent them from seeing the illuminating light of the gospel of the glory of Christ, who is the image of God."

In the dream the Lord gave me, I was in a VCU campus building I'd never been in before at 3 a.m. A woman walked up to me and handed me her jacket with the Virginia Commonwealth University symbol on it. I received the jacket and I went into a classroom where I began talking in depth with a strange man about pictograms and psychology.

The following morning, I asked the Lord to interpret my dream. Then, I started researching the pictogram on the jacket I received in the dream, as this pictogram represented the university. I discovered, the Virginia Commonwealth University pictogram is a building named the Egyptian building. I began to discover the history of this building and the medical school birthed from it.

The Egyptian building at VCU gives homage to the ancient Egypt's discoveries relating to health and medicine. In my dream, when the woman handed me her jacket or "cloak" to put on, it symbolized being clothed in unrighteousness, lies, and deception. I was clothed apart from God, and without God, as Adam and Eve attempted to do. The Bible says to be clothed in righteousness. We can clothe ourselves through God and His righteousness, through Christ, or we can clothe ourselves in the demonic, personal ambition, and human self-worth, apart from our Creator.

"I put on righteousness, and it clothed me; my justice was like a robe and a turban" (Job 29:14).

Isaiah 64:6 says, "For all of us have become like one who is unclean, and all our righteous deeds are like a filthy garment, and all of us wither like a leaf, and our iniquities, like the wind, take us away."

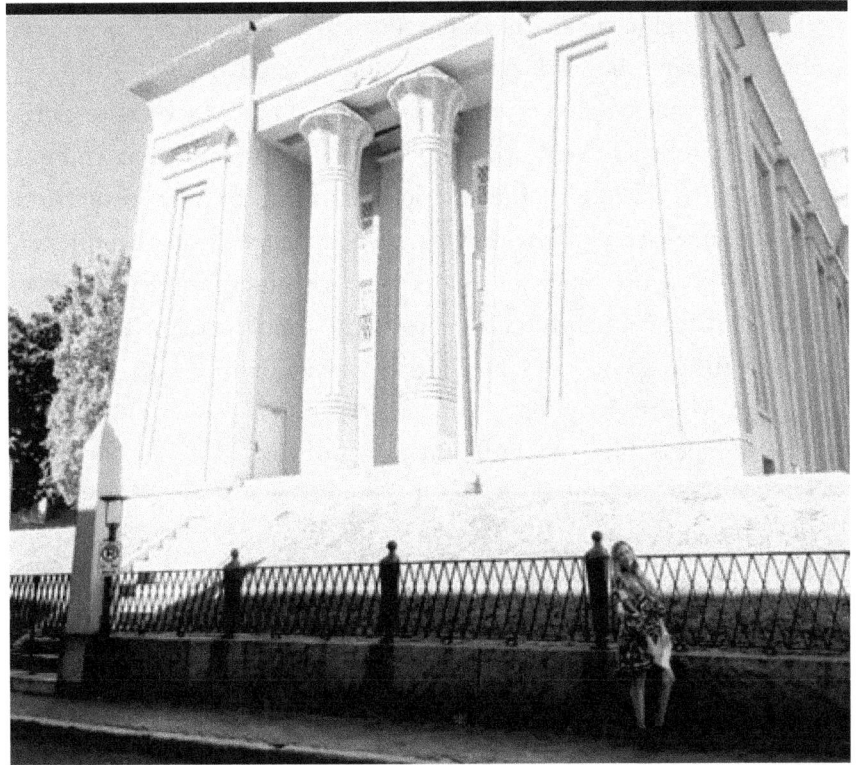

Ashton Bohannon outside of the Egyptian Building in Richmond Virginia

The Egyptian building is revered by many and is viewed as a place of supernatural influence by schools leaders. Virginia Commonwealth University is proud of the influence given to them by the Egyptians. A former Virginia Commonwealth President noted, "This really is sacred ground, I thank all of our students, faculty, staff and alumni who work to preserve our history."

Sacred is formally defined as: being connected to God or the gods, being dedicated to a religious purpose. By definition, sacred means as religious and not secular, including the writing of text embodying the laws and doctrines of a religion. In this case, the former president of VCU noted the Egyptian building is sacred, godlike, and embodies laws and doctrine of Egyptian religion. Thus, many VCU beliefs appear to be religious in nature, stemming from the gods of Egypt, even when they assert they are secular and non-religious.

The Egyptian religion is and always has been contrary to the Christian/Jewish religion. Many young people in America who attend universities within the field of medicine, counseling, or other professions are often unaware of what they are partnering with in the spiritual realm. Without the Spirit of God giving me supernatural revelation, I would have remained blind to these very important spiritual truths myself. Without God and His mercy, I would have been deceived about the origins of my former university.

"The oracle of him who hears the words of God, who sees the vision of the Almighty, falling down, yet having his eyes uncovered" (Numbers 24:4).

Virginia Commonwealth University was erected in 1846, before the Rockefellers' infiltration of medical education, and the American healthcare system. No doubt this school survived the mandates and compliance measures placed within the system of control, because they submitted to the rules of the elitist organizations. Standing strong, training and teaching the next generations doctors, physicians, and health professionals, is Virginia Commonwealth University, influencing best practice for the population.

The Holy Spirit produces supernatural life. Believers see, hear, and experience life in a unique way someone without God cannot experience. Light lives within Christians, and our light illuminates and straightens our path. God leads us to the path of life, and He leads us away from the paths of destruction. Psalm 119:105 says, *"Your word is a lamp unto my feet, and a light unto my path."* When God shows us the truth, we must believe Him, because God knows everything, and without God, man does not.

The Church will not be accepted by the world. Jesus was not accepted by the religious system, or governmental system. The Church shows people a different way, and we free people from manipulation by showing them the truth of God. The devil doesn't want us to liberate humanity, because this frees them from his domination. As the Church allows the Holy Spirit to flow through us, the world will see God through us. We will bring hope, healing, and peace setting the captives free.

For thousands of years the Church has created positive changes, influencing the societies they are a part of. We don't need to be overwhelmed by the world's system, because with God's help, we can overtake it. We can change the world we live in if we only believe and stand with the Lord. David was a shepherd boy, tending sheep, and then He became the king of Israel, because he stood against God's enemies in his land. He wasn't afraid of the giants, he challenged them. "Do not be overcome by evil but instead overcome evil with good" (Romans 12:21).

The Church is responsible to implement God's plan to defeat the enemy. We choose not to be swayed to the left or to the right by worldly concepts, ideas, or any other unholy persuasions or philosophies. We choose to stand against evil and defend God's name on the earth. The Church of Jesus Christ separates itself from the world and remains faithful to God. The Church hates evil and turns from it. The Church has an intentional plan to conquer the forces of darkness, to establish God's kingdom on the earth, because God gives us instructions.

Proverbs 4:27 instructs us, "Do not turn to the right or the left; keep your foot from evil."

Exodus 34:12 says, "Be careful not to make a treaty with the inhabitants of the land you are entering, lest they become a snare to you."

Colossians 2:8 warns us, "See to it that no one takes you captive through philosophy and empty deception [pseudo-intellectual babble], according to the tradition [and musings] or mere men, following the elementary principles of this world, rather than following [the truth-the teachings] of Christ."

To be a captive is to be enslaved, controlled, and confined. A person who is captive is at the mercy of the other person, deity, or power.

God never desired for His people to be without the power of choice, thought, imagination, or free will. God made us with a conscience, and He made us to operate from a place of freedom. When the world's system, backed by the forces of evil, wants to take us captive and into bondage, we must refuse to go. Goliath believed he could make the Israelite army his slaves, but his plan failed, and God's plan prevailed because David challenged him in the name of our Lord.

In a war, we must make wise decisions so enemy forces never overtake us. We must fight the giants who live on our land. By revealing things to come, God preserves our lives. He keeps us ahead of our enemies, and He ensures that those who want to overtake us in battle never conquer us. God trains us in wisdom and in strength, and He shows us how to navigate. The inner witness of the conscience and the Holy Spirit were specifically given to us to help us make righteous decisions. Relying on the Holy Spirit gives us the ability to make the right decision every single time.

"The Spirit of truth, has come, and He shall guide you into all truths, for He will not speak for Himself, but whatsoever He hear, that He shall speak, and He will show you things to come" (John 16:13).

"God will guide His people with a voice behind them saying, 'this is the way, walk ye in it'" (Isaiah 30:21).

Healthcare companies such as hospitals, pharmaceutical companies, and other health services benefit from the population being sick and needy. Holding the power and dictating the terms of any verbal or contractual agreements is beneficial for them, not us. Many wicked individuals enjoy being in control and having people need their help. Physician-patient relations are intentionally built to benefit doctors, nurses, hospitals, insurance companies, pharmacists, and pharmaceutical companies, not patients.

The educational system has also become corrupted and run for profit, not for free thought, and freedom. This system doesn't benefit our children, and it doesn't benefit us. We don't want our kids to grow up with limited opportunities if they don't conform, so we must fight against it, even if it currently influences the land. Children are entitled to a safe and nurturing environment for learning. They deserve an education that fosters free-inquiry rather than mere indoctrination.

To an unsuspecting American populus, higher education and healthcare are in place for society's well being, but through intentional research, we can determine the origins of the corruption and infiltration of evil. If education and healthcare remain controlled and beneficial primarily for the elite, they will be full of every evil thing. James 3:16 tells us, "For where jealousy and selfish ambition exist, there is disorder [unrest, rebellion] and every evil thing and morally degrading practice."

Holding ourselves responsible for our health and our family's health allows us to disconnect from the world's system and lean into God's system. As we connect to God and investigate the world around us, we perceive right and wrong, and we know what we are to do and what we are not to do. We receive clear vision as to the right and wrong path for our families.

Satan often gets people stuck into cycles of captivity by presenting evil as good, but when we stay connected to God, we will never be deceived. Sin is a seed, and seeds take time to grow. Some seeds grow faster than others, but sin always has a reaping season. Procedures and medications are often presented as good and convenient. They appear to help at first, but many people get stuck in the medical system quickly or unexpectedly, and before they know it, they depend on drugs, doctors, or procedures to even stay alive.

God will keep us from ever taking the first addictive or harmful substance by informing us ahead of time. When we heed the Spirit's guidance, we will be kept out of Satan's traps and schemes.

"Drug overdose is the leading cause of death for individuals younger than 50 years in the United States and accounted for 13.1% of all deaths in 2016" (CDC National Overdose Deaths). "Deaths due to opioid overdoses accounted for 66% of overdose deaths, and 40% of the opioids used in these deaths were legally prescribed" (Osmundson,

Min, & Grijalva 2019). Some women schedule surgical births and leave addicted to opioids. "Exposure to opioids after surgical procedures increases the risk of chronic opioid use" (Osmundson, Min, & Grijalva 2019).

At first, the medication alleviates the pain until the unsuspecting patient becomes dependent. "It is estimated that more than 80% of women fill opioid prescriptions after cesarean birth and about 54% of women after vaginal birth, although these figures vary greatly by geographical location and setting. This exposure leads to an increased risk of chronic opioid use" (Osmundson, Min, & Grijalva 2019).

Prevention of cesarean births and a prevention of the need for pain medications would keep women from being addicted and harmed by opioids; thus we as a nation concerned for public health should aspire to prevent unnecessary cesarean births.

A cesarean birth also makes the risk for continuous cesarean births much higher because many doctors will not allow for subsequent vaginal births. One surgery then leads to another surgery, and before women know it, they depend on their doctors for help birthing their child. Pregnant women and their children are not exempted from being duped and trapped in the medical system's grip in fact, they are regularly victimized by it. It often doesn't take long for Satan's traps for domination to manifest within the lives of unsuspecting victims when the victims are not diligent and watching for potential attacks.

Consider a child who is a few days old receiving surgical circumcision. From a circumcision failure, immediate and negative effects can follow. These effects can cause long-term consequences as serious as death. In less severe cases, a botched circumcision can cause infection, a deformity of sexual organs, psychological trauma, excessive bleeding, and unnecessary pain. Children who are harmed in circumcision may need lifelong medical intervention. Yet, a parent who asks the Lord if his or her child should receive this procedure, may be instructed to refrain from the procedure, and therefore will bypass any negative repercussions.

God will give us a plan, and often His plan is opposite of the medical recommendations. The Center for Disease Control and Prevention (CDC) asserts the benefits of surgery outweigh the risks, even though their focus for recommending circumcision comes from the chance of contracting HIV. However, if a male child is raised in a Christian home and is instructed to refrain from sexual activity outside of a safe marriage relationship, he can avoid contracting HIV without a surgical procedure. When we consult with God, and He gives us insight, and we implement the plan of the Lord, we are safeguarding our children. We are ensuring that the enemy cannot harm them or gain a foothold into their lives, because God warns us ahead of time.

Plans for success do not have to be complicated, if they are precise and intentional God-ordained plans. Our plans for birth, childrearing, and optimal health do not need to be extensive, and they do not need to make sense to world leaders. Planning to raise our children in a way that honors the Lord will shield them from all the fiery darts of the enemy. Having a plan to discuss the dangers of sin and sexual immorality with our children will protect their sexual health. By intentionally instructing my son to remain abstinent until marriage, I protect him God's way.

Plans help us to ensure that we receive our desired outcome. Birth plans help women to have the labor and delivery experience they want. Birth plans let our medical team understand preferences, so they can respect and facilitate them.

First Corinthians 6:20 says, "For you have been bought with a price; therefore, glorify God in your body." When making a birth plan, we must consider what the Holy Spirit leads us to do. Leaning on secondhand information or the opinions and experiences of others will often lead women to make decisions they are not comfortable with. Our plans must be determined within our hearts, and we must not be indecisive or double-minded.

Second Corinthians 3:12 tells us, "Therefore, since we have such a hope, we are very bold." God will provide clear answers for women who ask Him. There is no guesswork with God. God delights in informing and preparing His people for success. If you want to know what to do to protect your body or your child, then go to God and ask Him for direction. Once we receive our direction, we commit to the path and we do not stray from it, no matter what. Deuteronomy 4:29 promises us, "If you seek the Lord with all your heart and soul, you will find Him."

Mothers should consider their labor plans, birth plans, and postpartum plans, and consider newborns care. We need to know exactly where we stand on healthcare decisions, so when we face a question or pushback, you will not sway or be coerced into a different decision. Birth is an incredibly emotional experience. A lot of overwhelming feelings occur during labor, delivery, and postpartum. It is vital to respect your own needs, desires, and plans when you are giving birth to your baby.

No one has the right to alter, intercede, or try to negate a woman's preferences for herself and her babies. "Decisions about where, how, and with whom to give birth are meaningful reproductive health decisions. For many, they involve intimate considerations about the experience of bringing life into the world and meeting one's baby, connection with one's partner, self-empowerment, and connection with the divine" (The Legal Infrastructure of Childbirth).

Two important decisions a woman must make are: where she will birth and whom she will have at her birth. Most American women chose physician-attended births in the hospital, but midwife-attended births, whether in the hospital, a birthing center, or at home, are also options. The midwife vs. the physician approach to birth is fundamentally different. Acknowledging the differences and being comfortable with your choice is essential to control your birth.

"The medical model approaches birth as a pathological medical condition, requiring hospitalization and medical supervision, as well as frequent intervention. Technology is dominant and perceived risk is central. The process is doctor centered, with physicians direction the process and making the decisions. The midwifery model of care, on the other hand, understands birth to be a normal physiologic process. Care supports "the physical, psychosocial and spiritual health, well-being and safety" of the birthing dyad. The fetus and pregnant woman are an "interdependent whole." Midwifery emphasizes individualized care, built on an "egalitarian relationship" of "trust, honesty, and respect" between midwife and client. The pregnant person is "autonomous and competent to make decisions regarding all aspects of her life." Finally, midwifery care seeks to "minimize technological interventions" (The Legal Infrastructure of Childbirth).

"A recent phenomenon is the choice to have an unassisted birth (UAB) with no midwife or other professional maternity care attendant (Sperlich & Gabriel 2022). Unassisted births are also called free births. In a free birth, a woman chooses to birth unassisted by any professional and relies on the help of their husband, partner, or other support person. Every woman must decide whom she wants present during her birth. Women are free to choose how they want to birth their children, and some women want to freebirth.

For the birth of my third child, I chose an intimate home birth experience that allowed me to feel safe and comfortable. I let my husband, my midwife and my doula be present. I knew I didn't want to have any family members or friends present at my son's birth; I only wanted my husband, my chosen team, and my other children present.

I knew privacy would help me to experience a healthy and satisfying birth. I made sure everyone was aware of my plan, so it was not violated. In my first and second births, nurses, doctors, family members, and friends impacted my pregnancy, my birth, and my postpartum experience negatively. For my third birth, when I realized I had the power to change my birth experience, I was committed to keeping unsafe people, interventions, and medications away.

With my second child, COVID-19 restricted visitors from visiting me in the hospital, and this was a blessing. Despite having a c-section and being medicated, I could breastfeed and rest on the days after my birth. The COVID-19 pandemic also limited visitors when I came home from the hospital. I didn't feel the pressure to entertain family or friends during my recovery process with my second baby, and I could relax and bond with my husband and my baby. I had no issues breastfeeding my second child because I was given a safe space to practice.

My first and second birth experiences in the hospital allowed me to compare what I liked and disliked about my birth experiences. I understood how much the medications (opioids), the visitors, and the cesarean births impacted my mind, my body, and my baby bonding time. So, when I prepared for my home birth, I elected to give birth in private, away from medical interventions and with my chosen safe people. The decision to not use medications, birth at home alone, and to limit visitors had such a big impact on my birth experience.

Throughout my labor and birth at home I felt comfortable and safe. I was in control of my birth, and no one had access to me during one of the most intimate moments of my life unless I chose them. Within my birth plan, I also decided I did not want anyone to visit Gianni and me at home. I wanted to spend time with my new baby, my husband, and my kids in private. I wanted time to rest and recover.

After all my hard work preparing for a home birth, staying healthy, and creating a birth plan, I had a beautiful birth. But on my second day of recovery, my children told me a family member was there to visit me. I began to cry, and my peaceful bubble burst because I felt violated. I felt like my autonomy was being breached, because it was. My plan for recovery was not followed.

A visitor without respect for my boundaries showed up to my house unannounced, knowing I did not want visitors. I had a beautiful experience of laboring, birthing, and recovering, but during my postpartum recovery, my birth plan was violated. It did take me some time to process this violation, and I separated from this individual for some time afterwards. However, the space appears to have benefited the relationship between us, because my boundaries are now being respected more.

As a former survivor of sexual abuse, domestic abuse, and institutionalized medical abuse, my homebirth was healing, rewarding, and empowering. Being in complete control, without pressure to compromise strengthened me as a person. Learning to control your life and set boundaries is freeing, especially when you have always lived in a state of bondage in relationships. "Previous studies show that women who have experienced childhood physical or sexual abuse may prioritize having a sense of control and autonomy during their birthing experiences" (Sperlich & Gabriel 2022).

My birth plan prepared me to have Gianni without any pain medication, ointments, vaccines, or procedures. When women use a midwife in a birthing center or at home, the options for pain management are limited. I wanted a holistic birth, and I didn't want medical interventions. I wanted to be as natural as possible. When Gianni was born, as we had planned, my husband caught him, because I didn't feel comfortable doing it! We also decided ahead of time that we would not clamp or cut the cord until it had stopped pulsing. My husband was the one to cut his cord after the blood had finished transferring to Gianni.

During labor, women need to make many decisions, such as if they want to move around, be able to eat, play music, light candles, or dim the lights. We can decide if we want to use birthing and labor props such as squatting bars, birthing balls, birthing stools, or birthing chairs. We can birth in water or on land. Knowing what we want to do is key to ensure we get what we want. When women give birth at home or in a birthing center, they have more options and control. Hospitals have regulations about what is and isn't allowed, and that is why I gave birth to my son in my bedroom!

My birth didn't go exactly as I planned, but the things that really mattered to me were all implemented. The things that were most important to me were: where I birthed (at home), how I birthed (no medications, interventions, or surgeries), who was at my birth (just my chosen team), and what I allowed after my birth (no separation of me and baby—and no medical procedures or interventions for my child).

My husband and I gave Gianni his first bath and held him and bonded with him after he was born. We kept him with us, and he didn't go to a hospital nursery for any time away or for procedures. My son Gianni didn't leave our home for a month after he was born because the midwife came to us, and she performed his newborn appointments. Gianni adjusted to the world in the safety of his home, with the love and protection of his parents and his older siblings. He was able to adapt to the world around him and bond with his family. Gianni knows he is loved and is safe, and he has known it from the moment he entered the world. He is securely attached to us as his family.

The trivial things about our birth experiences won't matter if we get the things we really need and want. During my labor, the candles never got lit, and the music never got played. The birth pool never got blown up or filled with water. A birth plan is not exact, but it does help us to know what things matter most to us. Knowing what we need and what we want ensures that we are positioned to not be violated. Ultimately my main desires for my pregnancy and my birth were protected and respected. My midwife and doula never forced me to do anything I didn't feel comfortable with; instead they validated my plan, and me and provided me with safety and security.

When we go into labor, we don't know how we will respond if we've never given birth before. As believers, we know God will get us through it, giving us the help we need to successfully reach our goals. God designed our bodies to birth our children, and He will take care of us if we put our faith in Him. Know the things that are essential to you with your birth and your pregnancy. Then, delight yourself in the Lord. Psalm 37:4 says, "Delight yourself in the Lord, And He will give you the desires and petitions of your heart."

God will help us to receive what we want from our births as we walk with and trust Him. The medical establishment and the educational system manipulate it; know what they are doing, why they are doing it, and how they will accomplish their goal.

Rockefeller and his associates wrote a very detailed plan, explaining how and when they would annihilate groups opposing their plan—and what we see in medical education and the medical system today is a product of that plan. So, let us be wise and not foolish. Let us accomplish our plans with strategy and position. Let us know what we want so we can go get it.

10

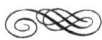

The Weapons of our Warfare: Prayer and Oil

As we submit to Jesus, we become eligible to be baptized in the Holy Spirit. The baptism of the Holy Spirit is required if we are going to become agents of positive change within our society and the world. God's Spirit is mandatory if we are going restore and replenish the earth. The anointing is the supernatural assistance enabling us to set the captives free from their oppression and drive out darkness from the land. Without the anointing of God, we can do nothing.

After Jesus was crucified and resurrected, He spent forty days with His disciples on the earth. During this time, Jesus instructed them to continue to carry out His mission on the earth. He promised they would have what they needed to do this. Jesus vowed the new covenant Church would continue to perform the good works He began, and we would even do greater works, after He sent our helper, the Holy Spirit.

John 14:12 says, "I assure you and most solemnly say to you, anyone who believes in Me [as Savior] will also do the things that I do; and he will do even greater things than these [in extent and outreach], because I am going to the Father."

Approximately 120 people were in the upper room when the Holy Spirit was first poured out on the believers. The outpouring of the Holy Spirit was the beginning of the fulfillment of the establishment of the new covenant. Since that time, hundreds of thousands of believers all over the world have been filled with the Holy Spirit. With the inner dwelling of the Holy Spirit, the Church today is performing many signs, wonders, and miracles on the earth. With Jesus' delegated power and authority, we are seizing the works of the devil and influencing the world.

As we partner with the Holy Spirit, we can show the world that our God is alive and willing to change their lives, communities, and the world at large for the better. As we near Christ's return, we expect to see more miracles and manifestations of the Spirit of God. God wants to see people saved, and He wants to reap a harvest in the land. The world will come to know Jesus personally through the Church, because of the demonstration of power working within us.

Mark 16:17–19 teaches, "These signs will accompany those who have believed: in My name they will cast out demons, they will speak in new tongues; they will pick up serpents, and if they drink anything deadly, it will not hurt them; they will lay hands on the sick, and they will get well." So then, when the Lord Jesus had spoken to them, He was taken up into heaven and sat down at the right hand of God."

In the world are two kingdoms: the kingdom of God and the kingdom of the devil. God has given us kingdom jurisdiction. Jurisdiction is the official power to make legal decisions and judgments. God assigned us with jurisdiction to orchestrate change and influence the world where we live, and He gifted us with the anointing to ensure our work comes to pass.

As we rise to the occasion, and we believe what the Lord has spoken to us, we can make a difference in the community, the nation, and our world. We are appointed to bring good news and change the pattern of the world. We have delegated jurisdiction. Matthew 10:8 says,

"Heal the sick, raise the dead, cleanse those who have leprosy, drive out demons. Freely you have received; freely give."

Within the devil's kingdom is bondage and corruption. Abuse, distortion, torment, and pain, are elements of Satan's work on the earth. Many large human systems, such as the healthcare system, the judicial system, and the education system, are infiltrated by Satan because these systems impact large groups of people. Satan wants to steal, kill, and destroy, and he can implement his mission through influencing the choices and lives of human vessels.

Sin is necessary for Satan's system to remain. Without sin, Satan cannot continue his work. Satan needs people to cooperate with him through sin, such as selling drugs, stealing money, telling lies, taking bribes, or killing others, if he is going to prosper and elevate his kingdom. Without sinful human cooperation, Satan's kingdom loses ground. Satan wants to reduce God's influence and raise his. He wants to remove God's leadership and introduce a new leader: himself. But Satan can only exalt his kingdom when people yield to sin.

As the word of God is taught, the Spirit goes forth healing those who hear and receive the word. As we speak the word, it helps people and sets those free who need to be delivered. Light is always stronger than darkness. As soon as the light enters a room or a person's heart, the darkness must go. Satan knows when God is present, sin is driven out of the land and the lives of those who are impacted. When God is present, Satan's plans are thwarted, and that is why he works so hard to keep God out!

A person who is not under the submission of Christ will always lead others into bondage, but a person who is submitted to Christ will lead people to freedom. Through our public confession and our intentional intercession, we bear witness to God's word and teaching, and we pull people out of the kingdom of darkness and into the kingdom of light. We show them the way to the cross and to their Healer, and we release them from their captor, Satan.

Spirits are behind everything we see in the physical world. There are antichrist spirits and the Holy Spirit. We will either allow the Holy Spirit to guide our actions, or we will allow the spirits of the Antichrist to determine our choices.

When we don't obey God, we restrict the anointing. The devil wants to create traitors to God's kingdom. He wants to influence people to violate God's laws, so he can steal what doesn't belong to him. But, when we restrain ourselves from sin, and we keep ourselves from engaging with sin through a life of righteousness and truth, the curse leaves our life, and we are endowed with supernatural power. If we want to increase in the anointing, we must submit ourselves to God and His laws and refuse to cooperate with our enemy.

Second Corinthians 5:14 says, "For the love of Christ constraineth us; because we thus judge, that one died for all, therefore all died."

The word constraint means to limit, restrict, or inhibit. As members of God's kingdom, we are constrained from behaving in ways that oppose the King we serve because of our love for our King. Our King has established laws, policies, and expectations for the kingdom residents. We do not determine the laws of the land, but we submit to them willingly, because we respect our King, and we know He will keep us safe from our enemy.

Spirits of hate, racism, alcohol, greed, and abuse are antichrist spirits. These spirits work in opposition to God's laws and his kingdom. Antichrist spirits attack the anointing, through attacking the people who carry the anointing. If antichrist spirits can influence us to gossip about someone we should be praying for, then they will restrict the anointing. Satan himself was once anointed. If Satan cannot get someone to completely walk away from the anointing, then he will try to limit the anointing.

Ezekiel 28:14 says, "You were the anointed cherub who covers and protects, And I placed you there. You were on the holy mountain of God; You walked in the midst of the stones of fire [sparkling jewels]."

One of the primary ways Satan harms the Church is through polluting the anointing. If he cannot stop the message from going forth, then he will try to dilute it, or water it down. Many people are afraid to stand up for God and the kingdom because they are afraid of what others will think or do to them. However, this fear causes them to submit to an antichrist spirit, and this dilutes the anointing in their lives or ministries.

We are not to be ashamed of the gospel or of the anointing. We should be joyful about the anointing we carry because we know we are cherished by God. Satan will try to corrupt the anointing through allowing impurity to come into a person or a church. Pure water is the only water that is fit to drink. When a water source becomes impure, it can cause serious problems for those who drink it. Not all water is the same, and we are to be assured we are drinking pure unpolluted water, and that we are not diluting the oil or limiting the Holy Spirit.

The United States Justice System is one of the human systems Satan has targeted. The criminal justice system in America influences a lot of people. In the United States, we do not have a king, but we do have many leaders who represent us. In the Bible, Satan targeted kings and rulers of the land, and in America, he also targets leaders. God instructs us to pray for all leaders and our leading organizations, because praying for them is right in God's sight. As we pray for our leaders and authorities, we submit to God's standard. We limit the power of Satan, and we distribute the Spirit of God.

"First of all, then, I admonish and urge that petitions, prayers, intercessions, and thanksgivings be offered on behalf of all men, For kings and all who are in positions of authority or high responsibility, that [outwardly] we may pass a quiet and undisturbed life [and inwardly] a peaceable one in all godliness and reverence and seriousness in every way. For such [praying] is good and right, and [it is] pleasing and acceptable to God our Savior, Who wishes all men to be saved and [increasingly] to perceive and recognize and discern and know precisely and correctly the [divine] Truth" (1 Timothy 2:1–4).

Satan wants us to submit to antichrist spirits of hate and personal vengeance, so we become polluted and limit God's Spirit from dominating in our lives, consequently losing our influence. Satan wants us to lose our power through submitting to antichrist spirits and corruption. Many large groups and organizations today attempt to fight evil with evil. When faced with injustice, these groups attempt to avenge themselves through violent and ungodly means. Although their pain may be valid, they separate themselves from receiving God's help when they partner with the devil, because they surrender the anointing.

Partnership with Satan will always lead to more bondage. Without knowing it, many align themselves with Satan and perpetuate the problem. When they perpetuating sin, Satan remains in control and people continue to be hurt by further injustice and abuse. The only way to create change in our society is through the pure anointing and the Spirit of God. If God is on our side, we will be successful despite human or demonic attempts to stop us.

The way we stay on God's side is through submitting to God's standards and laws. God will elevate us into a place of influence as we submit to Him. God is the ultimate judge, and we know He hates injustice. He wants to eliminate evil, and He wants to establish righteousness in the world, but He needs our cooperation with His laws, to bring forth positive change, as Satan needs our cooperation to bring forth destruction.

Martin Luther King Jr. understood peaceful protest, prayer, and the vengeance of God. He understood the power he held as a man of God, and he cooperated with God to bring positive change within his society.

As a victim of legitimate societal and personal abuse, Martin Luther King Jr. felt justified anger and pain. However, King refused to give into the antichrist spirits in the world. Instead, he submitted himself to God and used the anointing to gain influence. Martin Luther King Jr. is quoted as saying, "Darkness cannot drive out darkness; only light can do that. Hate cannot drive out hate; only love can do that." When given the opportunity to hate, he chose to love, because he understood the spirit of love was superior to the spirit of hate.

Martin Luther King Jr.'s life was not easy and void of pain, but he understood the power of an alliance with God. He understood when he stood with the Holy Spirit, no one could stop him from spreading God's truth. He knew God would prosper his cause, because he knew was standing for pure justice. He said, "May I stress the need for courageous, intelligent, and dedicated leadership. Leaders of sound integrity. Leaders not in love with publicity, but in love with justice. Leaders not in love with money, but in love with humanity. Leaders who can subject their egos to the greatness the cause."

Martin Luther King Jr.'s anointing was evident in his words and his actions. He spoke powerfully through the anointing. God gave him a dream and a message, established in righteousness and justice, and he chose to stand with God even when the spirits around him wanted to pull him out of the anointing. A refusal to compromise with the devil caused him to be one of the greatest leaders to ever change law within the United States of America. The Holy Spirit equipped him to lead others into justice and truth, because he refused to compromise with the devil.

The only way to change the problems we face in our culture, as in days past, is through the anointing. The Church is the most powerful institution to ever exist, and we can put the devil out of business if we stand firm in the truth and refuse to give into antichrist spirits. We can have no place within our hearts for hate, greed, or any other antichrist spirit. We must hate what God hates, and love what God loves, to be used mightily of Him.

Romans 12:9 says, "Love is to be sincere and active [the real thing—without guile and hypocrisy]. Hate what is evil [detest all ungodliness, do not tolerate wickedness]; hold on tightly to what is good."

Many people throughout history have been mistreated for standing with God. Martin Luther King Jr. was imprisoned and ultimately killed for his refusal to tolerate evil. Some within the government and within society hated what he was doing, and they wanted to stop him from doing it. However, Martin Luther King Jr. was successful anyway. The darkness could not overcome the light. He was able to establish policies that have impacted so many Americans, and his influence within our nation continues far beyond the grave.

Genesis 4:10 tells us, "The LORD said, 'What have you done? The voice of your brother's [innocent] blood is crying out to Me from the ground [for justice].'" The murder of Martin Luther King Jr., even from the grave, cries out for God's justice, and the sovereign and just judge hears the cries. God sees all who are abused or mistreated, and He stands with those who uncompromisingly stand with Him, even when they have gone to eternity. When evil people shed innocent blood, they violate God's laws, and God will repay for the unrepented evil that has been sown.

Proverbs 6:16–19 reveals, "These six things the Lord hates, indeed, seven are an abomination to Him: A proud look [the spirit that makes one overestimate himself and underestimate others], a lying tongue, and hands that shed innocent blood, A heart that manufactures wicked thoughts and plans, feet that are swift in running to evil, A false witness who breathes out lies [even under oath], and he who sows discord among his brethren."

God calls for us to love His word, speak His word, and pray. All these characteristics were present in the life of Dr. Martin Luther King Jr. He loved God and His word, and he submitted to it. He spoke the truth boldly, and he refused to tolerate evil. He also prayed for those who were against him, and he prayed they would see the truth and see his God-given dream.

To become great men and women of influence, we are instructed imitate the men and women of God who have achieved the things we too hope to achieve. If we want to change anything in our society or within our lives, we must love God and His word, speak boldly without compromise, and pray for our enemies. Matthew 5:44 declares, "But I say to you, love [that is, unselfishly seek the best or higher good for] your enemies and pray for those who persecute you,"

God hears the prayers of the righteous. He promises to answer righteous prayers. Prayer allows us to talk directly to God. When we pray in according to God's word, we know that our prayers have power and will produce things in our lives and the lives of others. We know prayer can influence things on the earth. Mark 11:24 promises, "Therefore I tell you, whatever you ask for in prayer, believe that you have received it, and it will be yours."

When we pray, we talk directly to our Father, who is sovereign over the whole earth. We present our case to God, and we know He takes the case. In the United States court system, cases are taken before a judge, so the judge can rule in favor of the party deemed to be on the side of justice and truth. When people take cases to the court system, they pledge to allow the judge and the court system to handle their case, instead of trying to handle the case themselves. When the judge is brought into the situation, he or she determines the outcome of the case.

As we pray to our Father in heaven, we present Him with our case. Unlike human court systems and judges, God knows all the evidence. God knows exactly how to rule in favor of justice. When God is given the opportunity to stand with us, He will show us what to do, and He will be with us, as our helper and our advocate in times of abuse or injustice. Isaiah 33:22 says, "For the Lord is our judge, the Lord is our lawgiver, The Lord is our King; He will save us."

An advocate is someone who supports or speaks in favor of someone or a plan or action. Advocates defend people in court, helping make sure they receive the justice they deserve. The Holy Spirit is our advocate and our helper, and he stands with us, bringing forth justice. John 14:26 says, "But the Helper (Comforter, Advocate, Intercessor—Counselor, Strengthener, Standby), the Holy Spirit, whom the

Father will send in My name [in My place, to represent Me and act on My behalf], He will teach you all things. And He will help you remember everything that I have told you."

If we want help from the advocacy of heaven, we must remain pure in the sight of the law, and we must take our case to the judge. Remaining holy and pure ensures that when we stand before the judge, He finds favor with us and our behavior in reference to the law. Then, after remaining pure in the sight of God, we talk to God, and we bring him into the spiritual court system through prayer.

Matthew 5:20 explains, "For I tell you that unless your righteousness exceeds that of the scribes and Pharisees, you will never enter the kingdom of heaven."

We cannot entertain Antichrist spirits operating in the world and expect to get to heaven or produce serious change on the earth. If we desire to be used of God and operate in God's Holy Spirit, we must remain pure and restrain ourselves from unholy alliances with evil spirits. The curse operating in the devil's kingdom can overtake any of us if we do not carefully obey and follow God's commands.

Authority and leadership must be respected, and we must realize God has put people into leadership, and He can take them out of their positions. Challenging leadership, in the wrong way is dangerous and ungodly. As believers, we are to respect authority and leaders, and not come before our leaders as rebellious, indignant, unruly, residents. Daniel 2:21 tells us, "He changes times and seasons; he deposes kings and raises up others. He gives wisdom to the wise and knowledge to the discerning."

In the book of Esther, we learn of an evil man named Haman who worked for the king and conspired to destroy all the Jews. Haman devised a plan to deceive the king into harming innocent people. Mordecai, Esther's cousin, asked her to go as a protector and deliverer of the innocent people and to reveal the agenda of the enemy to the king. Esther agreed and boldly faced her enemy who was working to cause harm and oppress God's people.

Esther 4:8 tells us, "[Mordecai] also gave him a copy of the decree to destroy them, that was given out in Shushan, that he might show it to Esther, explain it to her, and charge her to go to the king, make supplication to him, and plead with him for the lives of her people."

As Esther went before the king she prayed and fasted, eliciting God's help and anointing before she approached the king's throne. Esther did not approach king in an overbearing, disrespectful manner; instead she was respectful and honored his position of authority. Esther could have been killed for approaching the king without being invited to do so. However, the king ruled in Esther and the Jew's favor because Esther was on God's side, and God gave her favor with an anointing.

Many times, the devil wants to work through the legal system or legal authorities. He will plant evil people around leaders to deceive them to harm people. We see this same theme in the book of Daniel, when evil men working for the king wanted to create a law to harm God's servant, even when the king was innocent from wanting to inflict harm. God wants us to pray for the leaders, because the leaders need discernment to see the truth so they can make the right decisions.

Martin Luther King Jr. acknowledged that if he was going to be successful, he needed to remain in the truth. He knew he needed to stay on God's side and within God's kingdom to see justice established. Like Esther, he didn't follow the unjust laws of the land, but he went before the authorities in a respectful way. Peaceful protest and elegant speech and behavior flowing from the anointing were the ways both Martin Luther King Jr. and Esther, secured justice for their people. Even when they needed to challenge unjust laws, they did so respectfully and showed honor to authority.

Nonviolence was the way Jesus conducted Himself on the earth, and when Jesus interacted with unjust authorities, He confronted them with his words, rebuking the evil, while refusing to use violence to assert dominance. Jesus knew He was anointed and He didn't need to use human means to gain power. We must be willing to present the truth of God's word in a way that is wise and doesn't bring us or God's kingdom to shame. There is a right and a wrong way to advocate for change.

Abuse, violence, and injustice should be addressed through the court system or legal authorities when possible. When we go before the authorities, we should always ask God for favor, like Esther, Daniel, and Martin Luther King Jr. If there is injustice, abuse, or problems within the systems and organizations in our communities, we can take the challenge, knowing God is already on our side. If we are anointed and given the mission, God will go with us. But we must distinguish when we need to fight and when we need to get away from those who seek to do us harm.

Jesus did not allow anyone to dominate him, but He did not use violence to establish His kingdom on the earth. Jesus got away from people who wanted to do Him harm, but He also continued His work, regardless of anyone who tried to stop Him without the use of the criminal justice system. Luke 4:29–30 tells us, "and they got up and drove Him out of the city, and led Him to the crest of the hill on which their city had been built, in order to hurl Him down the cliff. But passing [miraculously] through the crowd, He went on His way."

Both Jesus and Martin Luther King Jr. changed their countries using public speeches. Our words have power, and when our words are anointed, we will inspire those we are called to lead and serve. Martin Luther King Jr. often discussed the concept of true pacifism, also known as nonviolent resistance, and this approach was the foundation of his activism. Martin Luther King Jr. organized and motivated many to stand and fight for the truth using only his anointed tongue.

Oil is a symbol that represents the Holy Spirit. Oil represents the anointing. Acts 10:38 teaches, "You know of Jesus of Nazareth, how God anointed Him with the Holy Spirit and with power, and how He went about doing good and healing all who were oppressed by the devil, for God was with Him." We can only operate in our authority and rule over the devil, if we have been anointed, and to be anointed, we must remain in Christ and be baptized in the Holy Spirit.

If you do not know Christ, and Christ does not know you, then you will not be able to do His work. There is difference between knowing Jesus and hearing about Jesus. The people who are baptized in John's baptism know about Jesus. The people who are baptized in the Holy Ghost know Jesus. Matthew 7:22–23 tells us, "Many will say to Me on that day [when I judge them], 'Lord, Lord, have we not prophesied in Your name, and driven out demons in Your name, and done many miracles in Your name?' And then I will declare to them publicly, 'I never knew you; depart from me [you are banished from My presence], you who act wickedly [disregarding My commands].'"

When you spend time with Jesus, other people can tell. Something is surprisingly different about us after we have communed with God. Acts 4:13 tells us, "Now when the men of the Sanhedrin (Jewish High Court) saw the confidence and boldness of Peter and John and grasped the fact that they were uneducated and untrained [ordinary] men, they were astounded, and began to recognize that they had been with Jesus."

Anyone who attempts to pretend to carry the anointing without the baptism of the Holy Spirit is walking on dangerous ground. Religion and traditions don't hold any power against the devil. Knowing about Jesus doesn't produce the anointing. The only way to be anointed is to be hungry for the words and truth of God. We must regularly be hungry and thirsty for righteousness if we want to be filled. We must desire God as we desire our food and drink!

Acts 19:13 teaches, "Some Jews who went around driving out evil spirits tried to invoke the name of the Lord Jesus over those who were demon-possessed. They would say, 'In the name of the Jesus whom Paul preaches, I command you to come out.' Seven sons of Sceva, a Jewish chief priest, were doing this. One day the evil spirit answered them, 'Jesus I know, and Paul I know about, but who are you?' Then the man who had the evil spirit jumped on them and overpowered them all. He gave them such a beating that they ran out of the house naked and bleeding."

The men who were religious and knew about Jesus tried to fight against demonic forces in their own strength. These men could cast out some lower-ranking spirits using the name of Jesus. However, when they came against high-ranking authority in the spirit realm, the devils overpowered them because they did not have the Holy Spirit working within them. Devils vary in their strength and authority, and being connected with God's power is the only way to overcome some high-ranking devils. Mark 9:29 teaches, "He replied to them, "This kind [of unclean spirit] cannot come out by anything but prayer [to the Father]."

The Holy Spirit rests on those who are one with Jesus Christ. To become one with Christ, a person must make a vow to Him and then remain true to the vow. As in a marriage, a vow to Christ requires commitment. It is not to be taken lightly. Jesus does not force anyone to walk with Him, but when someone vows to be His bride, then they shouldn't go back on their promise. Matthew 5:33 explains, "Again, you have heard that the ancients were told, 'You shall not make false vows, but shall fulfill your vows to the Lord.'"

When we tell the Lord we are going to be married to Him, we should be faithful to our word. Faithfulness shows God that we love Him and proves we mean what we have spoken. The new covenant that God established with people established Christ as the bridegroom and the Church as the bride. Like in any traditional marriage, Christ proposed to His bride by offering His life for her and vowing to provide her with all the things she will need. When a person says "yes" to Christ, he or she is accepting Jesus's invitation for marriage and pledging his or her life to Him. The heart's allegiance to marriage is important because love and allegiance are sometimes the only things keeping the couple together when life tries to separate them.

In betrothal ceremonies, the covenant is established when the two parties agree on the terms of the marriage. In traditional Jewish marriages, couples are betrothed or engaged to one another for a period, such as one or two years. Unlike modern American engagements, betrothal periods for Jewish couples involved the man, the groom, preparing a home for the future family, while the woman, the bride, would prepare herself to be a wife and a mother.

Scriptures tell us Jesus has gone to prepare a place for us, so we should likewise prepare to be His wife and a mother to our spiritual children. John 14:3 says, "And if I go and prepare a place for you, I will come back again and I will take you to Myself, so that where I am you may be also."

The Church is waiting for Christ's return so we can be with Him for eternity. As we wait, it is important to keep the oil of the Holy Spirit full. To be full, we must be hungry and thirsty and eat and drink from heaven. Jesus gave us the gift of the Holy Spirit as a betrothal gift. Similar to an engagement ring, a betrothal gift is a symbol of the relationship. As a woman sees her engagement ring, it is a reminder that she will be getting married soon. The gift of the Holy Spirit, likewise, is a reminder to us, as the Church, that Jesus will return, and He will take the faithful to the marriage supper of the lamb to begin our new life in eternity.

Then the kingdom of heaven will be like ten virgins, who took their lamps and went to meet the bridegroom. Five of them were foolish [thoughtless, silly, and careless], and five were wise [far-sighted, practical, and sensible]. For when the foolish took their lamps, they did not take any [extra] oil with them, but the wise took flasks of oil along with their lamps. Now while the bridegroom was delayed, they all began to nod off, and they fell asleep. But at midnight there was a shout, "Look! The bridegroom [is coming]! Go out to meet him."

Then all those virgins got up and put their own lamps in order [trimmed the wicks and added oil and lit them]. But the foolish virgins said to the wise, "Give us some of your oil, because our lamps are going out."

But the wise replied, "No, otherwise there will not be enough for us and for you, too; go instead to the dealers and buy oil for yourselves."

But while they were going away to buy oil, the bridegroom came, and those who were ready went in with him to the wedding feast; and the door was shut and locked. Later the others also came, and said, "Lord, Lord, open [the door] for us."

But He replied, "I assure you and most solemnly say to you, I do not know you [we have no relationship]."

Therefore, be on the alert [be prepared and ready], for you do not know the day nor the hour [when the Son of Man will come] (Matthew 25: 1–13).

People are unprepared for Christ's return if they are not continuously full of the Holy Spirit. True preparation for heaven requires the Holy Spirit. Believers must rely fully on God and have the ongoing indwelling of His Spirit to be prepared. Christians who have been called by God, and then choose to live carnal, careless, thoughtless, and silly lives, paying no attention to God or the Holy Ghost, will be unprepared for Christ when He returns to get His bride.

Five of the women in the parable of the ten virgins made a commitment to marry Jesus Christ. These women were once engaged, but they could not make it to the Marriage Supper of the Lamb. Five of the women in the parable will make it to the marriage supper because they were wise with what they had been given. These women wanted more oil in their lives. The desire for the oil for their lamps made the difference in these women's lives. Desire is a strong feeling of longing for something. When people desire something, they are hungry for it. John 6:35 tells us, "Jesus said to them, "I am the bread of life; he who comes to Me will not hunger, and he who believes in Me will never thirst."

We must regularly decide to continue to follow Jesus, and we need the Holy Spirit to remain faithful and patiently wait for Jesus' return. Some people begin following Jesus and cannot follow all the way through to the return of Christ. God gives us a grace to follow Him, and He helps us and strengthens us through His Spirit. Without the Spirit of God, we will stop following Jesus, and because of this, we must desire the Holy Spirit to be alive within us. John 6:65–66 tells us, "And He was saying, "This is the reason why I have told you that no one can come to Me unless it has been granted him [that is, unless he is enabled to do so] by the Father. As a result of this many of His disciples abandoned Him, and no longer walked with Him."

People who receive things from God are those who intentionally pursue righteousness and relationship proving their love. We must desire to know God and to do the things God asks us to do with our whole hearts. Just as we desire to eat and to drink, we must desire to live as people connected to our source and our substance in heaven. Matthew 5:6 says, "Blessed [joyful, nourished by God's goodness] are those who hunger and thirst for righteousness [those who actively seek right standing with God], for they will be [completely] satisfied."

Jesus is going to marry the people for eternity whose hearts are committed to Him. As in any marriage, it would be wrong to force a marriage with someone who doesn't desire the relationship. When someone isn't committed to the relationship, God allows them to make that decision, and He doesn't force the Holy Spirit upon them. Eternity is forever, and if someone cannot commit himself or herself for a short period of time within the engagement phase of the relationship, he or she is not eligible to spend eternity with Jesus in heaven.

James 4:3-4 says, "You ask and do not receive, because you ask wrongly, to spend it on your passions. You adulterous people, don't you know that friendship with the world means enmity against God? Therefore, anyone who chooses to be a friend of the world becomes an enemy of God."

Adultery is an extramarital affair. When people commit adultery, they fail to fulfill their vows with their spouse. They are not being true to what they have committed to. If infidelity happens during the engagement, there is a legitimate reason to call off the marriage. As we pledge our lives to Christ and wait for His return, we must remain true to Him alone. We must hate sin and evil and remain pure and holy, full of the Holy Spirit. We cannot love or lust for the world, because our main desire must be a desire for the Holy Spirit alone.

Jealousy is an emotion stemming from a feeling of loss. God is jealous when the world occupies the people He created to have a relationship with Him. Love for the world shows a lack of love and desire for Him, and it shows God they are not committed. When people love or tolerate the things of the world, they indicate to Jesus that He has lost their hearts. We can prove to God we are faithful to Him when we desire Him alone. When we are excited to talk to Him, we want to actively obey and learn His words. We can prove to Jesus that He has our hearts, and He is all that matters to us, or we can prove to Him that He doesn't and isn't our everything. First Corinthians 4:2 tells us, "Now it is required that those who have been given trust must prove faithful."

When God anoints people, He has shown them favor because of their actions stemming from their faithful heart. The religious leaders could not receive anything from God, His Spirit, or from Jesus, because they were proud and unbelieving people. They didn't love God or His word, even though they vowed to. The faithful Church fights to be around Jesus because they are hungry for the power of God. The faithful Church knows with absolute certainty that Jesus is their everything, and they prove it through both words and deeds.

In the Old Testament, many men and women of God would be anointed with oil so they could perform the works of God. The anointed oil permitted the Old Testament believers to move in power and operate in spiritual gifts. When David was anointed as the king of Israel, Samuel, a priest took a horn of oil and anointed him in front of his brothers. Samuel was able to anoint David because God gave him access and permission to pour out a blessing upon David. First Samuel 16:13 says, "Then Samuel took the horn of oil and anointed David in the presence of his brothers; and the Spirit of the Lord came mightily upon David from that day forward."

Today, with the new covenant, Jesus has been given access to pour out the blessing of the Holy Spirit upon the Church. Jesus is the high priest forever, and He pours out the oil for those who were eligible for the anointing of the Holy Ghost. It is not by might or human effort, symbolic oil, or religion that we are able to prosper. We are endowed with the Holy Spirit, which is the oil from heaven, as we accept Jesus as our Savior and keep the statues of the kingdom we have vowed to keep.

Philippians 2:12–13 teaches us, "So then, my dear ones, just as you have always obeyed [my instructions with enthusiasm], not only in my presence, but now much more in my absence, continue to work out your salvation [that is, cultivate it, bring it to full effect, actively pursue spiritual maturity] with awe-inspired fear and trembling [using serious caution and critical self-evaluation to avoid anything that might offend God or discredit the name of Christ]. For it is [not your strength, but it is] God who is effectively at work in you, both to will and to work [that is, strengthening, energizing, and creating in you the longing and the ability to fulfill your purpose] for His good pleasure."

Sacraments are religious signs and symbols that represent a spiritual reality. Sacraments illustrate a spiritual principle in the natural realm. When we anoint people with oil, we are illustrating a spiritual principle with our physical bodies. At the last supper, Jesus called His disciples together and had them eat bread and drink wine to symbolize His body and His Spirit. The last supper was sacramental because it represented the new covenant and the reality of the kingdom that was to be established through His sacrifice.

The Church should use oil as a symbolic representation to signify the work and the Holy Spirit as we pray for others or for ourselves, because scripture instructs us too. Yet the oil itself is not what holds the power of God and brings healing. The anointing oil is a symbol representing God's presence living within us. It represents what who we have joined to us. Let us prove to Jesus that we love Him through our hunger and our thirst for righteousness. Let us carry the pure oil and drink unpolluted water, so we can demonstrate to the world, the God we are one with, now and forever.

Luke 22:17–22 declares, "After taking the cup, he gave thanks and said, 'Take this and divide it among you. For I tell you I will not drink again from the fruit of the vine until the kingdom of God comes.' And he took bread, gave thanks and broke it, and gave it to them, saying, "This is my body given for you; do this in remembrance of me.' In the same way, after the supper he took the cup, saying, 'This cup is the new covenant in my blood, which is poured out for you. But the hand of him who is going to betray me is with mine on the table. The Son of Man will go as it has been decreed. But woe to that man who betrays him!'"

11

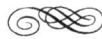

Development and Dedication

God made people out of the dust of the ground, and then He breathed His Spirit into them. Genesis 2:7 tells us, "And the Lord God formed man of the dust of the ground and breathed into His nostrils the breath of life; and man became a living soul." God designed us to live life joined to Him in our spirits. He intended for us to partake in the spirit realm as His heirs. People have been spirit beings from creation, because God is our Creator and He is a spirit.

Babies are human from the time they are conceived. When a sperm meets an egg, life is established. Development begins as soon as the sperm and egg combine. Life begins at conception and the development of the created life continues throughout the individual's life. Many assert development is the process of growth between birth and death, but biblically and scientifically we know this is false. Birth is not the beginning of human development, conception is.

As men and women reproduce, they have been permitted to create life and cultivate life. In the Garden of Eden, Adam and Eve were commanded to protect and care for the garden and every living thing within it. They were given the job of stewardship. Genesis 2:15 says, "So the Lord God took the man [He had made] and settled him in the Garden of Eden to cultivate and keep it."

Cultivation is the promotion or improvement within the growth of a plant or a crop by labor and attention. Adam and Eve were to cultivate the proper growth and development of all life forms, as they were assigned to be stewards over the earth. Genesis 2:19 says, "Now the Lord God had formed out of the ground all the wild animals and all the birds in the sky. He brought them to the man to see what he would name them; and whatever the man called each living creature, that was its name."

Cultivation enables life to progress from one stage of development to another. As we cultivate gardens, we must prepare the soil, plant the seed, and then grow the seed to maturity if we are going to reap the fruit. There is a process of involving yourself and ensuring the garden is healthy and thriving and receiving everything it needs to continue to grow.

Parents are responsible to cultivate, and properly manage, the lives of their children. We are mandated by God to help them to develop by involving ourselves in their lives and watching for the things they need to grow from one stage to the next.

Without accepting Christ and being filled with inner dwelling of the Holy Spirit, people are carnal beings. To be carnal is to be controlled by the flesh, the body, or physical components. Animals do not act reasonably, and they do not behave in ways that are morally or socially acceptable because they are ignorant of proper thinking and behaving. Animals act on primality, not intentionality. Humans who live life apart from their Creator will live a subpar and animalistic life. They will never experience life as God's superior creation, as men and women created in the image of God.

Evolutionary theory is a primal theory because it asserts that people are nothing more than animals. All evolutionary theories, whether they attempt to study the psychological, sociological, physiological, or other areas, study human beings solely from the primal worldview. Apart from Christ and the teachings of the Bible, people study humanity from this animalistic perspective because they do not view humanity as superior to other life forms.

However, creationists know there is more to the human being than primal instinct alone. Creationists study everything within the world from the framework of the Bible. All science, when it is studied from a creationist perspective, confirms the authenticity of Scripture. God asserted in His word that men and women are not created to live animalistic, carnal lives. Instead He commanded us to do the opposite—to live with intention and walk in authority, cultivating all of other life forms living on earth. Humans were created to rule over the other animals. Humans hold more authority, more understanding, and more power because God gave them a unique place within the world.

Satan disgraces people by luring them to behave animalistically. He wants humanity to be removed from the position God gave them. Satan works to humiliate and degrade God's most powerful creation by deceiving them to act in ways that are beneath them. When Satan has an opportunity to take over a life, people are violated and weaker than they are created to be, and thus, they do things they were never created to take part in.

Drug addicts who are in the later stages of addiction may talk to themselves, eat out trash cans, or lose their teeth. These same humiliating characteristics can be identified within any people who continuously yield themselves to Satan. Women who are prostitutes or strippers are humiliated and degraded publicly in front of others, and a glutton is consistently humiliated for his or her failure to exert self-control.

Once sin takes root in the life of a man or a woman there are noticeable disgusting and humiliating consequences that become visible to others. Satan lures humans to sin, and he creates a mockery of them for their sin. He publicly broadcasts humans' weakness relating to sin through embarrassment and dishonor.

God will take a man or a woman who was once humiliated and disgraceful, and He will honor him or her. God's Spirit living and operating within a man or a woman brings noticeable admiration and respect. God gives us power over sin, and He gives us self-control. Self-control is a discipline of the Holy Spirit, allowing us to defend ourselves from Satan. As we operate in self-control, we keep Satan from being able to harm us or humiliate us, and we refuse to be animalistic and carnal only, because we know that is beneath us. Proverbs 25:28 tells us, "A man without self-control is like a city broken into and left without walls."

Degradation and honor are both noticeable to others after a season or a period of sowing and reaping. Sin takes time to grow and develop as a seed takes time to grow and develop. The first drug, or the first drink a person consumes, does not generally cause him or her to become a disgrace. Women do not become porn stars overnight. Satan lures people deeper into sin through telling them they are not experiencing anything negative, even though God said they would. Satan causes people to slowly become comfortable in sin as he eases them to believe there is no danger in sin. This allows for a gradual but consistent sowing and reaping of evil in the lives of those who are undiscerning and unaware of seedtime and harvest.

Relating to holiness and honor Satan flips the script, and he tries to cause us to become impatient in our sowing and our reaping. As we sow righteousness and goodness, Satan wants to get us to believe we are sowing, and it isn't working. When we plant godly seeds, the devil wants us to be in a hurry, not patient and slow. He works to limit our growth in any way he can, attempting to restrict the blessings of God so we will not continue to plant good spiritual seeds but will give up and quit.

All seeds, whether good or evil, will grow after being sown, because God's word tells us so. We cannot see a child's developmental changes if we observe them minute-by-minute. Even if we watched our children every hour of the day, we would not immediately see them grow an inch or gain a pound. Our children grow and change little by little, progressing to the next stage of development. We know our children are growing because we observe the growth, but the exact measure of growth only becomes noticeable over time through larger increments, and we cannot measure it through a second-by-second analysis.

When we grow plants, we can do extra things to cultivate and speed the growth of our seeds. Our decisions to provide meticulous care for the seeds we plant aids the growing process. We water the plants and provide extra food and set them in conditions with the right light and humidity to help them flourish.

Likewise, we can involve ourselves in our children's lives to help them grow well and flourish. If we sow into our children seeds of righteousness and goodness, then we can expect to see the growth of what has been sown. Consistent sowing of righteousness and truth will produce a harvest of righteousness and truth within our children. The more we sow into their spirits, and we aid in their cultivation, the quicker we will see their spiritual growth come to fruition, producing an outward harvest.

Often, when parents experience a behavioral problem with their children, it has developed gradually through impure seeds. If a seed starts to take root in a child's life and it is not corrected immediately, then it will become larger and harder to deal with later down the road. Weeds are undesirable plants that grow and try to harm other thriving plants. If left unattended, weeds will choke out the plants' growth and production. Whenever we notice weeds growing in our lives or our children's lives, we must immediately rip them out and destroy the root. A failure to address the problem will cause the weed to grow in strength and magnitude.

At around 18 months, babies begin to learn to exert dominance and influence their environment through their interaction with others. Many young toddlers begin to throw temper tantrums if they do not get their way. Temper tantrums during the early stages of child development are normal. Babies are accustomed to being pampered. In their former stage of development, they needed to be given everything they requested because they were developing at a lower level, and this change in routine causes some emotional disturbance.

When children reach the age of 18 months and enter a new stage of development, they must learn through proper parental cultivation that they are members of a larger group. If parents do not correct bad behavior in their 18-24-month-old child and continue to treat the toddler as a baby who needs to get everything they want, then they are sowing seeds they will reap during the years many parents call the terrible twos. Child cultivation requires parents to interact with their children through teaching the children to properly relate to the world at the exact time they need it. Neglecting to respond when the child needs to be cultivated will lead to insufficient growth.

It would be inappropriate for a parent to teach a newborn baby behavioral management technique. Newborn babies are not yet at the stage of development to understand or respond to this type of teaching. Windows of cultivation opportunities are presented to parents, and we must evaluate our child's growth to determine what the child needs to advance to the next level. Parents must see and properly respond to the child's needs to reap the benefits of a healthy, thriving child.

My son, who is 17 months old, recently started climbing onto the kitchen table. This behavior is unsafe and improper. On one occasion, he had a ginormous temper tantrum after I removed him from the table. He screamed for about five minutes, and he then tried to do it again. I consistently took him off the table and kept him from going back into the kitchen for a few minutes, because he needs to learn this behavior is not allowed. Through repetition and reinforcement, he eventually learned mommy would not allow him on the table.

However, if I gave into his behavior and let him continue to climb on the table simply because he screamed and wanted on the table, then I would teach or reinforce to him that temper tantrums work and are beneficial to him! He would implicitly learn to do whatever he feels like doing- an evolutionary concept. Permitting behaviors to develop and become ingrained leads to significant challenges during the latter years of a child's life. If left unaddressed, these issues will persist and escalate further into childhood. Parents must diligently address the child's needs at a developmental level or they will face consequences down the road. We must perceive that correction brings forth health and wellbeing in our kids. We correct because we know we are driving out weeds and bad behaviors from our children.

Proverbs 22:15 explains, "Foolishness is bound up in the heart of a child; the rod of discipline [correction administered with godly wisdom and lovingkindness] will remove it far from him." Children are born with a sin nature. From the time they are young, they need to be taught spiritual truths so they can become spiritually wise and discerning. The earlier a child is born again, the better the child's life will be. Very early in a child's life, we can plant seeds of God's truth and God's kingdom laws. Our sole intention should be to train our children in the way to go, so they will never separate themselves from God or His kingdom.

Jesus was conceived through the Holy Spirit. With a spiritual father as opposed to a human father, Jesus was not from the lineage of Adam. Thus, Jesus was not imparted with the sin nature of man. Jesus received the Spirit of His heavenly Father from within the womb of Mary, and He became the first of a creation never created before. First Corinthians 15:45 tells us, "So it is written [in Scripture], 'The first man, Adam, became a living soul (an individual);' the last Adam (Christ) became a life-giving spirit [restoring dead to life]."

Jesus was first a baby and then He was a boy. Jesus was truly incarnate, experiencing both worlds—the Spirit and the flesh. He knew what it was like to be human, and Jesus operated in self-control while He grew spiritually and physically as a man. All people grow physically and spiritually, but physical maturity happens naturally, and spiritual maturity must be developed. Spiritual growth is a deliberate process that requires the guidance of the Holy Spirit. While instilling self-control in our children is of utmost importance, it is crucial to ensure that they receive the Holy Spirit, because only the baptism of the Holy Spirit will enable them to take their rightful stand against sin and the devil. Luke 2:52 explains, "And Jesus grew in wisdom and stature, and in favor with God and man."

As parents, we can dedicate our children to the Lord. As we use our own faith, acting and responding to their ever-changing needs, we can have confidence that the Lord will protect our children and guide them into all truth as they age and progress into the next stage of development, if we have sown good seeds into their lives. A decision to dedicate a child to God is a decision to involve ourselves as a parent, as a guide and a teacher, instructing, correcting, and driving out all improper behavior and thought. We cultivate, watch, and encourage development in the lives of the beings God has entrusted within our care. Second Timothy 3:15 says, "And how from childhood you have been acquainted with the sacred writings, which are able to make you wise for salvation through faith in Christ Jesus."

Each person is given the opportunity to become a new creature in Christ and to die to the old self. This regeneration process allows us all to be adopted into God's family, regardless of the situations and problems in our family of origin. Children who are raised in homes separated from God are not without hope, because Jesus loves them and wants them to learn the truth. God has a purpose for every life. He will deliver and restore the life of the child when the child wants to discover the truth, even if their parents refuse to teach him or her. Ezekiel 18:20 teaches, "The person who sins [is the one that] will die. The son will not bear the punishment for the sin of the father, nor will the father bear the punishment for the sin of the son; the righteousness of the righteous shall be on himself, and the wickedness of the wicked shall be on himself."

However, parents who fail to instill the principles of faith in their children from an early age hinder their development. Children who are not raised with an understanding of spiritual truths will face a more extensive healing process, as they must rewire their cognitive frameworks and acquire fundamentally new ways of engaging with others and the world around them. We need to take every possible measure to ensure that children are raised and nurtured in righteousness, enabling them to maintain their health and well-being throughout their lives.

The advancing stages of life development inside the womb are a miracle and should be protected throughout every stage. In the womb at four weeks old, babies are smaller than a poppy seed. Size does not determine human life, and babies are as alive and human at four weeks as they are at 10 weeks. The development may be more physically observed, but the creation was alive all along.

In vitro fertilization (IVF) has become popular in recent years, and many parents feel they should use fertility treatments if they have had problems conceiving naturally. In vitro fertilization is also known as assisted reproductive technology, and it refers to artificially fertilizing ovaries with sperm. Medical professionals remove a woman's eggs through a surgical procedure, and they collect the semen from the man. They combine the semen with the eggs in a lab to create an embryo. After numerous embryos are created, they are either placed inside the woman, frozen, or discarded.

Prolife Christians must assert that in vitro fertilization is not acceptable, if we truly believe life begins at conception. Scientists and medical professionals are manipulating life and then disposing of what they deem it to be less qualified or viable life forms. IVF allows humans to assert value to specific human life based on their personal analysis of worthiness. Although babies may be created and born from successful IVF treatment, many babies are left to die and are abandoned once created in a lab.

From a secular worldview, people may argue that these human lives are not truly viable without the mother, but from a biblical perspective, we must understand that life begins at conception without exception. We must resist IVF and artificial creation of life because we know babies are being created and then disposed of at the medical provider's sole discretion. All embryos created within IVF treatment who are frozen and never allowed to live are humans created and disposed of as if they were never alive, even when we know they were.

In vitro fertilization is a failure of proper stewardship. As we received authority and power on the earth, we were entrusted to cultivate life, especially human life. If God wanted us to care for plants and animals in a responsible manner, how much more would He expect us to care for the lives of human beings.

Babies should never become science experiments. They should never be created and discarded as if they were invaluable, even if we have medical advancement and the understanding to provide the service.

IVF is one way Satan humiliates women. He degrades women by causing them to suffer with their fertility, and then he insinuates that God is making them wait on their harvest. Satan tries to slow down the growth of God's blessings. If God wants a woman to have a baby and to be fruitful, Satan will try to keep the woman from receiving her miracle by hijacking her faith and reducing her fertility. Satan insists that God is too slow, or that God's plans and words of fruitfulness don't exist. This lie causes women to take matters into their own hands to create and dispose of their children's lives. How embarrassing, and how disgraceful, to not be able to conceive and to need interventions, and child sacrifice to "produce" life.

Hebrews 11:11 tells us, "And by faith even Sarah, who was past childbearing age, was enabled to bear children because she considered Him faithful who had made the promise." God opens a woman's womb. When a woman has not yet conceived, she can ask God for a baby, and then she can stand on His word in faith, expecting to get her miracle. Sarah was living in a stage of life far beyond childbearing years, but God supplied her with her baby, even when it took a long time for her to conceive.

God has appointed a special time for babies to be born. God gave many babies in scripture a purpose before their parents knew who they were. God knows who babies are and who He wants them to be, even before babies are named by their parents. Isaiah 49:5 says, "And now says the Lord, who formed Me from the womb to be His Servant, to bring Jacob back to Him, so that Israel might be gathered to Him (For I am honored in the sight of the Lord, and My God is My strength)."

God has a unique purpose for every life. As scientists remove ovaries or pick and choose who is to be born through procedures like IVF, they are altering who lives on the earth. They are determining who is created and who is disposed of, and they are practicing a great evil. God knows each baby created and killed through IVF. He knows their names and their purpose. Isaiah 43:1 tells us, "But now [in spite of past judgments for Israel's sins], thus says the Lord, He Who created you, O Jacob, and He Who formed you, O Israel: 'Fear not, for I have redeemed you [ransomed you by paying a price instead of leaving you captives]; I have called you by your name; you are Mine.'"

Carnal people rely on evolutionary perspectives, and theories are elementary in their thinking. They live below the standard for success, because they are intellectually incapacitated. They do not have the proper understanding within their minds or their spirits to operate at the level they should be operating at. Galatians 4:3 says, "So also we [whether Jews or Gentiles], when we were children (spiritually immature), were kept like slaves under the elementary [manmade religious or philosophical] teachings of the world."

To have an advanced understanding of the world in which we live, we must receive kingdom revelation and kingdom knowledge. In the kingdom, newly converted believers need guidance and support from older believers, because they are babies. Over time, people will be able to eat solid food and will progress in their development, but in the beginning, people must start with milk. First Corinthians 3:2 explains, "I gave you milk to drink, not solid food; for you were not able to receive it. Indeed, even now you are not yet able."

Babies begin their lives through drinking milk. Guidelines recommend exclusively breastfeeding for a baby's first six months. Breastmilk will continue to be a part of the baby's diet beyond the six-month period, but babies are gradually introduced to eating solid foods. Believers who never progress from milk to other teachings are delayed in proper spiritual development. Hebrews 5:13 teaches, "For everyone who drinks only of milk is not accustomed to the word of righteousness, for he is an infant."

Believers grow in spiritual truth. There is a period of development from the conversion of a new believer transitioning into healthy adulthood. Over time, people become capable of digesting much deeper principles and truths of God if they are properly cultivated and nourished as they are developing. However, when believers fail to receive the proper cultivation, they will struggle and fall behind when they should be thriving.

When babies are born, they are vulnerable and rely on other people to take care of them. They trust their caregivers because they wouldn't survive without help. New believers need older believers to train them in righteousness and truth.

It would be very abnormal if babies never stopped nursing and drinking breastmilk. Breastfeeding is a beautiful part of a baby's life, but eventually that season closes and a new season begins. Knowing when a child is ready to move to the next level requires us to use attentive observation. Abraham knew moving from milk to meat was a blessing, and we are told he celebrated his son's progression when he perceived he was ready to move on. Genesis 21:8 explains, "And the child grew and was weaned: and Abraham made a great feast the same day that Isaac was weaned."

The Church has been warned to beware of false teachers who forbid the eating of all foods. Spiritual food and spiritual meat or substance should be celebrated. When a child has developed and is ready for spiritual meat, we should celebrate with him or her. Some ministers within the church seek to stop the child or believer from going to the next stage of development with God and intend to keep the person underdeveloped, living in the elementary teachings of the law. First Timothy 4:3 says, "Who forbid marriage and advocate abstaining from [certain kinds of] foods which God has created to be gratefully shared by those who believe and have [a clear] knowledge of truth."

Children who are introduced to God early can go through the process of accepting Jesus Christ and becoming a member of the Church much earlier than those who never are exposed to the gospel. As children are developing they must start by learning the elementary teachings of God. They are exposed to the Bible, and they learn to digest the food. Then they will grow up in their behavior and in their knowledge. Over time, they will be weaned from elementary teachings and will continue to progress in the faith. The age of accountability should be celebrated with feasting.

Isaiah 62:5 says, "For as a young man marries a young woman, so shall your sons marry you, and as the bridegroom rejoices over the bride, so shall your God rejoice over you."

When we accept Jesus, we become the bride of Christ. God intends for the engagement period with Christ to begin when people are still young. Ideally, children will grow up with parents who teach them the religious customs. Children will learn about the scriptures and begin to understand them. Then, in time, they will be of age and can accept the bridegroom's invitation to marriage. This acceptance of the bridegroom's invitation enables the child to progress from elementary teachings of milk and law and move on to the teachings of meat and grace. It is possible for very young children to learn deeper truths and to operate in ministry gifts, as David and Samuel did, if they are properly cultivated.

Some parents do not want children to grow up. They try to keep their children at a former stage of development. There is a parental process of letting go. The parents must instruct the child but also allow the child to establish an identity as he or she becomes his or her own person.

God wants us to do our part as parents and instruct children, but as they get older, they need to learn to talk to God, hear from God, and receive from God with their own faith. If we always use our faith to safeguard them, even when they are old enough to begin to do this for themselves, then we are enabling them to stay weaker than they are supposed to be.

In the time of adversity, only the soldier who has been properly trained can win the fight. It is humbling to acknowledge that we cannot win our fight, because of our own lack of training in the word, but we must be willing to take responsibility if we are not prepared to win our battles. The only way to become equipped is through personal training and responsibility. The older children get, the more responsibility they should receive in their upbringing. This is the way we prepare them to win in the fights of life.

Ten-year-old children should be able to get dressed and clean their room without their parents, because they are developmentally capable, where a one-year-old child is not. In all things regarding our children's psychological, spiritual, physical or interpersonal health, children need to learn to take responsibility for themselves. Learning to take care of our teeth or bodies and learning to pick up after ourselves if we make a mess are very important components of successful adulthood. Children who never learn to take responsibility because their parents do everything for them will suffer in their development.

In faith, we can believe God has a plan for our children to develop as people progressing from one stage to another. By allowing our children to grow apart from us, we allow our children to begin to long for more than just milk. We must allow for them to grow up and become strong, healthy, independent people who need God—but not humans—for their health and survival.

Within the Church, some leaders refuse to teach congregants the elements of faith and personal responsibility because they are afraid the congregants will grow up and separate themselves from the family unit. But true godliness acknowledges that we are to train and teach, and then we are to let go and love from a healthy distance, when the time is right. Healthy children will become leaders modeling after those who led them.

When I first became a mother, I tried to be a perfect mother by doing everything for my kids. I thought I could make my children successful by doing the work for them. I intended to make my children's lives void of problems. I assumed that by focusing on their happiness I would raise strong, healthy children. Yet, this parenting style is in direct opposition to God's word and plan for children, because children must be cultivated, and they must learn personal responsibility.

Holding on to a child who is ready to move forward will ultimately cause the child to not properly develop without the parent's interference. These children will remain dependent instead of developing independence, because their growth has been stunted. Many people grow up learning this dysfunctional parent/child interaction, and they reproduce it in their own parenting. Others are unhealthy because they have not healed from trauma or personal wounds, such as divorce, and they cling to the child for personal affirmation and thus, refuse to properly separate and parent from a distance.

Believing that as mothers we are to do everything for our children is not the correct way to honor God in our parenting. We cannot keep kids too close and think they will develop properly. Children who are overparented are hindered in their decision-making abilities and fall behind psychologically and emotionally. When these children reach physical maturity, they are mentally and spiritually handicap and are prevented from growing in statue and favor with God and humans. Some adults continue to let their parents dictate their choices, even when they are grown. The healthy differentiation never occurred, and the child—who may be 50 years old—still allows his or her mom or dad to dictate his or her life because he or she never learned how to make decisions apart from parents.

Jacob's mother kept him too close. He didn't separate properly and leave his family's tent. Jacob's mother babied him and tried to make his life easy because she loved him. Jacob's brother and twin, Esau, moved onto meat while Jacob lingered behind. Genesis 25:27 teaches, "When the boys grew up, Esau was an able and skilled hunter, a man of the outdoors, but Jacob was a quiet and peaceful man, living in tents. Now Isaac loved [and favored] Esau, because he enjoyed eating his game, but Rebekah loved [and favored] Jacob."

Rebekah still controlled what Jacob did when Jacob should have been making his own decisions. Rebekah dictated all of Jacob's actions when he should have already progressed past this stage of parenting. When a child is very young, a mother is to lead a child, but at a point in every person's life, he or she must leave the tent and become separated from their mother and father, making his or her own decisions. Genesis 27:8–9 explains, *"So now, my son, [listen carefully] to me [and do exactly as I command you].* Go now to the flock and bring me two good and suitable young goats from there, that I may prepare as a savory dish for your father, such as he loves."

Esau was not pampered by his mother and he was not her favorite. This allowed him to separate from his tent and develop more quickly because he learned to survive outdoors without an overbearing mother. Esau enjoyed eating wild game when his twin was still interested in vegetable soups. Rebekah knew God's promise for Jacob that had been prophesied before his birth, and this knowledge caused her to favor her youngest son. But she harmed him because she did not allow him to separate from her.

Jacob was kept too close, and Esau was not kept close enough. Esau should have never been able to eat wild game' he should have been kept from straying too far from the tent when he was not prepared to enter the world. Rebekah could have asked God to bless both of her children. She could have asked Him to help her to raise two children who served the Lord, and God would have honored her request.

Rahab was a woman who was destined for destruction. The Lord had spoken He was going to destroy everyone in her town. But Rahab wanted to live, and she made choices that influenced her and her family's future. God approved of Rahab's faith because she believed God would help her if she simply believed and requested to live. Thus, we can conclude that the Lord would have honored a request to bless both of Rebekah's sons, just as He did for Rahab in the book of Joshua.

God also answered Abraham's prayer to bless both of his children Issac and Ishmael even when the circumstances were unfavorable. Intercession on behalf of our children is of paramount importance. While God designated Jacob as the blessed son, this does not imply that Esau would have been disqualified had his heart been appropriately nurtured by his mother. God did not say Esau was doomed in the womb. He said the boys would form two nations.

Genesis 25:21–24 tells us, "Isaac prayed to the Lord for his wife, because she was unable to conceive children; and the Lord granted his prayer and Rebekah his wife conceived [twins]. But the children struggled together within her [kicking and shoving one another]; and she said, 'If it is so [that the Lord has heard our prayer], why then am I this way?' So she went to inquire of the Lord [praying for an answer]. The Lord said to her,'[The founders of] two nations are in your womb; And the separation of two nations has begun in your body; The one people shall be stronger than the other; And the older shall serve the younger.'"

Esau reverted to a formal stage of development. Esau experienced a regression, and he traded his spiritual birthright for a bowl of vegetable soup because he was too enamored with the things of the world. Esau became complacent, no longer desiring meat. Instead, he began to long for the things he had already progressed away from. Hebrews 5:12 explains, "For though by this time you ought to be teachers, you need someone to teach you again the basic principles of the oracles of God. Yet, you still need milk not solid food."

When children are placed into ungodly situations and exposed to things too early, it harms them. Introducing children to something they are not ready to receive information about can lead them towards destruction. Esau was placed into the world prematurely. He was not properly shielded, loved, and protected by his mother.

In recent years, many educators have fought to teach elementary school children about sexual education. Yet, we know young children should not be taught about gender and sex and deeper revelation, because they are not prepared to hear that lesson. If young children learn advanced information when they are not ready, it damages their health.

Children who have been weaned from milk should not want to go back to drinking milk. If a baby has been weaned from milk, he or she is to remain eating meat. If a five year old refused to eat solid food and only wanted breastmilk after eating solids, it would be a serious regression.

Regressions occur when there is a traumatic event or a Satanic interference. Satan often causes developmental regressions in children by introducing them to things they are not ready for. The children naturally shrink back in fear because they are intimidated by the information. Regression is known to follow trauma, and all trauma is the work of Satan. Regression is a sign of distress. It is a sign that the child needs help understanding something he or she been exposed to but is not yet ready to learn about. A child who is abruptly exposed to sin through a divorce, to pornography, or to violent crime, drugs, or sexual abuse will exhibit signs of regression.

Some common childhood symptoms of regression are bed-wetting, temper tantrums, or thumb sucking. Many times, when professionals see a child who is acting irrationally or out of control, they see a child who has been given too much information and personal control of his or her life when he or she is not yet prepared to handle it.

God designed people to move forward. He designed people to grow instead of remaining in a former stage of development. Parents must foster their children's growth, so children can separate and become the strong people God intends for them to become. We limit our children's exposure to things they are not ready for, and we bring in new concepts they are prepared to receive. Isaiah 28:9 says, "They say 'To whom would He teach knowledge? And to whom would He explain the message? Those just weaned from milk? Those just taken from the breast?'"

Jacob longed for the spiritual blessing, even though he had never tasted the meat of the blessing. Jacob was hungry, and he saw his brother was not. Jacob purchased the birthright legally from Esau, and although Jacob was emotionally delayed because of his mother's parenting, he was spiritually wise, because he desired the blessings of God. Genesis 25:33 tells us, "Jacob said, 'Swear [an oath] to me today [that you are selling it to me for this food]'; so, he swore [an oath] to him, and sold him his birthright."

Jacob did not need to lie to or trick his father, because his brother had legally traded his birthright and his blessing. Jacob was not stealing. He had received the birthright, because he longed for it and his brother willingly traded him for it. Jacob could have chosen to be confident. He could have stood up to his mother's plot of deception, because he was old enough to do so, but his emotional weakness and underdevelopment allowed him to be controlled by his mom. He did what his mom said instead of making his own righteous decision, and the failure to confront his mom caused him to deceive his father unnecessary.

Jacob was naive and vulnerable. After being separated from his mother, he remained emotionally handicap for quite a while. Rebekah's led Jacob to not being able to stand on his own feet when he went into the world, because he never learned how to stand on his own two feet at home. This eventually led Jacob to be tricked by other people outside of his household. Jacob was still being controlled, manipulated, and dictated to by people in his life, even when he was a father. His mother's failure to prepare him for independence and success apart from her led to Jacob struggling socially for quite some time, even with the blessing pronounced over his life.

Genesis 30:25–30 tells us, "Now when Rachel had given birth to Joseph, Jacob said to Laban, 'Send me away, that I may go back to my own place and to my own country. Give me my wives and my children for whom I have served you, and let me go; for you know the work which I have done for you.' But Laban said to him, 'If I have found favor in your sight, stay with me; for I have learned [from the omens in divination and by experience] that the Lord has blessed me because of you.' He said, 'Name your wages, and I will give it [to you].' Jacob answered him, 'You know how I have served you and how your possessions, your cattle and sheep and goats, have fared with me. For you had little before I came and it has increased and multiplied abundantly, and the Lord has favored you with blessings wherever I turned. But now, when shall I provide for my own household?'"

Codependency is an unhealthy relationship pattern that causes people to stop growing emotionally because they aren't challenged or expected to carry their own load. Codependent relationships lack very important components that exist in healthy relationships, because one of the two parties exerts the effort, love, and contribution to the relationship, trying to force a specific outcome to occur. Within a codependent relationship, one person picks up the other person's responsibilities, obligations, consequence, efforts, and decisions, to "help" the other individual become successful. Yet, over time, this becomes crippling, because one individual does all the heavy lifting, and the other fails to do anything for himself or herself.

Rebekah wanted to help Jacob. She believed by keeping him close to her, pampering him, and telling him what to do, he would become who God wanted him to become. She made life easy for Jacob, and she did too much for him. Jacob didn't learn how to make good decisions. He relied on his mother, even as an older boy, and he was stuck emotionally at a much younger child's developmental level. Until Jacob separated from his mom, he could not properly grow. Genesis 29:10 say, "Now Jacob left Beersheba [never to see his mother again] and traveled toward Haran."

Jacob experienced another personal development and growth situation when he finally parted ways with his uncle Laban. Until he was able to separate and take his wives and his children away from Laban he was not able to tap into his full potential. Both parties within codependent relationships need to be healed because codependency causes dysfunction within families for everyone who is involved in the relationship.

Consider what happens when a person stops walking or using their muscles for a time. In the medical world, this phenomenon is called disuse atrophy. Disuse atrophy occurs when a muscle is not as active as it should be. Often muscle atrophy comes from a season of immobility, such as because of a broken arm or leg. When the limb is not used, it progressively becomes weaker. This type of atrophy can be prevented by muscle movement. People with muscle atrophy must exert effort, energy, and force, even when they experience discomfort, in the hope that they will not lose the function of their limb.

For codependent relationship patterns to be broken, a person must face his or her own consequences of poor behavior. The person must do his or her part, without relying on someone else. People must learn to confront others and face their problems, even if it is challenging or if it hurts to become healthy.

It would be unjust of the health professionals involved in a disuse atrophy case to continue to pamper and stop movement of the limb, even if it stopped the pain of the patient. The only cure for people in this situation is effort, exercise, and movement. The more the person does for himself or herself, the better the long-term outcome. As we teach our children to do things for themselves, we strengthen them and prepare them to succeed with or without us.

Muscles, as well as people's abilities, can be rebuilt. Healing is possible, as we saw in Jacob's life. Yet prevention is best. If we can prevent our children from developing emotional or spiritual atrophy, that is ideal. The mom who does everything for her kids will cripple them. The mom who doesn't teach her kids lessons through trial and error, pain, and suffering will stop her child from feeling the weight of his or her behaviors. The mom who tries to help a child experience utopia ultimately prevents the child from the opportunity to learn from mistakes.

The codependent mom carries far too much. Her codependency effects her as much as it effects her child. She will feel overwhelmed, anxious, and worn down from all the extra weight she is carrying in her life. God does want us to carry each other's burdens, but He does not want us to carry things for those who can carry them for themselves. God can help with codependency. If you ask Him for help, then He will show you parent in an appropriate and healthy manner. There is no situation too far gone that God can't do something about it.

God restores children's lives even when mothers fail to fully prepare their children for the world. As mothers, this is encouraging, because even when we fail, if we are doing our best and partnering with God, God never fails. Rebekah failed to prepare her child emotionally, and she contributed to his developmental failure, but God's word still came to pass in Jacob's life. When we love the Lord, and we operate in faith and love, God will fill in the gaps for us.

Second Corinthians 12:9–10 teaches, "but He has said to me, 'My grace is sufficient for you [My loving kindness and My mercy are more than enough- always available-regardless of the situation]; for [My] power is being perfected [and is completed and shows itself most effectively] in [your] weakness.' Therefore, I will all the more gladly boast in my weaknesses, so that the power of Christ [may completely enfold me and] may dwell in me. So, I am well pleased with weakness, with insults, with distresses, with persecutions, and with difficulties, for the sake of Christ; for when I am weak [in human strength], then I am strong [truly able, truly powerful, truly drawing from God's strength]."

Jacob was tricked, manipulated, and dominated for many years of his life. His control came from his mother at first, and then he was controlled by his fear of his brother and then eventually by his father-in-law. Jacob's failure to stand up to his mother, brother, and his father at home led to him being dominated again by other family members. If we don't face our challenges, they will never go away. They will come back with different people and have different relationships, because the problem is with us.

Jacob lied when he should have confronted his dad with the truth. Jacob ran instead of facing his brother. Jacob deceived instead of telling his mom no. God had already promised Jacob the blessing and the birthright before he was ever born. He had a legal right to it, because Esau sold it to him. Jacob never needed to lie; he simply needed to be honest with his mother, his brother, and his father. He needed to stand up to the people in his household and walk in his blessing.

Many church members are afraid of what others think of them. If we are successful because of our blessing, unhealthy people often try to stifle our growth. But we cannot allow anyone to intimidate us or control us if we are going to walk in our blessing. We must love our church family, but we must be confident to declare the truth when God is with us. Someone else's emotional dysfunction can only become our problem if we allow it.

Until Jacob took emotional responsibility for his life, chaos reigned. But as soon as he stood in his blessing and in his authority proudly, he was delivered from the bondage he had been living in.

Genesis 30:32–24 says, "Let me pass through your entire flock today, removing from it every speckled and spotted sheep and every dark or black one among the lambs and the spotted and speckled among the goats; and those shall be my wages. So my honesty will be evident for me later, when you come [for an accounting] concerning my wages. Every one that is not speckled and spotted among the goats and dark among the young lambs, if found with me, shall be considered stolen." And Laban said, "Good! Let it be done as you say.

God gave Jacob an opportunity to prove he had matured. He gave Jacob an opportunity to be honest, and that was when everything began to turn around. Jacob learned to rely on God alone. He learned to not be controlled by people in his life. God was never absent from Jacob when he was learning the emotional lessons he should have learned as a child. And God took a bad situation of an emotionally crippled boy and turned it around for His glory when Jacob finally decided he wanted to be free.

People can influence our decisions during certain seasons of our lives. We should have voices that we trust around us to help us to make good decisions, especially when we are young in the faith. God allows us as parents to influence young children because they need our influence to learn and become who they are destined to be. By living a pure Christian life, we influence and consecrate our children to the Lord. We commit to showing them the truth and shaping their perspective of God and others while they are still learning in their childhood.

Consecration is the act of declaring something holy. As mothers we can consecrate that our children are to be holy by ensuring we cultivate them. We teach, model, and influence their choices. We also correct and discipline when we find there is error. By pulling the weeds out of their garden, we help them develop properly, unhindered by demonic forces. We set them up to thrive beyond our time of cultivation, and we prepare them to go to the next level in their walk of faith with God.

Samuel's mom, Hannah, dedicated Samuel to the Lord, before she conceived him. She realized if she was going to have a child, he needed to come from God and be given back to God. She asked God for a son, and then she let her son go when the time was right. She dedicated her son to the Lord's purposes, even when it was hard for her to let him grow up and go into the call on his life for ministry. First Samuel 27–28 says, "For this child I prayed, and the Lord has granted me my request which I asked of Him. Therefore, I have also dedicated him to the Lord; as long as he lives he is dedicated to the Lord." And they worshiped the Lord there."

As mothers, we know God will call our dedicated children to Him when it is time. God was faithful to Hannah's prayers and the dedication of her son to Him. God called Samuel, and He used him to do many amazing things. Samuel was not old when he began to hear and talk to God personally. He was able to do that early because of the strong foundation his mother put in place. First Samuel 3:8 teaches, "So the Lord called Samuel again for the third time. And he arose and went to Eli and said, 'Here I am, for you have called me.' Then Eli discerned that the Lord was calling the boy."

Dedication services permit pastors and elders pray for children and anoint them with oil. Baby dedication is separate from baptism. In baptism, a person chooses to accept the Lord and be baptized in water in the name of Jesus. In a baby dedication, parents commit to raising their baby according to scripture, giving them milk, believing God will transition them into meat at the proper time in their lives. By faith, parents offer their children to God, agreeing to cultivate them until they are old enough to make the personal decision to join God's family.

Hannah nursed Samuel and provided him with the milk he needed during the season of his life when he needed it. Then, she trusted that Eli the priest would provide care for him when he needed more than her milk.

Today, Jesus is the high priest, and He is the one who will take our children into his loving care, instructing them into more and more truth. Yet, we must do our part by sowing seeds of righteousness and training our children in the adoration of the Lord through correction that provides them with an understanding of right and wrong.

As the time comes for children to progress, no longer receiving the milk and the elementary teachings of the word, we must let them go, knowing they are in the hands of Jesus. We must celebrate when we see our children's progression away from us as parents. To be healthy, children must accept responsibility for their lives and must separate from their parents, personally accepting the call on their lives, and talking to God themselves. First Samuel 2:11 explains, "Elkanah [and his wife Hannah] returned to Ramah to his house. But the child [Samuel] served the Lord under the guidance of Eli the priest."

Samuel was positioned and trained to love the Lord and to hear God's voice by those who were in his life. The church and the family work together to teach kids to hear from God. Adults are responsible to teach children that the Lord speaks and they can hear and respond to God's voice, even during their childhood. God will impact, speak, and talk to children! Children are ready and eager to learn about God. Matthew 18:3 explains, "I assure you and most solemnly say to you, unless you repent [that is, change your inner self—your old way of thinking, live changed lives] and become like children [trusting, humble, and forgiving], you will never enter the kingdom of heaven."

A mother can influence her child and ensure the child's salvation. Trying to force a child into his or her blessing prematurely will hinder the child, as it did with Jacob, but it is far better to be involved than distant and uninvolved. If we do not involve ourselves in our children's destiny, children can become an Esau, separated from God for the rest of their lives. It is better to keep a child close and to overly cultivate than it is to allow the weeds and the world to choke out our kids' lives. Be a watchman of your home. Watch your kids, cultivate their health, and don't allow the enemy to sow evil into their hearts.

Ephesians 6:4 teaches, "Fathers, do not provoke your children to anger [do not exasperate them to the point of resentment with demands that are trivial or unreasonable or humiliating or abusive; nor by showing favoritism or indifference to any of them], but bring them up [tenderly, with lovingkindness] in the discipline and instruction of the Lord."

12

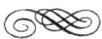

The Importance of Names

Names are incredibly significant. Names identify who we are. A child's name needs to be considered thoughtfully, because a name will speak to our life's purpose. Names establish us and explain to us who we are and where we come from, and they tell of what we will do and where we will go. A name describes, identifies, and prophesies over our future.

Names were traditionally associated with a family's occupation. When John baptized Jesus in the Jordan River, a voice from heaven said, "This is my son with who I am well-pleased." From that day forward, Jesus was known as the "Son of God," instead of the son of Joseph the carpenter. Before Jesus's baptism in the Holy Spirit Jesus was referred to as Jesus the carpenter, because of the family he was raised in.

Jesus was entering a new season of His life, and He received the baptism of the Holy Spirit. Jesus was fully separating himself from his family of origin and accepting the mission of His heavenly Father. As His mission changed, so did His name.

After Jesus' name changed and His ministry began to explode, many people were perplexed. Some wanted to continue to address Him as Jesus, the son of Mary and Joseph. These people refused to acknowledge the change that the Holy Spirit had brought forth in Jesus. Matthew 13:55 tells us, "Is not this the carpenter's son? Is not His mother called Mary? And are not His brothers, James and Joseph and Simon and Judas?"

Some parents pick a name for their child without considering its importance. Yet, when we read the Bible, we see that names hold meaning. If parents are open to hearing from the Lord when they are naming their children, God wants to inform parents whom their children will be and what their children will do. As we are receptive to hearing the names God has chosen for our children, we are given a prophecy about our children's purpose. We know what our children's personalities, characteristics, and outlooks will be because of the names the Lord gave them.

Parents are free to choose a baby's name without asking the Lord, but when parents believe that God has a special name for their child and ask Him to give them the correct name, God will respond. God specifically told many pregnant women and their husbands the names of their children. Mary and Joseph were instructed separately about Jesus's name. Jesus's name identified who He was and what He would do.

Matthew 1:20–21 says, "But after he had considered this, an angel of the Lord appeared to him in a dream, saying, 'Joseph, descendant of David. Do not be afraid to take Mary as your wife, for the Child who has been conceived in her is of the Holy Spirit. She will give birth to a Son, and you shall name him Jesus (The Lord is salvation), for He will save His people from their sins.'"

Our names identify us in the spiritual realm. An angel addressed Joseph by his name, The angel recognized who Joseph was by his family linage and addressed him as "Joseph, a descendant of David."

Today, we are recognized in the spirit and in the world by our lineage. If we have been born into God's family, we are a part of the lineage of Christ, and we are known by our relation to Him, as Joseph was known by his relation to David, an heir of God's promises.

As we accept Jesus, our old bloodline is wiped out, and our new bloodline is established. Christians become new creations and join a new family. We are no longer identified by our family of origin. We become citizens of heaven, and we are given a new family. Our family is the family of believers and the family of God. We leave the family of sin and of Adam, and God's family becomes our family, and our previous biological family becomes insignificant to our destiny. Jesus' baptism in the Holy Spirit positioned Him out of the family of a carpenter and into a higher position within the family of the God. He was promoted and given a new title and a new job.

When a woman gets married, she leaves her family and joins her husband. In most cultures around the world, women take their husband's last name, and the woman no longer identifies herself with her maiden name after her marriage ceremony because she has been given a new name and a new identity. The new identity will continue in her life, as the old name becomes extinct. As people meet a married woman, they do not know her as the woman she was before she was married; they interact with her solely by her new name and new identity.

Children born to the mother will also receive the family name, not her maiden name, and this is what God intended. The father, mother and children walk into the future together, sharing one name, and children may not know their mother ever had a different name because her old name and identity have been erased from her life. The woman becomes one with her husband, sharing his family lineage, and she joins a new family tree, leaving the old family tree behind.

As we become one in union with Christ, we receive a new name, and a new purpose. People who knew us before we were saved will not recognize us, and they may be shocked when they see the transformation in our life. We are noticeably different, and the old life we lived before has been wiped out. There is no trace of our previous lifestyle before we married Christ, because we have changed and identify with a new family unit.

Many believers received a new name when the direction of their life changed. On the road to Damascus, a Pharisee named Saul was persecuting Christians. The Lord appeared to Saul and gave him a new purpose and a new direction. As Saul was blinded by the bright light, the Lord changed Saul's entire direction and his entire outlook. After Saul saw the light, he was never the same, and his name and his mission in life were forever altered.

Acts 9:1–6 tells us, "Meanwhile Saul, still drawing his breath hard from threatening and murderous desire against the disciples of the Lord, went to the high priest And requested of him letters to the synagogues at Damascus [authorizing him], so that if he found any men or women belonging to the Way [of life as determined by faith in Jesus Christ], he might bring them bound [with chains] to Jerusalem. Now as he traveled on, he came near to Damascus, and suddenly a light from heaven flashed around him, And he fell to the ground. Then he heard a voice saying to him, 'Saul, Saul, why are you persecuting Me [harassing, troubling, and molesting Me]?' And Saul said, 'Who are You, Lord?' And He said, 'I am Jesus, Whom you are persecuting. It is dangerous and it will turn out badly for you to keep kicking against the goad [to offer vain and perilous resistance].' Trembling and astonished he asked, 'Lord, what do You desire me to do?' The Lord said to him, 'But arise and go into the city, and you will be told what you must do.'"

Without light, people cannot properly see the direction they are walking in. Light is the illuminating force we need to ensure we are safely headed in a direction. Spiritual light is from heaven. As God illuminates spiritual truth, we can properly determine where we are and where we are headed. As God reveals Himself to us, we are enlightened, and we can perceive spiritual things we were previously blind to seeing.

When God appeared to Saul, He enlightened him in the Spirit. God showed Saul the truth, about whom He was, and He warned him about the path he was heading down. Saul recognized God and repented for walking down the wrong path. As Saul obeyed God and God's direction, he changed the trajectory of his life, and he began to walk in the light of God's word. This change of mission and direction, combined with the change of the group Saul associated with changed Saul's name to Paul.

As we accept Jesus, we receive a church family. We become part of a new group, and the sinners and our former connections may hate us if they are unwilling to receive the gospel message. Saul no longer identified himself as a Pharisee and a persecutor of Christians. He became new and he received a new group of people as his family. The people who were once against his mission were now his friends, and the people who used to like him now wanted to get rid of him. As we accept Jesus, our associations change.

To enlighten means to give greater knowledge and understanding about a subject or a situation. The truth about Jesus and the kingdom of God was always there, but Saul was blind to the truth. As Saul received enlightenment, he was blinded by light, and he could perceive God and his God-given mission. Paul, previously known as Saul, saw the light, so he could properly see and evaluate the truth in the Spirit realm. From the moment Paul's eyes were opened in the Spirit, his life's purpose and direction changed, and he was no longer known as Saul.

The mid- to late-1600s to the late-1700s was a time of European history called the enlightenment period. This was characterized by the rise of humanistic reasoning and the scientific method. Before the enlightenment period, religious and political absolutes were the standard for establishing law, ethics, and culture within society. The Church and monarchs were viewed as the supreme influencers in societies, and most citizens felt respect for the Church and the Bible.

During the enlightenment period, many misled people attempted to eradicate the Church using human reason and scientific revolution. God was replaced with evolutionary science and human thought. Satan behaved as he did in the Garden of Eden. He introduced satanic wisdom and knowledge to the world, and he exalted human consciousness, reasoning, and thought above God's laws, causing humans to sin and fall into error. Through deception and human pride people were led to separate themselves from the light and the truths of God.

During the enlightenment period, many people believed they were being shown deeper truth. Eve was the first human to fall into this deception of Satan, believing she was being enlightened and shown more knowledge, when she was, in fact, being tricked into following darkness. Satan wants us to believe we are smarter, stronger, and wiser if we separate ourselves from God and His laws. He wants us to believe we are receiving superior information when we are not.

The enemy's lies during the enlightenment period were the same old lies of the same old devil. It is not a coincidence that the movement that drew many away from God is called the enlightenment period, when the enlightenment period, for many, was the opposite of the illumination of the truth. Like Saul, many "enlightened" people assumed they were standing for the truth. They believed they were pursuing justice when they were persecuting God and the church, and rebelling against proper authority. Saul advocated for the persecution of Christians because he was walking in darkness, void of correct reasoning.

Today we see a resurgence of Satan introducing the same concepts of the enlightenment area. Many believe they have superior knowledge and information because of their own perceptions, feelings, and scientific methods. This false superiority is rooted in pride and deception. Satan has lured many humans throughout history and into the present age to separate themselves from their Creator and to believe they are wiser for doing so.

Many secular people feel Christians are ignorant of their viewpoints or their perceived superior knowledge, when that is simply not the case. Christians know what the world believes, and we don't envy it, because when we stand with God, we have a higher level of understanding than the world has.

God was involved in the lives of many people during the enlightenment era. Those who trusted God for their knowledge learned more truth and became wiser. Proverbs 9:9 explains, "Give instruction to a wise man and he will become even wiser; Teach a righteous man and he will increase his learning."

The United States of America was established in 1766, shortly after the beginning of the enlightenment movement in Europe. We can see a positive influence of the enlightenment period within our American society today, because enlightenment played a role in the foundation of the United States of America.

People who loved God and His word began to question corrupted authority. The wise in Christ Jesus knew they were made to become more, and they knew they were being treated unjustly by those who were supposed to lead them. Enlightened believers hated to be mistreated by the Church or government because they knew abuse and mistreatment were Antichrist spirits.

God will never stand on the side of injustice. As a holy, righteous, loving judge, God will always stand for those who are on the side of justice. Justice is not established on the earth and respected in Heaven. True justice is established in Heaven and is respected on the earth.

Christians who came to America and fought against King George III gained the courage to break away from ungodly leadership because they believed that God was a higher authority than the King. They knew they were acting justly to oppose corruption, and God stood with them because they were in the right.

Settlers leaving Europe were righteously inspired by the love of God. The love of God overruled the love of Great Britain. When the rulers of the land refuse to serve God, or attempt to separate us from fully serving God, they are behaving unjustly in the courts of Heaven. If there is a law, policy, or expectation of leaders to keep the Church from God, the leaders making the law should be warned about the dangerous ground they are embarking upon. No one has the right to weaken our relationship with our Creator. Time and again throughout history, leaders who have gone against God learned they were fools.

When Americans fought the war with Great Britain, they didn't fight alone. God inspired and helped them. The greatest country of the day was forced to retreat, losing its tight grip on God's people because of the Lord's blessing. In First Kings 13:4, a man of God stood before a powerful ruler. As the king went to cause harm to the man of God, his hand withered and was held in place supernaturally. This phenomenon caused the king to respond to the man of God with respect because he realized that the man was not working alone.

First Kings 13:4 says, "When the king heard the words which the man of God cried out against the altar in Bethel, Jeroboam put out his hand from the altar, saying, 'Seize him!' And his hand which he had put out against him withered, so that he was unable to pull it back to himself. The altar also was split apart and the ashes were poured out from the altar in accordance with the sign which the man of God had given by the word of the Lord. The king answered and said to the man of God, 'Please entreat [the favor of] the Lord your God and pray for me, that my hand may be restored to me.' So the man of God entreated the Lord, and the king's hand was restored to him and became as it was before."

The Church is the most powerful institution in the world. Governments who exalt themselves and position themselves against the Church are making a grave mistake. In America today, many attempt to remove God and to limit people from serving Him. When these people take that stance, they will meet with the Lord's vengeance. God will never leave His Church unavenged. He will never let His people be outdone by wicked people.

Zephaniah 1:17–18 explains, "And I will bring distress upon men, so that they shall walk like blind men, because they have sinned against the Lord; their blood shall be poured out like dust and their flesh like dung. Neither their silver nor their gold shall be able to deliver them in the day of the Lord's indignation and wrath. But the whole earth shall be consumed in the fire of His jealous wrath, for a full, yes, a sudden, end will He make of all the inhabitants of the earth."

Americans must be willing to stand with God above our national citizenship, no matter the cost. We are American citizens, but we are first citizens of Heaven. Without the proper understanding of this government hierarchy, people will unintentionally place government over God. The government, when it is following God and God's laws, should be honored. By no means should a Christian find fault with their government and pull away from proper authority out of rebellion. However, if the government or a leader ever breaks authorities or commands a violation of God and His word, then we are obligated to break the law of the land and stand with God's law.

During the enlightenment period, Satan inspired many men and women to buck all forms of government and authority, both good and bad. However, a wise and discerning man or woman of God realizes we must determine if our leaders are following God and His laws. We do not buck authority for rebellion's sake. We only resist ungodly authority when it positions itself against the Church or the truths in God's laws. Rebellion of God is not the same as rebellion to ungodliness. To rebel against wicked laws, evil, and injustice is to stand with the Lord. To hate and oppose evil is to stand on the side of justice.

If a leader follows God and makes laws that respect God's laws, then Christians need to follow and respect those laws. Refusing to submit to proper, God-ordained authority is a sin. Christians are held to a higher standard than the world. Our moral, intellectual, and spiritual understanding is superior to that of the world. We do not need ungodly men and women monitoring us and managing us into proper behavior, because we follow a higher standard. God's law is perfect, holy, and flawless. He holds us to these standards as His people, and if we are citizens of Heaven following the standards of Heaven, we are always pursuing and implementing a higher level of truth and justice than those operating without God.

Many times, governments persecute those who live according to God's standard. Jesus was perfect, and yet He was dragged into the court system and put to death unreasonably and unfairly. Daniel was thrown into the lion's den for refusing to compromise with a wicked government, as was Paul on many occasions. Paul was put into prison in various locations, and he was treated as an unruly citizen when he was following God's laws and doing nothing to violate justice or truth.

Being persecuted, thrown in prison, or even killed are often signs of a person's spiritual impact for truth and justice. Satan uses people who work in government to try to stop the truth from going forth. Satan alters the law regularly to harm those who are working for the Lord. If he cannot stop the message through the governmental system, then Satan often tries to inspire the murder of the individual.

Martin Luther King Jr. was thrown into prison and ultimately killed for his spiritual social justice work. The devil wanted to stop him because he was standing for higher moral and spiritual laws relating to justice of Heaven when he opposed the weaker moral laws in the United States justice system.

Paul was in the city preaching good news and healing and helping hurting people. He was inspiring people to turn from false gods and to walk in truth. Paul was performing kingdom work in Lystra. He was setting captives free and having an impact on the culture. As he changed the culture and healed those who needed to be delivered from demon spirits, Satan inspired unholy leaders to kill him.

Acts 14:7–19 explains, "And there they continued to preach the good news. Now at Lystra a man sat who was unable to use his feet, for he was crippled from birth and had never walked. This man was listening to Paul as he spoke, and Paul looked intently at him and saw that he had faith to be healed, and said with a loud voice, 'Stand up on your feet.' And he jumped up and began to walk. And the crowds, when they saw what Paul had done, raised their voices, shouting in the Lycaonian language, 'The gods have come down to us in human form!' They began calling Barnabas, Zeus [chief of the Greek gods], and Paul, Hermes [messenger of the Greek gods], since he took the lead in speaking. The priest of Zeus, whose temple was at the entrance of the city, brought bulls and garlands to the city gates, and wanted to offer sacrifices with the crowds. But when the apostles Barnabas and Paul heard about it, they tore their robes and rushed out into the crowd, shouting, 'Men, why are you doing these things? We too are only men of the same nature as you, bringing the good news to you, so that you turn from these useless and meaningless things to the living God, who made the heaven and the Earth and the sea and everything that is in them. In generations past He permitted all the nations to go their own ways; yet He did not leave Himself without some witness [as evidence of Himself], in that He kept constantly doing good things and showing you kindness, and giving you rains from heaven and productive seasons, filling your hearts with food and happiness.' Even saying these words, with difficulty they prevented the people from offering sacrifices to them. But Jews arrived from Antioch and Iconium, and having won over the crowds, they stoned Paul and dragged him out of the city, thinking he was dead."

As we follow Jesus and do kingdom work, we will experience persecution. In America, we have been blessed to have many laws supporting God's truth and justice. Our founding fathers tried to create a society that honored God. However, in recent years, many have turned away from God and have begun to follow a new wave of demonic darkness disguised as enlightenment. In America today, we see the same lies of Satan combining scientific method, human reasoning, and an attempt to remove God, the Church, and proper authority.

Demon spirits are using the same playbook and pushing the same agenda they did in the 1600s–1700s, but this time, there is no new land for Christians to flee too. If we lose control of our country, we will not have another uncompromised and unrestricted land.

The Bible was the foundation of our country. The Bible was used to ward off evil and to orchestrate the most successful, longstanding, and beautiful country that has ever existed. Many men died during the American Revolution and fought for the right to be free. To remain free and in a holy land, Americans must refuse to compromise with evil and must stand with God, the highest King, knowing He will honor us for our obedience to truth. Consider this verse of the song, "My Country 'Tis of Thee."

> *Our fathers' God to Thee,*
> *Author of liberty,*
> *To Thee we sing.*
> *Long may our land be bright,*
> *With freedom's holy light,*
> *Protect us by Thy might,*
> *Great God our King.*

The presence and the influence of God's word, the Bible, is prevalent in all of America's founding symbols and documents. A Bible verse is engraved on the Liberty Bell, and our first amendment in the United States Constitution was specifically made to protect the freedom of religion for the American people: "Congress shall make no law respecting an establishment of religion, or prohibiting the free exercise thereof; or abridging the freedom of speech, or of the press; or the right of the people peaceably to assemble, and to petition the Government for a redress of grievances."

When the United States became a country, we were to be united in our love for freedom and for God. We were to be united in the mission to keep freedom alive and thriving in the country. Mark 3:24 says, "If a kingdom is divided against itself, it cannot stand."

Satan wants to promote tyranny of the government and a hatred of God so he can stir up rebellion and hatred within citizens' hearts. When citizens begin to tear down the system and position themselves against the Church, then the system has been divided and without a remedy it will no longer stand.

We, the Church, were given the first amendment to protect us from a tyrannical oppressive government that wanted to dim our light. The attempt to manipulate the first amendment to abolish the

Church's influence and hide the Church in America is inspired by Satan. For ignorant citizens who are blind to the truth, the first amendment is a protection of the government or state from the Church. The first amendment was never created to protect the state or government. The first amendment was written to protect the Church from the government, and it was written for the Church by a man who loved the Church.

Tyranny is defined as cruel and oppressive government rule. Tyrannical governments impose themselves on others by limiting freedom through oppressive power. All tyrannical governments are Antichrist, and we know Satan will destroy all independent, thriving governments to be able to reign over everyone living in the world during the tribulation period. Although America is not mentioned specifically in scripture, we know America has been a beacon of light to the world, promoting the gospel far and wide to many who need to hear and see the truth of God. We know Satan hates America and wants to see it destroyed.

It is essential, now more than ever, that all Americans who love the Lord stand boldly for Christ and be Christian witnesses. We must refuse to tolerate evil within any governmental system, and we must fight for godly laws to remain. When we vote, when we refuse to cooperate with evil, we must know we are pursuing God's justice system. Satan needs to take America down if he is going to establish his kingdom on the earth. Christians may experience persecution, especially in this new age of demonic "enlightenment," but we cannot give up because if we do America will fall.

Romans 10:8 tells us, "Therefore, get rid of all moral filth and every expression of evil, and humbly accept the word planted in you, which can save your souls."

As Paul set people free from devils, the government came after him. As he cleaned up the city, the people who were against the truth raged. When we are removing filth and getting rid of moral decay and corruption, Satan inspires people to try to stop us. Don't be surprised when the wicked try to stop you; be surprised if no one opposes your stance for God.

Satan has already begun to infiltrate the American court systems. He has begun to change laws at the state and the national levels to imprison those who believe in justice and truth. During the Covid-19 lockdowns, some pastors were wrongfully imprisoned for refusing to shut down their churches. Some ministers have been threated for refusing to marry same-sex couples, even when same-sex marriage is clearly against the Bible. In the last days, we know we will face persecution, but we must remain faithful to Him who called us. We must do the work of the kingdom and have faith to establish God's system on the earth.

Revelation 2:10 explains, "Fear nothing that you are about to suffer. Be aware that the devil is about to throw some of you into prison, that you may be tested [in your faith], and for ten days you will have tribulation. Be faithful to the point of death [if you must die for your faith], and I will give you the crown [consisting] of life."

Martin Luther King was killed for his faith. He was killed for standing for God's court system more than he stood with the United States courts. When Martin Luther King was born, his name was Michael King, but his father changed his name because he was impacted by a Christian leader named Martin Luther, and he wanted to show honor to the man of God. The change of Martin Luther King's name is remarkable, because his name is now known all over the world. He is not known by Michael King, and if anyone called him by his former name, most would not be sure who they were referring to.

The name change in Martin Luther King Jr.'s life spoke to his destiny. His name identified him as a man of God. His name showed the world who he belonged to and who he was going to stand for.

God's kingdom and God's children will always be honored. Our work for God is never done is vain, and the world will see the great light and the great God who lives, if we vow to stand with the Lord against anyone or anything that wants to stop the truth.

Luke 1:13 says, "But the angel said to him, 'Do not be afraid, Zacharias, because your petition [in prayer] was heard, and your wife Elizabeth will bear you a son, and you will name him John. You will have great joy and delight, and many will rejoice over his birth, for he will be great and distinguished in the sight of the Lord: and will never drink wine or liquor, and he will be filled with and empowered to act by the Holy Spirit while still in his mother's womb.'"

Elizabeth and her husband, Zacharias, were instructed to name their child John. An angel told Zacharias what the baby was to be named and what the baby's mission was to be. We know John was given his mission within the womb because he had already been commissioned for kingdom work. He received the Holy Spirit from the womb, and he never had a different mission. His mission was established even before his parents saw him with their eyes.

People do not need ultrasounds, name generators, or personality tests to determine whom their baby is and what their baby is called to do. The Lord will still tell parents the sex, the name, and the prophecy of their children before their children enter the world if the parents set their children apart for kingdom work even before the children are born. In an age in which many rely on technology to tell them what to do and what will happen, we can still rely on God, and God will reward us for our faith in Him.

The family and friends of Zacharias and Elizabeth were curious as to what their child's name was to be, just as people today ask pregnant women what they are naming their baby. Luke 1:62 explains, "They made signs to his father, as to what he wanted his name to be."

Friends and family members couldn't understand why Elizabeth and Zacharias chose the name John for their son. Luke 1:61 says, "And they said to her, 'None of your relatives are called by that name.' But Elizabeth was adamant she knew the name of her son, refusing to compromise or be swayed to change her baby's name." Luke 1:60 tells us, "but his mother answered, 'No indeed: instead, he will be called John.'"

Elizabeth knew by the Spirit her son's name was to be John. She knew his gender, his name, and his mission because an angel of the Lord told her. Zacharias and Elizabeth's neighbors and relatives were confused because they believed that John's parents would name him after his father. But Elizabeth and Zacharias wouldn't change their John's name, because other people thought they should. Luke 1:59 says, "It happened that on the eighth day they came to circumcise the child [as required by the Law], and they intended to name him Zacharias, after his father."

Zacharias, Elizabeth, Joseph, and Mary were all parents who knew their children's names and their children's missions with God, because they were open to hearing God's message to them through an angel. When the angel Gabriel spoke to Zacharias, he told him that John would not drink liquor or wine, and that he would be empowered by the spirit within the womb. This was fulfilled in John's life. The Bible makes a point that John did not have a normal appetite for the foods of man, and he didn't clothe himself in the normal clothing of man.

Matthew 3:4 explains, "Now this same John had clothing made of camel's hair and a [wide] leather band around his waist, and his food was locusts and wild honey." John did not identify with the world, and he did not want the things of the world because he was born from above from his mother's womb. He never desired to fulfill the lust of the flesh, and he never craved natural things, because the Holy Spirit removed his desire of sin before he was ever born. From the time John was in the womb, John was separate from the normalcies of the world.

Luke 1:41–44 says, "When Elizabeth heard Mary's greeting, her baby leaped in her womb; and Elizabeth was filled with the Holy Spirit and empowered by Him. And she exclaimed loudly, 'Blessed [worthy to be praised] are you among women, and blessed is the fruit of your womb! And how has it happened to me, that the mother of my Lord would come to me? For behold, when the sound of your greeting reached my ears, the baby in my womb leaped for joy.'"

Pregnant mothers baptized in the Holy Spirit allow their babies to be in proximity to Jesus Christ. The closeness of Jesus to babies can impact the babies. Babies can recognize and accept Jesus as all-powerful one. They can worship even within the womb. Spiritual identities are born when the child recognizes Jesus as their Lord and Savior, and in John's case, he identified Jesus from his mother's womb, so he never had a love or allegiance to the world.

Abraham's name was changed from Abram, the name given to Abram by his biological parents before he decided to separate from them and to follow God. Terah didn't love the Lord, and God instructed Abraham to separate himself from his biological family and go into a land He would show him. Joshua 24:2 explains, "Joshua said to all the people, 'This is what the LORD, the God of Israel, says, "Your fathers, including Terah, the father of Abraham and the father of Nahor, lived beyond the [Euphrates] River in ancient times; and they served other gods."'"

Like John and Jesus, God used Abraham's name to prophecy over his future. Abraham used his new name many years before he saw the full manifestation of the promise. God also changed Abraham's wife's name to Sarah from Sari. God renamed Abraham and Sarah to show them where He was going to take them. He gave them new names to instill faith in the direction of their lives. Genesis 17:15–16 tells us, "Then God said to Abraham, 'Regarding Sarai, your wife—her name will no longer be Sarai. From now on her name will be Sarah. And I will bless her and give you a son from her! Yes, I will bless her richly, and she will become the mother of many nations. Kings of nations will be among her descendants.'"

God told me I was pregnant when I was in a church service the day after I conceived my son Gianni. I knew in the Spirit I was going to have a baby boy while I sitting in a church service on Sunday December 4, 2022. Gianni was conceived on December 3, 2022. The Lord gave me a private message to prepare me for what was going to come. There was no way in the natural that I would have known I was pregnant a day after I conceived. It was something I knew because of the Spirit's revelation.

The Lord also told me what Gianni's name was to be that day. The pastor was speaking on the story of Jesus and John, and I knew my son's name was to be John. The name Gianni is a form of Gian and is the Hebrew equivalent of John. Gianni, like the name John, means "God is gracious."

Like with Elizabeth, people have asked me why I named my baby Gianni. I am not Italian and neither is my husband. I explained to many people that I didn't decide on my baby's name, that the Lord gave it to me. The Lord wanted him to be named John: Gianni. I simply obeyed in giving him the name the Lord instructed me to give him.

God understands all the languages existing in the world. God knows what the name means, even if the name is from a different cultural or language background. Middle names are also important because they are a part of a child's name. God has a name—a first, middle, and last name—for each person. Names are significant to God. Our names determine if we will spend eternity with Jesus. Revelation 20:15 says, "And if anyone's name was not found written in the book of life, he was thrown into the fire."

God provided me with a middle name for my son Gianni, but in a different way than I received his first name. Months before I became pregnant, I felt I was to name my next son Andrew, but I didn't share that with my husband. After we found out about Gianni, my husband asked me one afternoon what I thought about naming him Gianni Andrew. When he asked me about the name, I told him that I had already felt like that was a good name for our son. Later that evening, after my husband and I had determined his name, my husband's grandfather's wife reached out to us and jokingly suggested that his name should be Andrew. The Lord confirmed Gianni's middle name to me in one afternoon.

Angels have names. Like human names, the names of angels give us insight into who they are and what they do. The Bible doesn't tell us the names of all the angels, but it does tell us at least two of the angel's names. Gabriel was the angel who appeared to Mary and told her the good news about her pregnancy. Gabriel brought Mary prophetic information from God. Gabriel also appeared before Zechariah, informing him prophetically about baby John. Luke 1:19 tells us, "The angel answered him, 'I'm Gabriel! I stand in God's presence. God sent me to tell you this good news.'"

We see Gabriel again when he helped Daniel to receive a message of prophecy from the Lord. Daniel 8:15-17 says, "When I, Daniel, had seen the vision, I sought to understand it; then behold, standing before me was one who looked like a man. And I heard the voice of a man between the banks of the Ulai, which called out and said, 'Gabriel, give this man (Daniel) an understanding of the vision.' So he came near where I was standing, and when he came I was frightened and fell face downward; but he said to me, 'Understand, son of man, that the [fulfillment of the] vision pertains to [events that will occur in] the time of the end.'"

Gabriel is a prophetic angel who gives God's people information. He provides God's children with insight from God's throne. He is a messenger angel, revealing spiritual and supernatural things, and he helps people to make sense of God's vision and God's plan for their lives. The name Gabriel means "God is my strength," "God is my strong man," or "hero of God," and that is exactly who Gabriel is. Gabriel stands with God, and he works for God, strengthening the Church through prophecy.

Michael is another angel who does the work of the Lord. Michael means, "Who is like El? Who is like God?" Michael's job is different than Gabriel's job, even though He works for God. Michael told Daniel he and Gabriel have different jobs when he appeared to him in Daniel 10:12-13. "Then he said to me, 'Do not be afraid, Daniel, for from the first day that you set your heart on understanding this and on humbling yourself before your God, your words were heard, and I have come in response to your words'. But the prince of the kingdom of Persia was standing in opposition to me for twenty-one days. Then, behold, Michael, one of the chiefs [of the celestial] princes, came to help me, for I had been left there with the kings of Persia."

Michael is a war angel and has a high-ranking position, because we are told he oversees many other angels. In heaven, angels hold various positions and rankings. Archangels are chief or principal angels. They are charged with overseeing other angels. An archangel will blow the trumpet of God when the Lord comes back for the Church. As a high-ranking military official in the kingdom of God, the archangel will sound the war siren announcing that the battle is about to begin.

Revelation 12:7 says, "And there was a war in heaven, Michael and his angels waging war with the dragon. The dragon and his angels waged war and they were not strong enough, and there was no longer a place found for them in heaven. And the great dragon was thrown down, the serpent of old who is called the devil and Satan, who deceives the whole world; he was thrown down to the earth, and his angels were thrown down with him."

First Thessalonians 4:16 explains, "For the Lord Himself will come down from heaven with a shout of command, with the voice of the archangel and with the [blast of the] trumpet of God, and the dead in Christ will rise first."

Before Satan's rebellion, he had a different name. Lucifer was a beautiful angel and before he was excommunicated, he was called a star of the morning or a light bringer. Lucifer indicates bringing light and being a bearer of light. When Lucifer's position to God and the kingdom changed, so did his name. Lucifer didn't want to do the job God assigned for him; he made his own assignment, so he lost his position in the kingdom of the Lord. Isaiah 14:12 tells us, "How you have fallen from heaven, O star of the morning [light bringer], son of the dawn! You have been cut down to the ground, you who have weakened the nations [king of Babylon]!"

Demons recognized Jesus by His name when He was doing kingdom work. Demons referred to Jesus the "Son of the Most High God."

Even the demons that lived in rebellion under Satan's leadership saw Jesus for who He was in relation to His Father. Jesus responded to the demon speaking to Him by asking the demon his name. Mark 5:6–10 tells us, "When he saw Jesus from a distance, he ran and fell on his knees in front of Him. He shouted at the top of his voice, 'What do you want with me, Jesus, Son of the Most High God? In God's name don't torture me!' For Jesus had said to him, 'Come out of this man, you impure spirit!' Then Jesus asked him, 'What is your name?' 'My name is Legion,' he replied, 'for we are many.' And he begged Jesus again and again not to send them out of the area."

A legion was an army unit of 3,000–6,000 men in the ancient Roman army. By responding to Jesus, the demon was speaking for many demons living inside of the man. We can accurately speculate that this one man had 3,000 to 6,000 demons living inside of him when Jesus cast the demons out. It would have been impossible for the demons to all identify themselves and their jobs as individuals, because the number of demons was too great, so a higher-ranking demon spoke for the group, answering Jesus' question.

Angels and demons have rankings, jobs, and missions to fulfill. When the fallen angels lived in heaven, they had different names and different jobs. As they changed in their assignment and position to God, their names changed too. Demons and angels know our names. Believers are recognized by their relationship to the Father. Some people are leaders, and everyone knows their name in the spirit, where others are unrecognizable because they don't produce or impact either kingdom. Acts 19:15 says, "But the evil spirit retorted, "I know and recognize and acknowledge Jesus, and I know about Paul, but as for you, who are you?"

As in human systems, some people who are known for doing good and everyone recognizes who they are. Leaders like Martin Luther King Jr. will have their names remembered on the earth and in eternity because they made a big impact for the Lord. Spirits and men and women alike know who Martin Luther King Jr. is and what he stood for.

Other names will identify people as evil and as a disgrace. By standing for evil, and yielding to evil spirits, these men and women are recognized for great evil spiritual influence and power. These are names that remind us of the devil and the hatred of God, such as the name of Hitler.

The more we do for the Lord and the more we advance the kingdom of God, the more our name will be recognized in the Spirit by angels and demons. Humans will also remember our names if we stood for God and made a difference in the world. What we do determines if we are respected. It determines what we are known for and how many people or spirits recognize who we are. Aspire to be a kingdom warrior who stands with Christ, setting people free and destroying the works of the opposing kingdom. Everyone should know who we are and what we stand for. We should be indistinguishably bold and set apart, made for a purpose and recognized by our position of power and influence within the kingdom of God!

13

Medical Witchcraft

Witchcraft uses supernatural powers to harm people. Witchcraft is often broken into two categories: white magic and black magic. White magic is assumed to benefit or heal others, where black magic involves intentionally harming others. Despite the label and the assumed benefits of either form of magic, all magic is deadly, even if it is packaged as safe and effective.

God forbids both white and black magic. Scripture commands us to stay away from all forms of magic and divination. King Saul sought help from a witch, even when he knew better. Saul had previously banned witchcraft in his kingdom, but he changed his stance out of desperation.

King Saul is not to be confused with Saul/Paul whose name was changed by the Lord due to his loyalty to God. King Saul's story is the opposite of Paul's, where King Saul started out doing great exploits for the Lord but later turned to serving false gods. First Chronicles 10:13–14 says, "So Saul died for his breach of faith. He broke faith with the Lord in that he did not keep the command of the Lord, and also consulted a medium, seeking guidance. He did not seek guidance from the Lord. Therefore the Lord put him to death and turned the kingdom over to David the son of Jesse."

King Saul was expected to set a standard for the people who were under him, and God held Saul to a higher standard because of his leadership position. God gave Saul responsibility for the lives of others, not just his own life.

When children are born, they begin to follow their parents as leaders. Without parents, children would not learn how to behave or how to survive in the world, and all parents are leaders in their home, whether they take responsibility for their position or not. This leadership should never be taken for granted or abused, because God has entrusted us with people to lead into all truth.

King Saul was chosen by God to lead God's people and protect them from enemy forces, but Saul failed to perform the work he was called to do. This led him to be rejected by God and replaced by David. The involvement of God's enemies in witchcraft and sorcery depicts the gravity of Saul's betrayal, as he formed alliances with opposing forces.

First Chronicles 10:9–11 says, "The next day, when the Philistines came to strip the slain, they found Saul and his sons fallen on Mount Gilboa. They stripped [Saul] and took his head and his armor, and sent [them] round about in Philistia to carry the news to their idols and to the people. And they put [Saul's] armor in the house of their gods and fastened his head in the temple of Dagon."

Believers are given specific missions by God. God created us to perform the work of the kingdom, and we are assigned a job to do. A failure to produce fruit and to perform the work we have been assigned shows a rebellious spirit and heart. If we do not obey God, we will not bear fruit, and we will be removed from our position. The position will be given to someone else who is obedient.

Matthew 7:19 explains, "Every tree that does not bear good fruit is cut down and thrown into the fire. Therefore, by their fruits you will know them."

As believers, we are called to be fruit inspectors. Jesus warned His followers to evaluate people's lives and to judge the fruit or the lack of fruit, so we can keep from trusting in people who are of the devil. Determining evil forces within our personal lives, our social lives, or within the Church requires us to pay attention and discern the spirits we are interacting with. We must never take our guard down, even within the Church, because there are counterfeits spirits that pretend to be holy.

Matthew 7:15–18 says, "Beware of false prophets, who come to you in sheep's clothing, but inwardly they are ravenous wolves. You will know them by their fruits. Do men gather grapes from thornbushes or figs from thistles. Even so, every good tree bears good fruit, but a bad tree cannot bear bad fruit, nor can a bad tree bear good fruit."

Judgment is often criticized in our modern society. Many people believe that judgment is reserved for God alone, but the Bible commands believers to judge fruit, and to be intentional in determining our associations. Matthew 7:21–22 explains, "Not everyone who says to me, 'Lord, Lord,' will enter the kingdom of heaven, but the one who does the will of my Father who is in heaven. On that day many will say to me, 'Lord, Lord, did we not prophesy in your name, and cast out demons in your name, and do many mighty works in your name?' And then will I declare to them, 'I never knew you; depart from me, you workers of lawlessness."

Lawlessness is a state of disorder that happens when we disregard the law. Saul believed he could violate God's laws and still receive God's help. When Saul sought help from the witch, even she was afraid the law would punish her if her work was discovered. First Samuel 28:9 tells us, "The woman said, See here, you know what Saul has done, how he has cut off those who are mediums and wizards out of the land. Why then do you lay a trap for my life to cause my death?"

Saul falsely believed he could consult a witch and different spirits while also communing with the Holy Spirit. Saul not only broke God's laws, but he also broke the laws he had created to govern his people. Saul was full of corruption, even when he previously committed to serving God. Behind closed doors, Saul was breaking the law and disobeying God, but to the world and the witch, it appeared he was standing for truth.

In the Church body, there is no room for corruption, pollution or unholy spirits. There can be no compromise or no intentional violation of the Lord's laws without repentance and remorse. Anyone who preaches, teaches, or testifies against these truths is working for a different spirit. The message of Jesus and the message of the gospel is a message of repentance and turning from sin.

First Samuel 15:23 says, "For rebellion is like the sin of divination, and arrogance like the evil of idolatry. Because you have rejected the word of the Lord, he has rejected you as king."

Today, many churches are unwilling to confront sin from the pulpit. A fear of being perceived as judgmental keeps some ministers from speaking the word. But without the word of God, the blood of Jesus, and the message of sin and repentance, there is no Church and there is no salvation. The apostle Paul warned the Church of those who would present a different gospel. He warned us of the people who would make light of sin and appear to be messengers of truth.

Sin will send people to hell. If you do not repent and turn from sin, it will destroy you. In the American church today, many pastors will tell you what you want to hear. They will tell you God understands and forgives sin indefinitely, and you cannot lose your salvation. The theory that we are all sinners who are saved by grace is a different gospel. This spirit is a lying, rebellious spirit of witchcraft that promises salvation without a changed and repentant heart.

Second Timothy 4:3 tells us, "For the time is coming when [people] will not tolerate (endure) sound and wholesome instruction, but, having ears itching [for something pleasing and gratifying], they will gather to themselves one teacher after another to a considerable number, chosen to satisfy their own liking and to foster the errors they hold,"

Many teachers, preaches, and counterfeits within the Church teach a demonic doctrine of continual grace. But if God allowed lawlessness in his leaders, his children, and in His house, then King Saul would have never been replaced, because he would have been permitted to continue in his lawlessness and sin. However, First John 3:4 declares, "Everyone who makes a practice of sinning also practices lawlessness; sin is lawlessness." And Jude 1:4 explains, "For certain men have crept in among you unnoticed—ungodly ones who were designated long ago for condemnation. They turn the grace of our God into a license for immorality, and they deny our only Master and Lord, Jesus Christ."

God is always watching people, and we cannot hide our deeds and our lifestyles from God. Being blameless before the Lord is a requirement if we are going to go to Heaven. We must live our lives in a manner that is pleasing to God. Matthew 12:36 explains, "But I tell you, on the day of judgment people will have to give an accounting for every careless or useless word they speak."

If we will be held accountable for our words, how much more will we be held accountable for our actions? The Lord will have everyone give an account for their words and actions when they stand before Him. We will be face to face with our Creator, and if we are disobedient, we will have to explain why we didn't do the things He told us to do.

When our lives are pleasing to God, we radiate a sweet aroma to the world and to Heaven. Second Corinthians 2:15 says, "For we are the sweet fragrance of Christ [which ascends] to God, [discernible both] among those who are being saved and among those who are perishing." The practice of sinning is the practice of witchcraft. The Church is commanded to live holy and distinctive lives that will even be noticeable to unbelievers. All sins are law violations, and if we practice sin, we put off a certain aroma by breaking the laws of God.

First John 2:1 declares, "My little children, I am writing these things to you so that you may not sin. But if anyone does sin, we have an advocate with the Father, Jesus Christ the righteous."

Sin should not be normalized or excused in our lives. Our prayer should be for God to help us and to strengthen us daily, so we can remain pure and holy, separated from lifestyles and patterns of sin. Sin is our enemy. Sin is an opposing force to God.

In the criminal justice system, repeat offenders are those who are convicted of multiple offenses over time. They are often given harsher sentences for their crimes because they refuse to repent and stop their bad behavior. Relating to sin and the laws of God, there will always be a higher level of accountability than the human court system. When people refuse to stop sinning, they become repeat offenders, and without a change in behavior, they will one day be held accountable in the courts of Heaven.

People do not get a pass from God to continue to sin. There is no such thing as a sin license. Within the criminal justice system, judges do not allow offenders to continue in their lawlessness. These judges operate at a lower level of excellence than God, so what makes anyone believe the Creator of the universe would permit lawlessness to continue unchecked without implications or judgment?

Sinners who have never accepted Jesus Christ are repeat offenders living lives of repetitive sin through law violations. If they don't turn from their sin and their lifestyles, they will go to hell when they die. Within the church there are not sinners, but "backsliders." Backsliders are people who once converted to the Christian faith, but have since reverted to previous habits, through sin or lawlessness. Backsliders can also be repeat offenders. Once God forgave their transgressions and granted them pardon, they unfortunately misused the freedom bestowed upon them, persisting in their lawlessness despite the divine mercy extended to them.

King Saul was a backslider. He was once a man who knew God and heard from God, but after repetitive sinning and disobedience to God, he was cut off from experiencing the Lord's presence.

Judges are public officials who hear and decide legal matters in the court of law. Judges know the law, and they decide if a person is guilty, and the punishment of the offender who has made law violations. To evaluate, judges must use their knowledge of the law and their discretion to form an opinion or a conclusion about the behaviors and the choices of the individual in front of them.

Isaiah 33:22 says, " For the Lord is our Judge, the Lord is our Lawgiver, the Lord is our King; He will save us."

The Lord is a judge, and He appoints us to work within His court system. God assists us to recognize and confront unrighteousness, helping to distinguish between lawbreakers and law-abiding citizens. However, He emphasizes the importance of approaching others with love, understanding that their opposition is directed toward Him rather than us. We cannot determine who will or will not face eternal judgment; however, we are compelled to warn individuals of their standing in relation to God.

Jude 1:20–21 explains, "But you, dear friends, by building yourselves up in your most holy faith and praying in the Holy Spirit, keep yourselves in God's love as you wait for the mercy of our Lord Jesus Christ to bring you to eternal life."

When people choose to turn from sin, then they will be pardoned, but when people continue to live as rebels, lawless, corrupted citizens, they will be charged with their crimes. The Church, as ambassadors for Christ, must be willing to proclaim God's truth, regardless of how it makes anyone else feel. Warning others of the need for striving for purity in their lives is compassionate because we are trying to position them to receive their salvation.

Treason is the most serious crime one can commit against their government. Treason is defined as betraying a person's country and alliance by the aiding enemy forces. A person who commits treason lets the enemy gain entrance into the camp of those who they are sworn to protect and align themselves with. King Saul committed treason against God and God's kingdom, by allowing the enemy and false gods to overtake him and some of the people he was to protect.

Believers who made a pledge to Jesus through a confession of sin and accept salvation must remain true to their kingdom, because those who pledge the kingdom of God but refuse to turn from sin remain in a treaty with the enemy forces. During a war, a treaty is a binding formal agreement. It is a contract or an alliance. An alliance with evil will cause a once-chosen and once-forgiven member of God's kingdom to become convicted of high treason against God.

Church leaders who refuse to stand boldly against evil and sin and let evil spirits enter places of worship that should be dedicated to the Lord alone commit high treason. Churches who permit homosexuality, drunkenness, cohabitation, witchcraft, or other sins and law violations, will be judged if they do not repent from their treaty with the enemy forces.

We are not permitted to sin. Sin will send anyone to hell if he or she does not get it out his or her life. Sin is not something to come into alignment with and must not be given any place within the life of a man or a woman of God. Faithful citizens of the kingdom refuse any alliance with evil. We don't make any treaty with enemy forces, because we have been sworn in to protect and serve our kingdom alone.

First Corinthians 6:9–11 warns, "Do you not know that the unrighteous and the wrongdoers will not inherit or have any share in the kingdom of God? Do not be deceived (misled): neither the impure and immoral, nor idolaters, nor adulterers, nor those who participate in homosexuality, Nor cheats (swindlers and thieves), nor greedy graspers, nor drunkards, nor foulmouthed revilers and slanderers, nor extortioners and robbers will inherit or have any share in the kingdom of God. And such some of you were [once]. But you were washed clean (purified by a complete atonement for sin and made free from the guilt of sin), and you were consecrated (set apart, hallowed), and you were justified [pronounced righteous, by trusting] in the name of the Lord Jesus Christ and in the [Holy] Spirit of our God."

God gives a new life and separates us from the world, apart from lifestyles of sin, so we can remain pure from corruption and lawlessness. Any minister, leader, or spirit who tells you God permits or understands sin is an agent of the devil. Repent and turn from your sin or you will have to give an account for your sin.

First Corinthians 6:3 says, "Do you not know also that we [Christians] are to judge the [very] angels and pronounce opinion between right and wrong [for them]? How much more then [as to] matters pertaining to this world and of this life only!"

It is foolish to not judge the lifestyles and behaviors of others. Without judgment we would align ourselves with people and things we are commanded to reject. God said to judge even the angelic realm, how much more the earth realm? A wise Christian is always evaluating fruit and determining which people and spirits are Antichrist and against us. A failure to evaluate the fruit and the spirits would be idiotic and unbiblical. It would allow the enemy to attack us as we sleep in ignorance.

We are God's ambassadors on the earth. We have been placed here to proclaim and work for God bringing justice within the land. We are called to separate good from evil, and we are called to proclaim liberty for all who are willing to hear. If we do not preach, teach, and proclaim the truth of God's word to the world, then the people who need to hear the message of repentance will never hear the words they need to hear to save their souls from an eternal state of hell and judgment.

Our biggest goal in our lives should be to behave and respond as Jesus did. We should model our ministries and our entire lives around Jesus Christ and His example. Jesus looked for the fruitfulness of the tree that was supposed to bear fruit, and when He saw no fruit, he cursed the tree. Jesus analyzed the tree, then He made a judgment, and finally, a rebuke for the lack of fruit in a tree intended to produce. Jesus wasn't afraid to call a cursed tree cursed. He knew what it was and He labeled it properly.

Matthew 21:13 declares, "He said to them, The Scripture says, My house shall be called a house of prayer; but you have made it a den of robbers." There are people within the house of God who should be refreshing others and helping to provide nourishment to the world. As the people who were called to bear fruit and to help others, they should have the fruit on their branches, but they do not, because of their lawlessness and rebellion towards God and His word.

The fruit of the spirit is love, joy, peace, patience, kindness, goodness, faithfulness, gentleness, and self-control. Those who do not teach self-control or faithfulness to God should immediately be identified as counterfeit spirits, hiding and pretending to be the Holy Spirit. Pray you never become one of the people who should have refreshed others but didn't. Ask God to help you remain faithful and pure before Him, so you will not become a backslider and a person who is removed from their position.

Matthew 21:19 teaches, "And as He saw one single leafy fig tree above the roadside, He went to it but He found nothing but leaves on it seeing that in the fig tree the fruit appears at the same time as the leaves]. And He said to it, 'Never again shall fruit grow on you! And the fig tree withered up at once.'"

Evil spirits want the undiscerning Christians in the Church to believe they are holy spirits. Remaining in hiding ensures that they are not resisted and rebuked and sent out of the Church. Snakes love to hide. People often do not see or recognize a snake because it silently blends into its environment and conceals itself. Satan, and the other snakes that work for him, operate within churches silently and quietly. They try to blend in to keep from being discovered and thrown out.

In the Bible, there were demons in the church. These same demons remain in many churches of today. We must discern which spirits are corrupted and lying spirits to walk in authority and dominion over the kingdom of darkness. If we have the gift of spiritual discernment, and we stay alert for the presence of potential snakes, then God will show us when a snake is around us. Luke 4:33 explains, "There was a man in the synagogue who was possessed by the spirit of an unclean demon; and he cried out with a loud and terrible voice,"

When Paul was performing his ministry, he encountered a girl with a spirit of witchcraft and divination. This woman followed a ministry and proclaimed to know the truth about Jesus Christ. The demon noted that Jesus was the Most High God, but the spirit was still a demon spirit and was not holy.

Believers cannot be deceived, and we cannot think everyone in church loves Jesus Christ and submits to Him. Scripture tells us evil spirits are operating in churches and near traveling ministries.

Acts 16:16–17 teaches, "It happened that as we were on our way to the place of prayer, we were met by a slave-girl who had a spirit of divination [that is, a demonic spirit claiming to foretell the future and discover hidden knowledge], and she brought her owners a good profit by fortune-telling. These men are servants of the Most High God! They are proclaiming to you the way of salvation!"

All believers must be committed to hearing and obeying the Lord's words for themselves. We are expected to be watchful and on guard against the enemy, no matter where we are. Misleading, misinforming, and misguiding, proclaiming false doctrines of demons using Jesus' name, these snakes come to mislead and steal the people who are ignorant to their scheme. Matthew 24:4–5 teaches, "And Jesus answered and said to them, 'See to it that no one misleads you. For many will come in My name, saying, "I am the Christ," and will mislead many.'"

We are not excused to disobey God simply because other believers give their personal seal of approval. In First Kings, we are told about a prophet who was instructed to tell the king a message and had a glorious future in God, but he never arrived where he was intended to arrive. This prophet was bold, standing for the word of the Lord in front of an unbeliever, but when he interacted with a lying church member, he disobeyed God and was removed from the ministry, losing his life to a lion.

First Kings 13:8–24 teaches: "And the man of God said to the king, "If you give me half your house, I will not go in with you, and I will not eat bread or drink water in this place. For I was commanded by the word of the Lord, 'You shall eat no bread or drink water or return by the way you came.'

So he went another way and did not return by the way that he came to Bethel. Now there dwelt an old prophet in Bethel; and his sons came and told him all that the man of God had done that day in Bethel; the words which he had spoken to the king they told also to their father. Their father asked them, "Which way did he go?" For his sons had seen which way the man of God who came from Judah had gone. He said to his sons, 'Saddle the donkey for me." So they saddled the donkey and he rode on it.

And went after the man of God. And he found him sitting under an oak, and he said to him, "Are you the man of God who came from Judah?" And he said, "I am." Then he said to him, "Come home with me and eat bread." He said, "I may not return with you or go in with you, neither will I eat bread or drink water with you in this place. For I was told by the word of the Lord, 'You shall not eat bread or drink water there or return by the way that you came.'"

He answered, "I am a prophet also, as you are. And an angel spoke to me by the word of the Lord, saying, 'Bring him back with you to your house, that he may eat bread and drink water.'" But he lied to him. So the man from Judah went back with him and ate and drank water in his house. And as they sat at the table, the word of the Lord came to the prophet who brought him back.

And he cried to the man of God who came from Judah, "Thus says the Lord: Because you have disobeyed the word of the Lord and have not kept the command which the Lord your God commanded you, But have come back and have eaten bread and drunk water in the place of which the Lord said to you, 'Eat no bread and drink no water'—your corpse shall not come to the tomb of your fathers." And after the prophet of the house had eaten bread and drunk, he saddled the donkey for the man he had brought back. And when he had gone, a lion met him by the road and slew him, and his corpse was cast in the way, and the donkey stood by it; the lion also stood by the corpse.

The central theme of this story is obeying God, not man. If the Lord has declared we are to not behave or go in certain places, and we ignore that command because a brother or sister within the church talks us into ignoring the commands of God, we are the ones who will be judged for our decision to disobey the Lord.

Leaders and members of the church should be loved, and they should be respected, but they should never be given authority over the Lord's word. If there is a word to refrain from sin, we must obey God. We cannot listen to a lying spirit or lying word from anyone, even those who are working in the church alongside us.

If the young prophet had used his judgment, discretion, and godly wisdom, he would have never returned to the place God told him to leave. A blind trust in another person who has claimed to have heard from the Lord through an angel led this young prophet to lose his life. To remain safe from the enemy, all of us must be on guard and obedient to God, regardless of the position of the person we are dealing with. We must discern lying and unclean spirits operating within and outside of the Church, because they are functioning in both domains.

Proverbs 29:25 says, "The fear of man brings a snare, But whoever trusts in and puts his confidence in the Lord will be exalted and safe."

If we have the fear of saying no or being perceived as harsh or judgmental, this allows the devil access into our lives. If we are to maintain in a victorious position, we must judge others' work and deeds. We must know what God has told us to do and refuse to compromise with anyone speaking a different word. If anyone, on earth or Heaven, attempts to lead us away from God's word, and they illustrate characteristics and behaviors of unrighteousness, then we must be strong enough to rebuke them from influencing our lives.

Samson was called to be a judge for Israel and to defend holiness and truth, even from the womb. Judges 13:3–5 explains, "The angel of the Lord appeared to her and said, 'You are barren and childless, but you are going to become pregnant and give birth to a son. Now see to it that you drink no wine or other fermented drink and that you do not eat anything unclean. You will become pregnant and have a son whose head is never to be touched by a razor because the boy is to be a Nazirite, dedicated to God from the womb. He will take the lead in delivering Israel from the hands of the Philistines.'"

Samson had a purpose in life. He was set apart and special to God from his mother's womb. But Samson compromised with the enemy. Samson chose to permit ungodly women to come near him which was something God specifically instructed him not to do. And his willingness to welcome the enemies' women was all the devil needed to take him out of his calling and take his life from him.

Compromise is a weakness. Compromise allows the enemy to harm us. Without compromise, the enemy cannot stop, hurt, or carry out his attacks against the Church or against God. Throughout scripture, we see how compromise with the enemy led to the Israelites being taken into captivity or killed. We see men who were called to set themselves apart from their countries or their communities but failed to and as a result were destroyed.

Judges 15: 20 says, "And [Samson] judged (defended) Israel in the days of the Philistines twenty years." Samson did many great things for the Lord. He was able to defeat many of God's enemies, because he knew right from wrong, and he had a relationship with the Lord. But it only took one compromise of sin to destroy the calling on Samson's life and lead him into the enemy's captivity. When God chooses us, the enemy tries to take us captive and keep us in bondage, if he cannot stop us from doing God's work. He is only successful when we cooperate with him through sin.

Judges 16 explains, "Then Samson went to Gaza and saw a harlot there and went in to her. After this he loved a woman in the Valley of Sorek whose name was Delilah."

Samson permitted Satan to destroy him because he did not stand in purity with the Lord. He let evil near him when he was called to be set apart from sin and ungodliness. No one is too anointed, called, or chosen to not be removed from their position if they give in to sin. Sin is bondage and sin is a destroyer. If Satan is presented with the chance to forge an alliance with a member of God's army, he will propose a deceptive agreement designed to undermine and ultimately remove them from their purpose.

All believers are called to live separately from the world and from the demonic family of the enemy. We are called to keep sin from entering our homes and our hearts. The book of Judges confronts God's people, challenging them to live holy lives and to stop cohabiting with the enemy. Joshua and Caleb instructed the people to live holy and to destroy all the false gods, and they warned the people of the bondage that would come if they disobeyed this instruction from the Lord.

Codependent people tolerate the behaviors of others, even when those behaviors are toxic. Ultimately, codependent people contribute to maladaptive and even destructive behaviors in others, enabling those behaviors to continue because they will not set appropriate, healthy boundaries. Christians who refuse to confront sin are codependent, unhealthy, and in need of deliverance. Only through strong boundaries with others who are doing evil will we ever truly be free. If Christians cosign poor behavior and limit the consequences of the poor behavior, those behaviors are increased. This concept is biblical and is why the Lord instructed us to drive evil from the land so it would not grow in magnitude and consume us.

Codependent people fail to properly identify right from wrong, because they fail to see their influence and the position God has given to them to be an ambassador and a spokesman of justice. God did make His people into court officials of the land, and an analysis of the book of Judges teaches us that. Many Christians suffer from codependency. These Christians believe they are helping others when, indeed, they are hindering them.

If we refuse to address evil, that doesn't make evil go away, it only increases the problem. We are to drive evil out of the land as the Lord commanded. We are not to sleep with the enemy and tolerate evil to reign in our lives and in our neighbors' lives. Preaching, teaching, and proclaiming the words of God and the remission of sin is the only way to deliver and heal our land.

Testing and proving God's will, combined with analyzing and determining other people's agendas, are foundational components of a Christian's life. If Samson had properly judged the women he was linking up with, he would have never been involved with ungodly women. Without proper analysis and judgment, we will become one with the world we were called to be set apart from. We allow Satan to take away our power and strength, because we refuse to identify and stand against evil.

First Peter 5:8 declares, "Be sober [well balanced and self-disciplined], always be alert and cautious. That enemy of yours, the devil, prows around like a roaring lion [fiercely hungry], seeking someone to devour." To be sober is to be aware. When we are sober, we are judging and watching everything around us. Sobriety is true self-control. A lack of sobriety is to be out of touch and out of control. Drunk people are unaware of their surroundings, and they lack understanding and perception necessary for their safety.

God's people, the Israelites, were taken into captivity many times in the book of Judges because they did not confront the demons and the wicked people from their culture. By allowing evil spirits and evil people in their midst, the Israelites became slaves in a land they should have owned. After realizing their sins against God, the Israelites repented and asked the Lord to help them regain control of their land.

Judges 2:1–3 teaches, "Now the Angel of the Lord went up from Gilgal to Bochim. And He said, I brought you up from Egypt and have brought you to the land which I swore to give to your fathers, and I said, I will never break My covenant with you; And you shall make no covenant with the inhabitants of this land; but you shall break down their altars. But you have not obeyed My voice. Why have you done this? So now I say, I will not drive them out from before you; but they shall be as thorns in your sides, and their gods shall be a snare to you."

Antichrist beliefs, policies, and laws become the norm if godly people do not confront evil. Determining something is a violation in God's kingdom requires us to judge and to be sober within our social environment. When we see a violation of God's law being promoted and pushed on society, we are commanded by God to resist it, because Satan is attempting to destroy the United States of America through the infiltration of wicked law and policies.

Throughout history, the devil has used kings, rulers, or political leaders to stop God's people from prospering and continuing in the standards of holiness.

American believers must have an objective standard of truth based on the Bible and not based on the norms of American culture. American believers must yield themselves to God's voice alone, while rebuking the devil's voice. It is not satisfactory or just to be quiet and endure evil, allowing the evil to reign. Daniel could have prayed silently, quietly, and hidden when the king's degree required him to, but Daniel refused to hide in his ungodly culture. Daniel prayed boldly to the Lord, for all to see.

Culture cannot be our guiding force to determine right from wrong. Norms of society should not determine what we do or don't do. In the 1900s, almost all births in America took place at home. Today, almost all births take place within hospitals. In the 1900s, society promoted and celebrated home birth, and today it celebrates hospital birth. We must hear from God ourselves and not let anyone or anything—within or outside of the Church—change what we do and where we go.

Psalm 119:105 says, "Your word is a lamp to my feet And a light to my path."

Delilah deceived Samson to undermine his strength, presenting herself as a trustworthy ally to achieve her goal. Medical professionals who are unethical and biased can easily yield unhealthy power and act as agents of oppression by preying on the young mother and father's vulnerability and lack of knowledge. They will present themselves as allies, and if the parents fail to perceive providers as a potential threat, they will unwittingly reveal their vulnerabilities, believing it to be a safe course of action.

Just because someone has gone to school, held a good job, or seems innocent to society at large, does not mean individuals are not dangerous. Research has shown us the opposite. Oftentimes evil people are charismatic and can fool others. Many abusers hold important positions, seem great to outsiders, and set the legal odds in their favor to win against their abusee, if the abusee every attempted to step outside of the person's control. Many outsiders are blind and unbelieving when a person reports an abusive individual, because abusers have intentionally mastered deception and can paint their victims as crazy or incompetent.

Many people trust their medical providers, and they believe they are being cared for, but they are not. Like Samson, some lose their strength by trusting people who do not have their best interest in mind, even when they pretend that they do.

Most of us probably know people who have pretended to care for us, just as Delilah pretended to care for Samson. They will let us share our hearts and our vulnerabilities with them, only to use them against us. When I was sharing information with one of my doctors, I was sharing information with an enemy. She learned where I was vulnerable because I opened my heart to her. Then, she used those things to coax me into another cesarean birth, even when she knew I wanted a v-bac.

One way patients lose their power in the relationship is through informed consent paperwork. Informed consent paperwork is required by medical professionals to keep the patient from having a legal right to sue and win in a court of law. This is an intentional manipulation of the law. Without informed consent paperwork, people would have the right to sue for damage done to them or their children, but many cannot rightfully sue because they signed the informed consent paperwork.

Children have been harmed from vaccines, but because of their parents' approval of these vaccines through their signatures on the informed consent paperwork, no payout or responsibility is claimed by the administering doctors, nurses, or even the pharmaceutical companies. In the documentary *VAXXED: From Cover-Up to Catastrophe*, Dr. William Thompson, a CDC senior scientist and whistleblower, discusses how the CDC intentionally omitted data that showed a causal relationship between the MMR vaccine and autism.

Money is often the primary motivator influencing many medical practices. When money began to control healthcare in America, it was the beginning of many sorrows. The potential loss of money or licensing in the case of a lawsuit or medical liability claim is very significant to medical professionals, but patient welfare is not as important. Ethics have taken a backseat to financial profit, where medical professionals and pharmaceutical companies do, indeed, have a dog in the fight.

Insurance companies similarly influence medical decisions, such as what brand of medications people are prescribed, what tests are required, and what treatment plan is to be performed. More concerning, the leading reason mothers cited for choosing their provider for their pregnancy was "accepted health insurance" at 96 percent (Declercq, Sakala, Corry, Applebaum, & Herrlich 2014).

If women allow doctors intimate access to their lives, their decisions, and their babies primarily due to their insurance companies' approval of the doctor or practice, they are being controlled by money, and are not free to making their own decisions based on the merit of a doctor who may or may not be an enemy. First Timothy 6:10 tells us, "For the love of money is the root of all evil: which while some coveted after, they have erred from the faith, and pierced themselves through with many sorrows."

Parents have spiritual, legal authority for their lives and the lives of their children. God enables people to make choices that will affect their future as well as the future of their offspring, and God will never tell us to do something that will put us in danger. It is impossible to fully commit to God when we find ourselves in unequal partnerships with unbelievers and those who oppose His teachings. Therefore we must determine through our observations of others who is and who isn't on our team.

In the hospital setting, 32 percent of women have a cesarean birth. Cesarean rates have climbed from 4.5 percent to 31.9 percent since 1965, and hospital births have not improved infant mortality, which remains higher in the United States than in any other comparably wealthy nation. Maternal mortality ranks fifty-fifth in the world, after Russia, and is climbing. (The Legal Infrastructure of Childbirth).

However, "among 16,924 women who planned home births at the onset of labor, 89.1% gave birth at home. The rates of spontaneous vaginal birth, assisted vaginal birth, and cesarean were 93.6%, 1.2%, and 5.2%, respectively." (Cheyney, Bovbjerg, Everson, Gordon, Hannibal, & Vedam 2014). The data speaks for itself: Midwives attending home births have a 5.2 percent cesarean rate and the hospital has 32 percent.

These numbers should raise some red flags to mothers. If women needed so many interventions in the hospital, why can so many women successful birth their children unassisted at home? Why do the numbers prove that the practice of women birthing at home is more successful for vaginal births and reduced cesarean births? A 32 percent cesarean rate vs. 5.2 percent cesarean rate indicates something is wrong in the hospital setting. While some women do need medical intervention, such as a cesarean, they do not need it at the rate the hospitals are performing it.

Also, in the hospital setting women are regularly forced to go into labor prematurely. "In hospital births, between 27% and 41% of labors are induced, many without medical indication" (The Legal Infrastructure of Childbirth).

There is no chance God created women to have babies but left our bodies incapable of knowing when we are supposed to go into labor. For thousands of years women all over the world have birthed successfully and safely without interventions and medications to speed up their labor process. Studies have shown negative repercussions for children and mothers from both inductions and the drugs that speed up the labor process. We know these interventions can bring health and safety concerns.

For instance, "Compared to all other study groups, women exposed to Pitocin in labor combined with an epidural demonstrated significantly lower oxytocin levels during breastfeeding. Several studies have linked exposure to synthetic oxytocin to reductions in lactation, and diminished feeding-related behavior in the newborn" (Bell, Erickson, & Carter, 2014).

Because of the testimonies and the studies done on women who have birthed in hospitals, we know doctors are suggesting these interventions against best practice in medicine. We also know mothers and babies have been and continue to be harmed through unnecessary and too many medical interventions. When studies were done to collect data on the providers' reasoning for inductions, "quite a few women selected an indication that is not supported by best evidence such as provider's concern about the size of the baby (16%). The most commonly cited medical reasons were a provider's concern that the woman was overdue (18%) and a maternal health problem that required quick delivery (18%)" (Declercq, Sakala, Corry, Applebaum, & Herrlich 2014)

Inductions and medications that speed the labor process alter the timing of the baby's arrival. By inducing a woman, the medical professionals determine when the woman's body progresses for delivery, and they determine when the baby is born. Inductions work in complete opposition to faith. When a woman gets an induction, her body, and her baby's body, are insignificant in the birthing process. She loses complete control of her birth.

In these circumstances labor and the baby's birth is controlled by the healthcare provider instead of the woman's body and God. God has a time for babies to be born. God has a special process for labor and delivery. When medical professionals force the time because of their own expectations they are performing witchcraft at the expense of the woman and the child. They are using medical witchcraft to harm women and children.

Ecclesiastes 3:1–2 tells us, "There is a time for everything and a season for every activity under the heavens. A time to be born and a time to die, a time to plant and a time to uproot."

Traditional witchcraft involves practices such as rituals or spells to alter and control the outcome of events. In medical witchcraft, providers perform their rituals and use their potions to alter and control the outcome of events. Inductions, synthetic medications to speed up labor, epidurals, unnecessary cesarean births, birth control, abortions, and vaccines for babies all fall under the category of medical witchcraft. These potions and rituals attempt to alter, control, and change the God-ordained outcomes for women and children's lives.

While some assert that these interventions and procedures are intended to assist women—similar to the claims of white magic—clear evidence indicates the detrimental effects they have on the lives of women and children. It is important to recognize that God does not require the assistance of medical professionals. God does not need doctors to consistently intervene and dictate the outcomes of other people's lives.

When medical professionals use intervention to control labor and delivery, they start a chain of events leading to more intervention. Epidurals keep women in labor longer and alter the labor process. "Epidurals are associated with lower rates of spontaneous vaginal delivery, and a higher rate of instrumental vaginal delivery, longer labors" (Lieberman 2002). By using the epidural, women are positioned to need instrumental vaginal delivery because their bodies are medically hindered from properly progressing through the stages of labor as God intended.

Epidurals come with many risks outside of the increase in instrumental vaginal deliveries. "Epidural drugs pose a potential threat of neurotoxicity and other side effects. Local anesthetics (LA) are the main component in most epidural mixtures used in daily clinical practice. LA toxicity after systemic absorption of high doses of LA can produce central nervous system excitation with seizures, central nervous system inhibition, loss of airway reflexes, respiratory arrest, hemodynamic instability, and in extreme cases, coma or cardiovascular collapse" (van Zuylen, Ten Hoope, Bos, Hermanides, Stevens, & Hollmann 2019). Before taking an LA, do women really know and willingly consent to the dangers they are agreeing to?

Epidural opioids are also popular and have been used for over three decades, after receiving their United States Food and Drugs Administrations (FDA) approval in 1984. "The first studies ranging back as far as 1979. Since the introduction of epidural opioids, it is well-defined that they all share, to some extent, the adverse effects as known from their systemic administration. These include, but are not limited to, hypotension, sedation, nausea, vomiting, pruritus, urinary retention and respiratory depression, whereby pruritus occurs more often after epidural opioid administration.

Morphine is one of the most frequently used opioids in epidural anesthesia. It has long-lasting analgesic effects, especially in combination with LA. Epidural morphine can produce delayed respiratory depression" (van Zuylen, Ten Hoope, Bos, Hermanides, Stevens, & Hollmann 2019). When women are receive LA combined with epidurals, they are being put in great danger and so are their children. Most women are unaware of the real, studied dangers of their providers' suggestions.

"Childbirth is a significant and memorable life event for a woman and her family. Women's experiences of birth have both short and long-term effects on their health and wellbeing for them and for their infants" (Healy, Nyman, Spense, Otten, & Verhoeven 2020). Forcing women to give birth before their bodies and their babies are ready, or using too many interventions, is harmful and most importantly, regularly unnecessary. The biggest problem is most women believe they are safer because they are listening to their providers' guidance when most would really be safer declining these unnecessary interventions.

Many medical professionals begin planning for inductions, cesareans births, and using medications as soon as possible. Many doctors intervene in a woman's birth process from start to finish, and they never allow women to be in control of their birth. while putting women and children's lives in danger. There are many health benefits of women waiting on their bodies and allowing labor to develop naturally. Limiting interventions and medications is ideal, especially when most women are capable of delivering without them.

A woman's birthing experience should be considered when they are delivering their children. "Normal physiological birth is associated with the non-use of an epidural or other pharmacological pain relief, as it may affect the natural course of labour and can lead to rare but potentially severe adverse maternal effects. The same accounts for induction and augmentation of labour. Especially high doses of synthetic oxytocin may cause more and longer painful contractions when compared to normal labour" (Healy, Nyman, Spense, Otten, & Verhoeven 2020).

Studies show children's health, including cognitive benefits, are one of the reasons to delay a birth, refusing an induction or cesarean at 38 weeks. "Children born at 39-41 weeks have higher cognitive outcome scores compared to those born at early term (37–38 weeks). This should be considered when discussing timing of delivery" (Murray, Shenkin, Mcintosh, Lim, Grove, Pell, Norman, & Stock 2017). Babies need to have the proper amount of time in the womb to prepare to enter the world. Even two weeks or a week can make a difference in a child's readiness for cognitive or physical survival outside of the womb.

Many women are kept from natural birth when they chose to use a physician. Most do not know what they are signing up for. "We asked mothers who made the decision concerning a cesarean and when they made it. Almost two-thirds of mothers (63%) with primary cesareans indicated the doctor was the decision maker. For mothers with a repeat cesarean, the decision typically had been made before labor by either the provider (47%) or the mother (30%)" (Declercq, Sakala, Corry, Applebaum, & Herrlich 2014).

Mothers should never have their birth decided on solely by a physician. Doctors will intercede throughout a woman's pregnancy and her birth from start to finish. Many doctors will even recommend abortions and termination of a pregnancy if they deem the baby unfit to live or "unwell" due to a genetic deformation in their testing process. Mothers often consent to things pushed on them, but they may not agree with everything, and if women are in the hands of unethical, controlling providers, they are in danger and so is their child.

I had two medically controlled births. I was out of control with my pregnancy and my delivery. I followed the providers' recommendations at my own detriment. Sometimes we're safer breaking the "norms." Sometimes what is normalized is unhealthy and ungodly. Knowing when we need to say no and when we need to refuse unholy things pushed on us will protect us and ensure that we are walking within God's will, not a humans.

It is a misconception that most women are incapable of delivering their children naturally without medical interventions. In reality, many women possess the ability to give birth without the assistance of medical professionals. When women recognize and embrace their inherent strength and capability to give birth independently, it fosters a sense of empowerment. Natural childbirth reinforces a women's strength and serves as a profound source of true empowerment.

Some people want to take our strength and they do not have our best interest in heart. These are unholy alliances. Then, there are those who encourage us to be strong. These are the people God uses to keep us walking on His intended course. With my third child, I found two people who helped me walk God's path; my midwife and my doula. Thankfully, they believed in me, and didn't push any medical interventions or unnecessary procedures on me. My birth was natural and the way that God intended it to be before the world of medical witchcraft—through an overemphasis on "science"—took over the birthing model.

By trusting God and returning to the basics of womanhood, I found a level of freedom I had never experienced. I was empowered during pregnancy, birth, and beyond. I have been forever changed because I realize I can say no to things that don't benefit me. And when we say no out of an obedience to God, we will always find heightened levels of freedom, even if the world doesn't understand or doesn't like it.

A few days before my birth, God gave me a verse to encourage me. Let it be an encouragement to you today. Isaiah 66:9 tells us, "'Shall I bring to the moment of birth, and not give delivery?' says the Lord. 'Or shall I who gives delivery shut the womb?' says your God."

I knew God would get me through my pregnancy and birth because He promised me He would take care of my baby and me. I trusted Him more than I trusted humans or medical science, and God rewarded my faith—and I will never be the same.

Things are not always as they seem. Witchcraft is a big illusion promising and pretending to be holy and good. We must watch and determine what is good and what is not. We must be judging everything by God's standards of truth and justice, regardless of what is expected in the culture around us. As we judge and stay sober, watching everything and everyone around us, God will show us who is for us and who isn't. He will guide us into all truth and show us the way He wants us to go. Who is telling you where to go? Is it God or is it someone else?

It is believed white magic originated in Egypt, where magicians used charms, spells, and rituals to harness power and influence people's health. We know Satan is behind all magic, and God warns us to stay away from witchcraft. Plenty of health professionals are practicing witches or warlocks. They harness "power" and use "spells, potions, and rituals" to change the destiny and the health of people. Be sure you know who is for you and who is against you. Be sure you stand with God and refuse to cooperate with demon spirits for your health and your well-being. *Your future and your children's future depend on it. Who is telling you your future?*

14

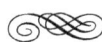

Dreams, Visions, and Trances

The Bible is supernatural book. All Bible stories became possible because of God's supernatural power. Jonah was swallowed by a whale and lived to preach; Jesus' walked on water and rose from the dead; people heard, saw, and were healed despite being blind or deaf from their mothers' wombs. All these situations required God's supernatural presence. The Bible is not natural, and believers' experiences have never been explainable by human reasoning and logic.

Our trust in God and His word permits us to see natural laws shift to make room for the supernatural. To experience God personally, we must tap into the spirit world while operating within the physical world. A very real spiritual world exists beyond the five human senses. If we want to see it, we must first believe it exists. John 4:24 tells us, "God is spirit [the Source of life, yet invisible to mankind], and those who worship Him must worship in spirit and truth."

Spirits are invisible. We cannot perceive them with the human eye. Wind is real and so is oxygen, but we cannot see these elements. We can see the effects of oxygen or the wind, but we cannot see the wind or oxygen.

Many things exist within the physical world that cannot be seen with the naked eye, but they can be experienced and proven to exist.

The spirit world is one of the things we can experience, and we can prove it exists, even if we can't always see it.

God started interacting with me and helping me before I got saved. God's voice drew me to the cross and to repentance, before I did anything to deserve His help. Seeing the kingdom of God and experiencing God comes after we hear about God. Bartimaeus was a blind man who heard that Jesus was coming. At first, he could not see or experience Jesus personally, but he used his faith to get close to Jesus so he could begin to see and know Jesus for himself.

Like Bartimaeus, we can know God exists and hear others talk about Him. We can hear in the spirit, and receive the testimonies of others through the spirit, even if we have not had a personal encounter with Jesus. If we want a personal encounter with Jesus we must hear the truth and decide if we want to interact with Him. Hearing is only the first part of the encounter.

Mark 10:47–52 teaches, "Then they came to Jericho. And as He was leaving Jericho with His disciples and a great crowd, Bartimaeus, a blind beggar, a son of Timaeus, was sitting by the roadside. And when he heard that it was Jesus of Nazareth, he began to shout, saying, 'Jesus, Son of David, have pity and mercy on me [now]!' And many severely censured and reproved him, telling him to keep still, but he kept on shouting out all the more, 'You Son of David, have pity and mercy on me [now]!' And Jesus stopped and said, 'Call him.' And they called the blind man, telling him, 'Take courage! Get up! He is calling you.' And throwing off his outer garment, he leaped up and came to Jesus. And Jesus said to him, 'What do you want Me to do for you?' And the blind man said to Him, 'Master, let me receive my sight.' And Jesus said to him, 'Go your way; your faith has healed you.' And at once he received his sight and accompanied Jesus on the road."

Spiritual senses are important. To be healthy spiritually, we need to hear, see, and experience God using our spiritual senses. The spiritual senses can be activated or deactivated in our lives, but we need all of them to be healthy. When we only utilize some of the spiritual senses, we do not properly operate in the spirit because we are hindered, just as someone is hindered physically without their physical senses. Without all five of our spiritual senses, we don't properly analyze our surroundings.

When we come to Jesus for full spiritual healing, we will operate on a higher level because we have everything we need to be successful in the realm of the spirit and the physical world. Everything that exists in the physical realm exists because of the spiritual realm. When people attempt to live as physical beings but are crippled in the spirit, they will never interact with the world in the way they were created to. They are disabled from fully participating with life.

Someone may describe a cake to us, but if we could never eat the cake ourselves, we would never truly know what cake takes like. People can tell us about Jesus, but if we have never experienced Him ourselves, we will never know who He is. There is no substitute for knowing Jesus and understanding who God is and what He wants us to do. Just like we can't have someone else eat for us, we cannot have someone else tell us who we are and what we are to do in the realm of the spirit. We must experience spiritual things ourselves.

Regardless of the context, our understanding is profoundly shaped by personal experiences. The interpretation of events by others is insufficient in comparison to our own revelations. Whether through taste, sound, sight, touch, or smell, the essence of someone else's lived experience cannot be fully conveyed to us. It is essential that we engage with the world directly. Hearing a song offers a distinctly different experience than simply being informed about it.

When God interacts with us, no one can convince us we didn't have an experience with God. An experience with the Lord is just as real as eating a sandwich or hearing a song. God meets with us, talks with us, and teaches us things, all within the realm of the spirit. We fully encounter and experience the supernatural when we come near to God, and He interacts with us.

Walking with the Lord as His child is a fully immersive experience. Once we learn to hear, see, experience, and taste the things of God, we can quickly identify things working in opposition to God. God's word tastes, smells, feels, and looks different than the devil's words. An interaction with Jesus is vastly different than an interaction with a devil.

In the same way we can taste, see, or smell rotten food, we can do the same in the realm of the spirit. First Corinthians 10:21 declares, "You cannot drink [both] the Lord's cup and the cup of demons. You cannot share in both the Lord's table and the table of demons [thereby becoming partners with them]."

Dreams, visions, and trances are ways God communicates messages to us. Through these, we can hear, see, and experience God through the spiritual realm. Dreams, visions, and trances are fully immersive spiritual experiences. When we are given a dream, a vision, or a trance, all our spiritual senses are activated. We can fully perceive and receive the will and the words of God or the words and plans of the enemy.

As we draw near to the return of Jesus Christ, we will see an acceleration of the supernatural, both the good and the evil. Some supernatural experiences pull people away from the truth and some will pull people towards it. The framework a person uses to determine what is happening to him or her and to the world will determine the person's response to the spiritual things increasing and revealing themselves within the earth. If you want to understand what is happening, and you want to perceive the truth, then that spiritual understanding can only come through Jesus Christ, the Son of God.

If we are going to properly understand what is happening in the supernatural realm, we must regularly have experiences with Gods' Spirit. Some experiences are auditory, visual, or through smell, and some are through taste. Others are through touch, like the woman who reached out and touched Jesus's robe for her healing. An understanding and proper use of the five spiritual senses allow us to fully immerse ourselves in the spirit realm.

Experiences are encounters or direct observations through participation. Experience comes from immersion. Relying on someone else's spiritual senses can only take us so far. Many things in the physical world, as well as the spiritual one, require us to take responsibility for our lives. Many times, if we want something, we must get it for ourselves. We are responsible for our lives and our health.

John 5:6–9 tells us, "When Jesus noticed him lying there [helpless], knowing that he had already been a long time in that condition, He said to him, 'Do you want to become well? [Are you really in earnest about getting well?]' The invalid answered, 'Sir, I have nobody when the water is moving to put me into the pool; but while I am trying to come [into it] myself, somebody else steps down ahead of me.' Jesus said to him, 'Get up! Pick up your bed (sleeping pad) and walk!' Instantly the man became well and recovered his strength and picked up his bed and walked. But that happened on the Sabbath."

When this man took responsibility for his healing, he was healed. Jesus was able to heal Him through word and auditory alone. Scripture tells us the man did not even know who had healed him, but he heard his commands, which means we can have and auditory experience and receive from Jesus before we fully know who He is.

John 5:12–13 says, " They asked him, 'Who is the Man Who told you, Pick up your bed and walk?' Now the invalid who had been healed did not know who it was, for Jesus had quietly gone away [had passed on unnoticed], since there was a crowd in the place."

When this man first received from Jesus, He was unsure of who Jesus was. He did not know the conditions of his healing. Later, Jesus revealed Himself on a deeper level to the man. He told the man what he needed to do to continue walking in his healing. John 5:14 tells us, "Afterward, when Jesus found him in the temple, He said to him, 'See, you are well! Stop sinning or something worse may happen to you.' The man went away and told the Jews that it was Jesus Who had made him well."

I can testify about my experience with Jesus in this same manner when He saved me and healed me. I heard about Jesus, and when I needed healing, I went to Jesus. I asked Him to help me and save me, and He did before I fully knew who He was. After He healed me, He began to instruct me in what I needed to do if I was going to stay well. He continues to show me how to keep my healing and remain strong. He regularly teaches me what to avoid and what to partake in.

If we have only eaten rotten or nasty food, we do not have proper perspective to identify how bad the food truly is. When we become used to eating healthy, whole foods and we are presented with a rotten fruit, we quickly identify the problem with the subpar food. Eve should have identified the fruit in the garden as rotten. She should have seen it was inferior to what she was accustomed to, and she should have refrained from eating it to remain alive. There are many foods in the spirit realm; there are heavenly angelic foods and there are demonic foods.

First Kings 9:5–8 explains, "He lay down and slept under the juniper tree, and behold, an angel touched him and said to him, 'Get up and eat.' He looked, and by his head there was a bread cake baked on hot coal, and a pitcher of water. So he ate and drank and lay down again. Then the angel of the Lord came again a second time and touched him and said, 'Get up, and eat, for the journey is too long for you [without adequate sustenance].' So he got up and ate and drank, and with the strength of that food he traveled forty days and nights to Horeb (Sinai), the mountain of God."

We are not supposed to eat demonic food as believers. However, there are also foods we need to eat to remain healthy and strong in spirit. Kings eat the best of the land but commoners or prisoners do not. When someone is in prison he or she will eat prison food, and when someone lives in the palace, he or she will eat the food of the kings and royals. We should know the difference between prison food and palace food.

Proverbs 31:4–7 explains, "It is not for kings, O Lemuel, It is not for kings to drink wine, Or for rulers to desire strong drink, Otherwise they drink and forget the law and its decrees, And pervert the rights and justice of all the afflicted. Give strong drink [as medicine] to him who is ready to pass away, And wine to him whose life is bitter. Let him drink and forget his poverty And no longer remember his trouble."

The best food and the best of the land is reserved for those who are in God's family. As believers, we have been set apart to be special, royal, and honorable. God wants us to eat the best of the land. Yet, we know not everyone called to eat palace food chooses to eat. Isaiah 1:19 says, "If you are willing and obedient you will eat the best of the land." This scripture informs us that if we are not willing and obedient we will not eat the best food even when we have been authorized to do so.

When Elijah was given the food from Heaven, he went higher into the heavenly dimension. He went to the mountain of God. We are positioned on a higher level than those who are not saved and sanctified by the blood of Jesus. With our position in Christ comes responsibility to refrain from eating and drinking things tainted by evil. We are to refrain from eating and drinking the same things the world eats and drinks, *while choosing to eat the supernatural food from Heaven*

We can eat angelic bread. We can nourish our spiritual bodies through our decision to eat in the way the Lord instructs us to eat. We have heavenly bodies, and our heavenly bodies are to be nourished by heavenly food. In the same way we can choose to eat whole, healthy foods on the earth for our physical health. We can choose to eat whole healthy foods in the realm of the spirit, and what we choose impacts our spirits. Psalm 78:25 explains, "Man ate the bread of angels; God sent them provision in abundance."

The Bible is the written word of God, and God's Spirit brings the Bible to life when we read it. When the Spirit of God illuminates or brings light to us through revelation knowledge, we connect with the scriptures in a powerful way. Scriptures will "jump out at us" or speak to us directly, even when we may have heard them or read them before, because God's Spirit is present and brings light to the scripture for us.

Seeing the truth is introductory to living a healthy spiritual life. Blindness can impact our entire bodies. When we are not able to see the truth and determine a lie from the truth, we are hindered in our entire spirituality. Matthew 6:22 says, *"The eye is the lamp of the body. If your eyes are healthy, your whole body will be full of light. But if your eyes are unhealthy, your whole body will be full of darkness. If then the light within you is darkness, how great is that darkness!"*

We need the Holy Spirit and the help of God's ordained angels to receive light and revelation. Anytime we see, hear, or experience God's word personally, we have been helped by the Holy Spirit or God's appointed workers. God shows us who He is through experiences, and He directs us into truth. When Paul saw the light, he saw the truth, and this was the beginning of his spiritual conversion. To see the truth, we must receive God's light and the lamp of God. We need healthy spiritual lenses.

The closer we are to Jesus, the more we will experience everything intimately in the supernatural realm. When we sit at the King's table and we live in the King's palace, we will regularly eat the King's food! As we spend time in the light, we will see everything more clearly. The voice of a stranger or enemy forces become noticeably different than God's voice. Rotten food becomes noticeably rotten, and heavenly food becomes what we crave.

First Peter 2:2 declares, "Like newborn babies [you should] long for the pure milk of the word, so that by it you may be nurtured and grow in respect to salvation [its ultimate fulfillment]."

Although dreams are a fully immersive spiritual experience, they are not exclusive to believers. Some in Scripture who were disconnected from God still received dreams from the Lord. God will allow all people to experience Him in a supernatural way, and anyone who rejects God does so willingly. Not one person on the earth can be excused from not knowing whom God is and that He exists.

Romans 1:20 says, "For ever since the creation of the world His invisible nature and attributes, that is, His eternal power and divinity, have been made intelligible and clearly discernible in and through the things that have been made (His handiworks). So [men] are without excuse [altogether without any defense or justification],"

Abimelech the king was warned in a dream not to harm Sarah when she was brought into his house. The dream God gave to Abimelech, an unbeliever, directed him and made an impression on him. Abimelech and all of his household knew the dream was supernatural and that God had spoken on behalf of Abraham and Sarah. Abimelech and his servants were all terrified by the supernatural occurrence. They were in shock and knew God had sent the dream.

Genesis 20:2–8 says, "Abraham said [again] of his wife, 'She is my sister.' So, Abimelech king of Gerar sent and took Sarah [into his harem]. But God came to Abimelech in a dream during the night, and said, 'Behold, you are a dead man because of the woman whom you have taken [as your wife], for she is another man's wife.' Now Abimelech had not yet come near her; so he said, 'Lord will you kill a people who are righteous and innocent and blameless [regarding Sarah]? Did Abraham not tell me, "She is my sister?" And she herself said, "He is my brother." In the integrity of my heart and innocent of my hands I have done this.' Then God said to him in the dream, 'Yes, I know you did this in the integrity of your heart, for it was I who kept you back and spared you from sinning against Me; therefore, I did not give you an opportunity to touch her. So now return the man's wife, for he is a prophet, and he will pray for you, and you will live. But if you do not return her [to him], know that you shall die, you and all who are yours (your household).' So Abimelech got up early in the morning and called all his servants and told them all these things; and the men were terrified."

Some intellectuals think dreams are insignificant or are just a happenstance occurrence. These individuals say dreams may come from eating too much before bed or from the unconscious mind but hold little weight as to their meaning or significance. However, scripture tells us people know dreams are supernatural, and when they have a personal and intimate dream from God, it will impact them, even if they pretend it doesn't.

We can put too much emphasis on dreams or put trust in a demonic vision or a demonic dream if we are not accustomed to identifying what we are experiencing in the spiritual realm. God is the source of wisdom and discernment. Without God's light shining into our spirits, we are blind to see the true nature or meaning of the things we see in the spirit realm. Daniel 2:21 teaches, "He changes times and seasons; he deposes kings and raises up others. He gives wisdom to the wise and knowledge to the discerning."

Living in a dream world and never properly analyzing, understanding, or applying our dreams is problematic. Many people have been given demonic visions and have birthed demonic dreams and visions into the world. A dream is given to us, and then we decide if we are going to act on the dream and bring it to life into the world. If we do not know which dreams are demonic and which come from God, we will be confused and birth things into our lives we were never meant to birth.

Babies and young children frequently explore their environment by placing objects in their mouths, including items that are not safe for ingestion. This behavior is part of their developmental process as they learn to identify food and engage their physical senses. Similarly, we must cultivate our ability to recognize and understand the supernatural realm. It is essential for us to learn and grow in our discernment of what we are experiencing.

Dreams are first conceived in the spirit. We see the dream, we experience the dream, and we nurture the dream inside our hearts. When a dream, whether good or bad, is allowed to grow and occupy our hearts it will be born, if it is not aborted. To abort a dream, we must discard it and not allow it to enter our hearts or influence our actions.

God-given dreams are aborted in some people's lives, and demonic-given dreams are birthed in others. We determine what we grow and what we receive from the spiritual realm. We determine what we conceive and birth.

Martin Luther King Jr. is known for his speech, "I have a dream." God gave Martin Luther King Jr. a dream in his heart and spirit, and he then acted upon this dream and brought it into existence through his decisions and his determination. Dreams begin in the spirit realm; they begin deep within the heart as a baby begins deep within the womb. His dream was born into the world because he held onto his dream, gave it time to grow and develop, and did the painful labor to see it come into existence.

The American dream is the belief that anyone, regardless of where they were born or whom they are, can attain their vision and dreams of success, and experience upward mobility in life if they are willing to believe in their dream and perform the work. The American dream begins in the heart, and then, through faith, hard work, and sacrifice, the dream can become a reality for the one who believes. The American dream is not an illusion or delusion, but a reality for anyone who wants to believe it exists and receive it.

Dreams and visions should always be in alignment with God's word if they are going to bring good things into our future. Meditating on God's word gives us dreams and visions, drawing us towards a place of success and prosperity. As Isaac went to mediate and pray to God, he supernaturally received a wife God had chosen for him. Isaac's future was impacted by what he saw after he spent time in mediation and prayer. Genesis 24:63 teaches, "Isaac went out to bow down [in prayer] in the field in the [early] evening; he raised his eyes and looked, and camels were coming."

When we meditate on God's word, we are dwelling in His presence. This dwelling place is an experience with God. When we are in God's presence, we know which way to go and what to do. We clearly see right from wrong, and we are so in tune with the Lord that we do not even need the written law to know truth from a lie. God's presence and His Spirit show us personally and intimately. We know because we are accustomed to spending time in God's presence. Galatians 5:18 explains, "But if you are led by the Spirit, you are not under the Law."

If we do not use our spiritual senses, we need the written word as a physical guide because it is all we have to use if we want to hear from the Lord. People who cannot see, hear, taste, or feel in the spirit need help knowing right from wrong and good from evil in a physical, natural, and tangible way. The Bible was given to help us, but when God created us, He didn't create us to need a Bible to talk to Him. He made us for personal relationship using our spiritual senses. Ephesians 2:6 explains we are seated with Christ in the Heavens. We have access to the throne of God.

God wants us to experience Him. It is possible for us to write God's word on our heart. It is possible for us to know what God wants us to do and to see what God wants us to see without the Bible revealing it to us first. Many times, I have dreams or see visions in the spiritual realm, and then I research the Bible, and I find the things I saw in the spirit. God has shown me things plenty of times, and I didn't know those things were in the word until I saw them using my spirit senses first.

Joshua 1:8 *teaches,* "This Book of the Law shall not depart out of your mouth, but you shall meditate on it day and night, that you may observe and do according to all that is written in it. For then you shall make your way prosperous, and then you shall deal wisely and have good success."

Dreams, visions, and spiritual experiences should lead us into a deeper relationship with God. They should lead us into God's truth for ourselves or for others. Aliens and demonic forces can hijack dreams or visions, and it is possible for someone to be led off course entirely by demonic influence through a dream or a vision. If a dream or a vision is in direct opposition to God and His word and His nature, then we know it does not come from God. All God-given dreams should pull us closer to God and should strengthen us in our relationship to God. Our dreams, visions, and spiritual experiences should testify of God's known character.

Men like Abraham did not have the written word of God. The Bible did not exist. They heard from God directly. They knew which dreams and visions came from God. They knew when God was speaking to them because they knew how to identify His voice . Spiritual senses help us to operate like our spiritual forefathers. We can interact with God, and we know God is speaking to us because we know how to use our spiritual senses to navigate the spiritual terrain.

Abraham did not question if it was the Lord who told him he would be the father of many nations. He didn't need the Bible to verify the word from God. He heard it from God directly and personally, so he believed God. We will not be confused or tricked by the enemy in the spirit realm if we are accustomed to using our spiritual senses. We will always know when something is foreign or when it is domestic. We know when the message is coming from the enemy or from our Commander and Chief.

Dreams and visions can come from the demonic realm. Unlearned spiritual people have a hard time determining the source of their visions and dreams. They are influenced by the demonic because they don't properly hear and see in the spiritual realm. Witches hear in the spirit, and they can see in the spirit, but the things they see are not clear to them because they do not see the truth in the spirit world; they have been taken off course by the enemy who tells them lies instead of truths.

Jeremiah 23:27 says, "Who intends to make My people forget My name by their dreams which they relate to one another, just as their fathers forgot My name because of Baal?"

Jeremiah 29:8 warns us, "For thus says the Lord of hosts, the God of Israel, 'Do not let your prophets who are in your midst and your diviners deceive you, and do not listen to the dreams which they dream.'"

Dreams and visions are revelatory gifts that give people understanding about God and the world beyond. Dreams and visions provide future information and prophecy. The futures of our lives are determined by the dreams and the visions we follow. The choice to pursue a God-given dream will produce a righteous and godly harvest within our lives. Yet, those who see visions and dreams from the demonic realm will produce demonic futures impacting their lives and others' lives.

Analyzing our dreams and visions is not hard when we are used to sitting in the heavenly realm next to God. Soldiers in battle spend no time differentiating a foreign threat. They know who is on their side and who is working for the enemy. The enemy's team is noticeably foreign. Development in the spirit realm provides us with wisdom in interpreting spiritual messages as development helps children to identify what is to be eaten and what is not.

Revelation and prophecy have been and always will be a part of how God communicates with humanity on the earth. We can always consult with God, and He will respond, to confirm and properly encode the message sent. Many times when I receive a word from the Lord, I ask the Lord to verify the word. God doesn't mind providing us with assurance; in fact He expects us to test the things we hear, see, or experience in the realm of the spirit. First John 4:1 says, "Beloved, do not believe every spirit, but test the spirits to see whether they are from God."

Gideon experienced God and angels. He interacted in the realm of the spirit. In Judges 6 he asked the Lord to verify he was hearing from Him. He asked God to verify what He heard and experienced. Judges 6:17–23 explains, "And Gideon said to God, If You will deliver Israel by my hand as You have said, Do not leave here, I pray You, until I return to You and bring my offering and set it before You. And He said,

I will wait until you return. Then Gideon went in and prepared a kid and unleavened cakes of an ephah of flour. The meat he put in a basket and the broth in a pot, and brought them to Him under the oak and presented them. And the Angel of God said to him, Take the meat and unleavened cakes and lay them on this rock and pour the broth over them. And he did so.

Then the Angel of the Lord reached out the tip of the staff that was in His hand, and touched the meat and the unleavened cakes, and there flared up fire from the rock and consumed the meat and the unleavened cakes. Then the Angel of the Lord vanished from his sight. And when Gideon perceived that He was the Angel of the Lord, Gideon said, Alas, O Lord God! For now I have seen the Angel of the Lord face to face! he Lord said to him, Peace be to you, do not fear; you shall not die."

Gideon had a custom of interacting with God and asking Him to confirm the message. Gideon wanted to be sure He was making the decisions the Lord wanted him to make. God would rather us ask Him for assurance than not ask Him at all. When we need assurance and help from God we should never hesitate to ask Him for a sign and a conformation as Gideon did. Judges 6:36–40 teaches, "And Gideon said to God, If You will deliver Israel by my hand as You have said, Behold, I will put a fleece of wool on the threshing floor. If there is dew on the fleece only and it is dry on all the ground, then I shall know that You will deliver Israel by my hand, as You have said. And it was so. When he rose early next morning and squeezed the dew out of the fleece, he wrung from it a bowlful of water. And Gideon said to God, Let not your anger be kindled against me, and I will speak but this once. Let me make trial only this once with the fleece, I pray you; let it now be dry only upon the fleece and upon all the ground let there be dew. And God did so that night, for it was dry on the fleece only, and there was dew on all the ground."

When Jesus communicated with God, we know He received visions from heaven. We know God showed Him future prophetic events. Jesus saw Nathanael under the fig tree in the spirit realm. Nathanael recognized Jesus as the Son of God and the King of Isreal, because he perceived Jesus' supernatural, spiritual vision. Jesus didn't need to see Nathanael in the natural to see him and know him in the spirit.

John 1:47–51 tells us, "Jesus saw Nathanael coming toward Him and said concerning him, 'See! Here is an Israelite indeed [a true descendant of Jacob], in whom there is no guile nor deceit nor falsehood nor duplicity!' Nathanael said to Jesus, 'How do You know me? [How is it that You know these things about me?]' Jesus answered him, 'Before [ever] Philip called you, when you were still under the fig tree, I saw you.' Nathanael answered, 'Teacher, You are the Son of God! You are the King of Israel!' Jesus replied, 'Because I said to you, I saw you beneath the fig tree, do you believe in and rely on and trust in Me? You shall see greater things than this!' Then He said to him, 'I assure you, most solemnly I tell you all, you shall see heaven opened, and the angels of God ascending and descending upon the Son of Man!'"

Jesus also instructed His disciples how to handle future events in the physical realm. He saw what would happen before it happened, because he perceived it within the spirit realm. Jesus' spiritual insight allowed Him to instruct the disciples on what to do next, and like Jesus, we can use these prophetic gifts to direct our lives and others' lives. We can see what is coming and warn or instruct others for their betterment or for their protection.

Matthew 21:1–6 teaches, "And when they came near Jerusalem and had reached Bethphage at the Mount of Olives, Jesus sent two disciples on ahead, Saying to them, 'Go into the village that is opposite you, and at once you will find a donkey tied, and a colt with her; untie [them] and bring [them] to Me. If anyone says anything to you, you shall reply, "The Lord needs them," and he will let them go without delay.' This happened that what was spoken by the prophet might be fulfilled, saying, 'Say to the Daughter of Zion [inhabitants of Jerusalem], Behold, your King is coming to you, lowly and riding on a donkey, and on a colt, the foal of a donkey [a beast of burden].' Then the disciples went and did as Jesus had directed them."

From Genesis to Revelation, men and women of God saw, heard, tasted, and experienced the spiritual realm from their natural physical bodies. The scriptures do not inform us that these gifts and experiences would cease to exist or diminish over time, so we can know the Lord is still using supernatural means to communicate with His people today as He has for thousands of years.

Revelation 1:10 explains, "On the Lord's Day I was in the Spirit, and I heard behind me a loud voice like a trumpet,"

John, living in the body of a man, was able to travel into the spirit and hear. John also saw and experienced His vision from the Lord. Revelation 1:1–2 tells us, "The revelation from Jesus Christ, which God gave him to show his servants what must soon take place. He made it known by sending his angel to his servant John, who testifies to everything he saw—that is, the word of God and the testimony of Jesus Christ."

When we are asleep, we exist in another realm that does not require our physical bodies to move. We taste, see, smell, feel, and hear, but we do so outside of our physical bodies. Dreams provide us with a glimpse of the spirit realm's existence, and they allow us to verify that we are more than our physical bodies. We do not need our physical bodies to experience the spiritual realm. In a dream, we verify the existence of the spirit realm.

Joseph, Jesus's earthly father, received protective dreams that impacted his family. An angel gave Joseph his first dream, and Joseph did exactly as the angel had commanded him in the dream. Joseph's quick obedience to his first dream from the Lord impacted his family's future. We saw the same quick obedience to God in the story of Abimelech. Both men, upon waking, knew what the Lord instructed them to do and proceeded to do it.

God-given dreams are straightforward and informative, providing us with direction or assurance. If our dreams bother or confuse us, then the dream originated from Satan, not from God. First Corinthians 14:33 states, "For God is not a God of confusion but of peace."

Joseph and Abimelech knew they had encountered God, and they knew what they needed to do. When God speaks, He doesn't bring confusion. He brings clarity and perspective. He guides us into all the truth by bringing light. Second Timothy 2:7 says, "Think over what I said, for the Lord will give you understanding in everything."

Dreams, visions, and prophecy are linked. God sends His people group prophecies and personal prophecy verifying His plans. Joseph's first dream provided Joseph with comfort. It helped him know his family's future, even giving him Jesus' name. Before Jesus was born, prophets could determine that a child would be born, and even where He would be born. But Joseph and Mary both needed the Lord to minister to them personally, through dreams and angelic visitations, to receive the personal, intimate prophetic guidance for baby Jesus.

Matthew 1:20–25 tells us, "But after he had considered this, an angel of the Lord appeared to him in a dream and said, 'Joseph's son of David, do not be afraid to take Mary home as your wife, because what is conceived in her is from the Holy Spirit. She will give birth to a son, and you are to give him the name Jesus, because he will save his people from their sins.' All this took place to fulfill what the Lord had said through the prophet: 'The virgin will conceive and give birth to a son, and they will call him Immanuel.'"

Joseph's second dream provided protection for Joseph and his family. God prepared Joseph by telling him what was going on where they were living and where he needed to go. King Herod attempted to get rid of the baby boys using his natural knowledge of the scriptures. If the scriptures had been all encompassing with the baby's location, then Jesus, Mary, and Joseph would have been in danger. So, God used personal prophecy to communicate with His people. He used the written word and the spiritual spoken word to speak to those who loved Him.

Some prophetic words from the Lord are intentionally hidden. God hides the personal message from the world to protect His people. He doesn't share all things will all people. He decides who gets information and when they get it. God speaks messages in private, and He communicates to individuals personally when He needs to. Amos 3:7 promises us, "Surely the Lord God does nothing unless He reveals His secret counsel to His servants the prophets."

King Herod wanted to kill the baby boys to protect his kingship. He tried to use the Scriptures to locate Jesus. Herod knew the Scriptures were the words of God, so He tried to use them against God and His people. The Scriptures did provide information about the birth and life of the baby boy, but God left out information, to hide a deeper truth from an evil man. Herod couldn't see, hear, or interact in the spirit, so He was blind, deaf, and unable to receive the supernatural information to be successful against God.

Matthew 2:13 tells us, "Now when they [the wise men] had departed, behold, an angel of the Lord appeared to Joseph in a dream, saying, 'Arise and take the Child and His mother, and flee to Egypt, and remain there until I tell you; for Herod is going to search for the Child to destroy Him.'"

God protects us and shows us things the world cannot see or comprehend, even when they try their best. Without spiritual assistance, people are limited to the natural realm. Many people in history tried to use God's prophets to learn secret spiritual truths, but wise prophets only speak what God wants them to, intentionally concealing deep spiritual plans from the wicked.

When King Herod died, an angel appeared to Joseph a third time in a dream. This time the angel told Joseph that it was safe to leave Egypt and to take Jesus to the land of Israel. Joseph again had supernatural, prophetic information. He knew the king was dead. He knew where he and his family would live safely in the future. Joseph's God-given dreams were necessary information about the plans of his enemy, and they guided Joseph into the places he needed to go on the earth.

Matthew 2:19–20 explains, "After Herod died, an angel of the Lord appeared in a dream to Joseph in Egypt and said, 'Get up, take the child and His mother and go to the land of Israel, for those who were trying to take the child's life are dead.'"

Matthew 2:22–23 tells us, "But when he heard that Archelaus was reigning in Judea in place of his father Herod, he was afraid to go there. Having been warned in a dream, he withdrew to the district of Galilee, and he went and lived in a town called Nazareth. So was fulfilled what was said through the prophets that he would be called a Nazarene."

Dreams provide parents with insight and protection for their children's lives. Without the prophetic dreams God gave Joseph, his family would have been in danger multiple times. Joseph, Mary, and Jesus would have been in the wrong places at the wrong times, instead of in the right places at the right times without God's prophetic instructions.

Prophets are a group of men and women in the church who regularly see dreams and visions. Prophets have a gift of prophecy. While not everyone is a prophet, everyone can receive dreams and visions from God when they need them. If God sent evil men like Abimelech dreams to warn them, He will send his children dreams and visions too. When we receive a dream or other message from heaven, we can receive help from prophets, if we are unsure of the meaning. But ultimately, God must give us the interpretation.

Genesis 40:5–8 says, "And they both dreamed a dream in the same night, each man according to [the personal significance of] the interpretation of his dream—the butler and the baker of the king of Egypt, who were confined in the prison. When Joseph came to them in the morning and looked at them, he saw that they were sad and depressed. So he asked Pharaoh's officers who were in custody with him in his master's house, 'Why do you look so dejected and sad today?' And they said to him, 'We have dreamed dreams, and there is no one to interpret them.' And Joseph said to them, 'Do not interpretations belong to God? Tell me [your dreams], I pray you.'"

God may give us a dream to start a business, to begin a church, to start a homegroup, or to join a ministry. He will guide us in our sleep and in our waking hours, if we come near to Him and dwell in His presence. When we are inspired to do something, and we know the dream or vision is coming from the Lord, we must know it is for our protection and never for our detriment. Through our spiritual experiences God is telling us where to go, whom to be friends with, who to stay away from, and what to do so we can remain safe from the schemes of the enemy.

We are instructed to be cautious living through others' dreams. We should never make our life's journey and our plans based on another person's dream. God will give us our own dreams. He will give us our own future and prophecy that future to us when we listen and choose to come close to Him. God had an interpretation for the butler and the baker. He had a prophetic word to give each person.

Expect God to give you the dreams you need for your own journey. Expect Him to show you where to go and what to do spiritually through dreams and your visions. When we expect to experience and receive Jesus, we will receive like blind Bartimaeus received the light. The light opens our eyes, and it allows us to illuminate the rest of our bodies, from the realm of the spirit.

We have a supernatural navigation system guiding us through life. We don't need to try to figure out the path and the way to go, because if we listen, see, and experience God He will make the way clear to us. Dreams and visions from God are prophetic. They are an illumination of the road, guiding us into all truth. Psalm 32:8 says, "I will instruct you and teach you in the way you should go; I will guide you with My eye."

The Bible is a lamp to our feet and a light to our path. God's word, regardless of the format through which it comes, is a light and a lamp to our path. God is His word. His Spirit and His presence are who He is, just as much as the Bible is who He is. To encounter God's Spirit is to encounter the light, and God will meet us anywhere and anytime, and sometimes people don't even ask for it! Unbelievers like king Abimelech didn't ask to hear a word from God, but got one anyway. God doesn't need our permission to speak to us.

Isaiah 55:11 declares, "So will My word be which goes out of My mouth; It will not return to Me void (useless, without result), Without accomplishing what I desire, And without succeeding in the matter for which I sent it."

Dreams have always been influential in my life. Before I was saved, I was led astray by dreams because I didn't have a point of reference to identify the origin of the dream. In the first phase of my life, I let any dream impact me. However, after I became a Christian, I realized the dreams I received were sent from God or they were sent from the enemy. I began to see patterns in my dreams, and I became able to identify the good or the rotten fruit presented to me while I was asleep.

When I became a parent, God began to reveal things about my children to me through dreams. One night I dreamed my child was having an issue with anger that got him into trouble when he was older. When I woke, I knew the Lord was telling me to focus on that child's anger outbursts and correct them. This dream was God giving me revelation about one of my children so I could prevent him from the trouble I saw in the dream. This dream was prophetic, and it prompted me to change my parenting style and focus on the weeds trying to grow in my child's life.

Once I had a dream that a minster I trusted approached me as I held one of my children in a church building. In the dream I was concerned about my child. The minister told me my child had a particular medical issue. God had revealed it to him. The minister prayed for us, and when I woke up, I knew I had received the blessing and the healing in the spiritual realm, even though I had not left my house or physically interacted with that minister. It is possible to receive things spiritually without physically receiving them.

God sent me supernatural help in the spirit realm. I was transferred with a blessing of healing supernaturally, and I never left my bedroom to receive it. At the time of the dream, I didn't see any physical manifestation of a medical issue. My child showed no symptoms of anything medically concerning. However, we know dreams are prophetic, and we know God gives us dreams to protect us and our children. My child must have needed prayer and healing in that area even when it didn't seem like anything was wrong. God provided me with the help I needed while I was asleep, and this help prevented a problem.

God will give us specific dreams, so we can get ahead of the enemy's attack. He will send us spiritual, angelic food while we are in the realm of the spirit. Dreams and visions allow us to always interact with the devil from an offensive position instead of a defensive one. Offensive fighting keeps our enemy away. When we fight in an offensive stance, we see the plot ahead of time so we attack the enemy before the enemy can attack us.

When people fight defensively, they respond to an attack that is already present. Defensive fighting usually results in defeat, because the person defending himself or herself is positioned as the weaker fighter.

When we are interacting with the devil or his demons God wants to ensure we are never defending ourselves as unprepared victims. Being victorious requires being prepared and positioned as the offensive fighter, not the defensive one. We need our spiritual senses to defeat the plans of the enemy.

With God's revelatory insight, I can protect my children before the enemy can even shoot his arrows at them. I can see clearly where we are to live, work, and be. I can see when someone is not who they pretend to be. Spiritual insight and senses keep us from ever being harmed by someone or something demonic because we are prepared and are wearing our armor, and the devil can't sneak up on us.

The spirits alive in the world are subject to the born-again believer; we are not subject to them. To be subject, means to depend upon another thing before it can happen. By law, Satan cannot take ground against the Church, because he is subject to us. He needs us to refuse the power of God and walk in ignorance and weakness if he is going to take ground. The Church has the authority to make Satan and every demon subject to us. We have the power to walk on top of every serpent and scorpion.

Luke 10:19 tells us, "Listen carefully: I have given you authority [that you now possess] to tread on serpents and scorpions, and [the ability to exercise authority] over all the power of the enemy (Satan); and nothing will [in any way] harm you. Nevertheless, do not rejoice at this, that the spirits are subject to you, but rejoice that your names are written in heaven."

Like dreams, visions and trances provide prophetic revelatory information about the future. In a vision or trance, people are not asleep; they are always awake. We do not see visions with our natural eyes. We receive them through a spiritual lens. Visions and trances operate like a projector. Projectors use rays of light to show moving images or slides, through images and videos. When the light comes in, the image is manifested.

When we have a vision or experience a trance, we are given supernatural light showing us moving pictures or still images. We see deeper into the spirit realm when God or his angels bring light portraying a message to us like we are watching a movie on a projection screen. Some visions and trances occur in a group format, like a movie theater experience. Others are given to individuals, and only one person watches the spiritual movie.

Daniel 10:7 says, "Now I, Daniel, alone saw the vision, while the men who were with me did not see the vision; nevertheless, a great dread fell on them, and they ran way to hide themselves."

The word of the Lord is separate from a vision of the Lord. Words from the Lord are auditory spiritual experiences. They are the lowest level of spiritual revelation. Visions, dreams, and trances operate on a higher frequency. They come from fully entering God's presence using many combined spiritual senses. Genesis 15:1 teaches, "After these things the *word of the Lord came to Abram in a vision*, saying, 'Do not fear, Abram, I am a shield to you; Your reward shall be very great.'"

Visions are motion pictures originating from the kingdom of God. God is the director, and He decides what is in the movie. Visual images can be projected as an image. These revelations are focused. When teachers use projectors to teach, they often go to one PowerPoint slide or image to demonstrate or teach a point. Likewise, God will use visions to focus on one thing, and thus, the image we see projected is a stand-still type of picture.

Motion pictures are separate from the fixed pictures given by God. A motion picture is a movie or story we watch in the spirit realm. Some people see angels or Jesus in visions. Some people see scripts, or performances acted out in front of their eyes, as if they are watching a show live through spiritual glasses. Regardless of the type of image or images we see, visions can teach us by allowing us to experience the supernatural.

Dreams, trances, and visions are immersive experiences. In recent years, immersive experiences through digital technologies have become popular. We understand how to manipulate light and use technology to powerfully communicate with one another. But God has always had this technology. He has always known how to make movies, stand alone images, and how to communicate messages through immersive spiritual experiences.

When we are given spiritual revelation, it is often so powerful that we experience physical side effects. We see the same things happen to people when they use some of the immersive experiences like virtual reality. Some people get physically sick after interacting with VR. As we learn more about virtual reality and projections, we know God already knew about them, because He created them to be used by His people, many years before we "discovered" them.

Luke 1:22 says, "But when he came out, he was unable to speak to them; and they realized that he had seen a vision in the temple; and he kept making signs to them and remained mute."

After Paul/Saul's first encounter with Jesus he was blind. He needed a believer to lay hands on him and help him process his spiritual experience. Paul had a physical manifestation requiring intervention after a spiritual encounter. Acts 9:12 tells us, "And he has seen a vision a man named Ananias come in and lay hands on him, so that he might regain his sight."

Sometimes visions don't produce physical side effects. People can be attending church services, driving in cars, or doing other things they normally do when God gives them a vision. Visions do not have to disrupt our lives. They can come as we work and do other things, and we can receive information from Heaven without ever stopping our regular lives. When we drive down the highway and see a billboard, we can process the information, but we don't have to stop moving to comprehend the message presented to us.

At least twice, Paul had a vision of the Lord that gave him information about his own life and the lives of others. These visions were while he was awake. Paul saw the visions with his spiritual eyes while he was in the physical environment. Paul's visions from God allowed him to continue walking in faith towards his calling, even within situations that seemed hopeless. They also protected him supernaturally and defended him from the attacks of his enemies.

Acts 22:17–18 says, "When I returned to Jerusalem and was praying at the temple, I fell into a trance and saw the Lord speaking to me. 'Quick!' he said. 'Leave Jerusalem immediately, because the people here will not accept your testimony about me.'"

Angels can appear and bring us messages from God as we are awake or as we are sleep. God sent an angel to provide Paul with an open vision. Paul "saw" the Lord speaking to him, he didn't only "hear" in the spirit realm. Paul's vision prophesied the future and told the people they would be okay. Paul saw the future before it happened, like Jesus saw the donkey and he saw Nathanael.

Acts 27:23–25 tells us, "But now I urge you to keep up your courage, because not one of you will be lost; only the ship will be destroyed. Last night an angel of the God to whom I belong and whom I serve stood beside me and said, 'Do not be afraid, Paul. You must stand trial before Caesar; and God has graciously given you the lives of all who sail with you.' So, keep up your courage, men, for I have faith in God that it will happen just as he told me."

While it is true that the Lord selects who receives the gifts, the gifts are available now as they were in the days of the men and women within the Bible. Just like we need to hear, see, taste, smell, and feel, we need all the gifts of the Spirit operating within the Church to be healthy and full of life. The revelatory gifts are special gifts that need to be appreciated within the Church of Jesus.

First Corinthians 12:18–31 teaches:

But as it is, God has placed and arranged the limbs and organs in the body, each [particular one] of them, just as He wished and saw fit and with the best adaptation. But if [the whole] were all a single organ, where would the body be? And now there are [certainly] many limbs and organs, but a single body. And the eye is not able to say to the hand, I have no need of you, nor again the head to the feet, I have no need of you. But instead, there is [absolute] necessity for the parts of the body that are considered the more weak.

And those [parts] of the body which we consider rather ignoble are [the very parts] which we invest with additional honor, and our unseemly parts and those unsuitable for exposure are treated with seemliness (modesty and decorum), Which our more presentable parts do not require. But God has so adjusted (mingled, harmonized, and subtly proportioned the parts of) the whole body, giving the greater honor and richer endowment to the inferior parts which lack [apparent importance],

So that there should be no division or discord or lack of adaptation [of the parts of the body to each other], but the members all alike should have a mutual interest in and care for one another. And if one member suffers, all the parts [share] the suffering; if one member is honored, all the members [share in] the enjoyment of it. Now you [collectively] are Christ's body and [individually] you are members of it, each part severally and distinct [each with his own place and function]. So God has appointed some in the church [for His own use]: first apostles (special messengers); second prophets (inspired preachers and expounders); third teachers; then wonder-workers; then those with ability to heal the sick; helpers; administrators; [speakers in] different (unknown) tongues.

Are all apostles (special messengers)? Are all prophets (inspired interpreters of the will and purposes of God)? Are all teachers? Do all have the power of performing miracles? Do all possess extraordinary powers of healing? Do all speak with tongues? Do all interpret? But earnestly desire and zealously cultivate the greatest and best gifts and graces (the higher gifts and the choicest graces). And yet I will show you a still more excellent way [one that is better by far and the highest of them all—love]."

As the body of Christ, we are positioned on the earth to do His will. We need the whole body to be healthy members of Christ's body. We should appreciate the different parts of the Church even if we hold a different function within the body. Jesus is the head, and He decides the parts of the body, but if we don't have all the parts, we will be unable to do the things we are supposed to do. A healthy body is made up of many parts working together to create perfect health and harmony.

Some men and women will experience more dreams, visions, and trances because Jesus allows them to. They have been given the ability to operate in this way as the eye is given the opportunity to see and let in light. Dreams visions, and trances are supernatural and come from the light entering the spiritual eyes. For the light to come, men and women must be in God's presence; they must be communicating with God in the spirit realm.

Peter was deep in prayer as he experienced a spiritual trance. The heavens opened to Peter through sound and sight. Peter heard, he saw, and he also spoke back to the spiritual vision. He was immersed in the trance. He was participating in the realm of the supernatural.

Acts 11:4–10 says, "Starting from the beginning, Peter told them the whole story: 'I was in the city of Joppa praying, and in a trance, I saw a vision. I saw something like a large sheet being let down from heaven by its four corners, and it came down to where I was. I looked into it and saw four-footed animals of the earth, wild beasts, reptiles and birds. Then I heard a voice telling me, "Get up, Peter. Kill and eat." I replied, "Surely not, Lord! Nothing impure or unclean has ever entered my mouth." Then the voice spoke from heaven a second time, "Do not call anything impure that God has made clean." This happened three times, and then it was all pulled up to heaven again.'"

Dreams, visions and trances are supernatural experiences that often change a person's life forever. As we read in some of the stories of people who experienced trances and visions in the Bible, God used these experiences to alter their view of where they should be, who they should be with, and how they should proceed through life. When God speaks to us, we know it, and we will never be the same.

Children who are born with a prophetic gift can be trained to operate in the revelatory gifts. Samuel was a child who needed to be instructed by Elijah as to how to hear, see, and interact within the spirit realm. Samuel's mother let Samuel grow up under the gifts of Eli the priest and so he was able to operate fully in the supernatural gifts of God, even from a young age.

If children are born with prophetic gifts and are not taught to use them, the enemy will try to pollute their gift and use it for his kingdom. Children born as prophets can see, hear, and experience in the spirit, but if they are not trained to identify and understand the things they hear, see, and experience, they will learn to trust other voices, or pictures. Prophets benefit from the leadership of other prophets who can help them to become who they are meant to become.

Amos 7:14 says, "Then Amos replied to Amaziah, 'I am not a prophet [by profession], nor am I a prophet's son; I am a herdsman and a grower of sycamore figs.'"

The son of a prophet is a young prophet who learns from an older prophet. Samuel was the son of Eli. He learned from the older, seasoned prophet, so he could properly use his prophetic gift for God's kingdom. Being a prophet is an occupation. It is the prophet's profession to prophecy and to train others who are new to the occupation so they can learn the proper ways to interact and respond to the supernatural spiritual world.

First Samuel 3:1 explains, "The boy Samuel continued to serve the Eternal One under the guidance of Eli. In those days, messages from the Eternal were rare, and sacred dreams or visions were given to very few. Eli, who was very old, had become almost blind. He was lying in his room; it was late at night but before dawn as the lamp of God still burned. Samuel was resting in the house of the Eternal One, where the covenant chest of the True God was located, and he heard a voice."

God wants us to develop our gifts in the spirit realm, just like a newborn baby develops physical senses. To develop gifts, we must ask the Lord to show us who we are in the body of Christ. We must ask God to reveal to us the things we need to know personally. If we do not know what we are called to do or who we have been created to be, we cannot train for the Lord's service. A prophet who never learns how to operate as a prophet, may serve in another capacity in the Church, even when this is not God's intended place for him or her.

As parents, we need the Lord's help to show us who our children are. We need God to tell us the role they will have within the body of Christ. God will show parents who their children are. He will tell us what our children have been called to do and where they need to be.

Like Hannah, we can position our children under the right leadership, and we can impact their ability to work for the Lord in the future because we know they are learning how to perform their job within the Church.

Ask God who your kids are in His kingdom, and then when He reveals it to you supernaturally, believe it and nurture it, so they can do what they have been ordained to do.

15

The Sons and Daughters of God

All babies are born into families. The family a baby is born into is his or her family of origin. In the family of origin, children watch and learn from the conduct and the expectations of the household. Children learn how to respond to the world. Parents are responsible for their children's health and well-being until the children get old enough to take care of themselves. Parents are responsible to model a godly lifestyle so their children learn God's truths effectively.

Not all children come from healthy families. Some children grow up in homes where their families are very sick emotionally and spiritually. Others grow up with families that try to serve the Lord but still make mistakes due to their human flesh. The further a family deviates from God's standards, the worse off a family becomes. Conversely, the closer the family is to the Lord, the healthier the family will be.

The Bible is transparent about problems existing in families. Through Scripture we learn about dysfunctional family systems. Some men have awful wives like Job's wife who told Job to give up, curse God, and die. Some women have awful husbands, such as Abigail's husband Nabal, whom God called a fool because Nabal almost had their entire household killed if Abigail hadn't intervened. Who we join ourselves to in marriage is important, and God's best for us is to be equally yoked with other believers.

Like adults, children can be dysfunctional and unhealthy. Children who are unhealthy have picked up sickness from people who live around them. Children can pick up problems from their parents or others who have been allowed access into their lives. In today's culture, many children pick up disease from the community around them. If parents do not shield children from the physical, social, emotional, and spiritual diseases plaguing the surrounding culture, then the culture can make children sick.

Our nuclear family, combined with our larger society, does impact us. By influencing our beliefs, attitudes, and mindsets, our family and society shape what we believe to be normal. Lot and his wife were believers, and they were expected to teach their children how to walk with the Lord. However, when they moved near Sodom, they allowed their children to pick up the norms of the city, instead of sheltering them from the evil.

It is possible to be raised and surrounded by evil and still serve the Lord. But the child's parents must attach the child to the house of God, and separate him or her emotionally and spiritually from the world, as Jochebed did for Moses. When God destroyed the cities of Sodom and Gomorrah, He gave Lot and his family a chance to leave. Some of Lot's children wouldn't listen to him, showing they had no respect for God's word. When the city was destroyed, Lot's children were also destroyed because they had joined themselves in the world/city around them, instead of joining themselves to God's family.

Lot's two daughters were plagued with the problems of the city even when they left the city. Scripture tells us they brought sexual immorality with them out of the city, because they had normalized the sexual immorality while living in the city. The community children are raised in, and how close they are allowed to get to the world, can impact them, even if they come from a godly home. Children do not naturally understand things of the spirit. To understand who God is and who they are, they must be taught.

Social, emotional, and demonic spiritual problems can be transferred like physical sickness can. When a child comes into close contact with a social, emotional, or demon spirit, and the child does not have a spiritual shield around his or her life, then he or she can catch the infections of the people around him or her. Exposure to infection leads to a personal infection when the child is not spiritually protected. Psalm 28:7 teaches, "The Lord is my strength and my shield; my heart trusts in him, and he helps me."

The cities of Sodom and Gomorrah were plagued with sexual immorality. The people had normalized very wicked lifestyles. When Lot's children were raised in the city, they picked up the customs and lifestyles of the wicked people around them and didn't realize how bad the sins truly were, because they had become conditioned to sin. Genesis 18:20 says, "And the Lord said, 'The outcry [of the sin] of Sodom and Gomorrah is indeed great, and their sin is exceedingly grave.'"

The normalization of sinful lifestyles caused the girls to carry those wicked behaviors into their futures, even when God spared them and removed them from the wicked people. The evil of the community penetrated their hearts and became attached to them. Lot knew the Lord, and he knew how to recognize the spirit, but he did not teach his daughters to do the same. Genesis 19:1 "It was evening when the two angels came to Sodom. Lot was sitting at Sodom's [city] gate. Seeing them, Lot got up to meet them and bowed down with his face to the ground."

When Lot saw the angels of the Lord, he recognized them, respected them, and welcomed them into his home. Lot was used to hearing from God and interacting with supernatural beings. Lot recognized them as angels, and He knew they were God's messengers, even when others in the city did not properly discern who the angels were. This depicts the intimate relationship Lot shared with God and the supernatural realm.

Genesis 19:5 explains, "But before they lay down [to sleep], the men of the city, the men of Sodom, both young and old, surrounded the house, all the men from every quarter; and they called out to Lot and said to him, 'Where are the men who came to you tonight? Bring them out to us so that we may know them [intimately].'"

If the men of the city had properly recognized the angels they wouldn't have tried to have sex with them. The other people in the city were spiritually blind. But Lot was very much aware of who he was interacting with, and he knew the difference between good and evil. Lot saw into the spiritual and physical because he was a citizen of Heaven, and he knew how to operate in the realm of the spirit. Genesis 19:7 tells us Lot pleaded with the men, "and said, 'Please, my brothers, do not do something so wicked.'"

Despite Lot's awareness of the spiritual realm, it is noteworthy that he did not take the initiative to protect his daughters by educating them about spiritual matters. In addition, his willingness to offer his daughters to the men of the city reveals that he, too, had internalized certain aspects of sexual immorality. Genesis 19:8 teaches, "See here, I have two daughters who have not known a man [intimately]; please let me bring them out to you [instead], and you can do as you please with them; only do nothing to these men, because they have in fact come under the shelter of my roof [for protection].'"

Lot had not properly trained his children to differentiate between good and evil, spiritual and physical. Lot's family did not know how to see in the spirit for themselves, and they did not know the significance of the interaction with the angels. The angels came into Lot's house, so the members of his immediate family should have identified who was with them. If they had been properly trained to see the realm of the spirit, they would have clearly seen the severity of the situation. They would have never mocked or ignored Lot's warnings.

Genesis 19:14 teaches, "So Lot went out and spoke to his sons-in-law, who were [betrothed, and legally promised] to marry his daughters, and said, 'Get up, get out of this place, for the Lord is about to destroy this city!' But to his sons-in-law he appeared to be joking. When morning dawned, the angels urged Lot [to hurry], saying, 'Get up! Take your wife and two daughters who are here [and go], or you will be swept away in the punishment of the city.'"

Lot allowed the city to expose the demonic to his house, and he failed to prepare and shield his family. Lot was compliant with evil, even though he did not participate in evil. Lot wanted to fit into the city. He wanted to be apart of the city, joining himself to the people who lived there, and his desire to be accepted by the ungodly caused him not to make any spiritual impact, even on those in his inner circle. Lot was called to be a leader in the city, but he chose to be a follower.

When Christians refuse to stand boldly against evil in our culture, choosing to try to be accepted by the world or the wicked people who live among them, they become worthless. If Christians know better and do not do better, it is the sin of omission. Matthew 5:13 says, "You are the salt of the earth, but if salt has lost its taste (its strength, its quality), how can its saltiness be restored? It is not good for anything any longer but to be thrown out and trodden underfoot by men."

The sin of omission is when we don't do something God's word teaches us we should do. Lot knew the men and the women around him were full of evil, but he didn't do anything about it. He lived amongst it, tolerating it instead of opposing it, and he allowed his wife and his children do the same. The result of Lot's sin of omission cost him most of his family and friends.

When we do not remain salty and full of quality and strength in our spirits, we will be trampled by the people of the world around us. When we are tramped by the world, we are bruised, injured, or pushed down, even to the point of death. Most of Lot's family was trampled by evil, and the two children who survived were unwell and plagued with the sickness of the city even after they were no longer exposed to the source of the disease.

Genesis 19:24–38 says,

Then the Lord rained on Sodom and on Gomorrah brimstone and fire from the Lord out of the heavens. He overthrew, destroyed, and ended those cities, and all the valley and all the inhabitants of the cities, and what grew on the ground. But [Lot's] wife looked back from behind him, and she became a pillar of salt. Abraham went up early the next morning to the place where he [only the day before] had stood before the Lord.

And he looked toward Sodom and Gomorrah, and toward all the land of the valley, and saw, and behold, the smoke of the country went up like the smoke of a furnace. When God ravaged and destroyed the cities of the plain [of Siddim], He [earnestly] remembered Abraham [imprinted and fixed him indelibly on His mind], and He sent Lot out of the midst of the overthrow when He overthrew the cities where Lot lived.

And Lot went up out of Zoar and dwelt in the mountain, and his two daughters with him, for he feared to dwell in Zoar; and he lived in a cave, he and his two daughters. The elder said to the younger, "Our father is aging, and there is not a man on earth to live with us in the customary way. Come, let us make our father drunk with wine, and we will lie with him, so that we may preserve offspring (our race) through our father." And they made their father drunk with wine that night, and the older went in and lay with her father; and he was not aware of it when she lay down or when she arose.

Then the next day the firstborn said to the younger, "See here, I lay last night with my father; let us make him drunk with wine tonight also, and then you go in and lie with him, so that we may preserve offspring (our race) through our father." And they made their father drunk with wine again that night, and the younger arose and lay with him; and he was not aware of it when she lay down or when she arose. Thus both the daughters of Lot were with child by their father. The older bore a son, and named him Moab [of a father]; he is the father of the Moabites to this day. The younger also bore a son and named him Ben-ammi [son of my people]; he is the father of the Ammonites to this day."

Lot's wife turned into salt, when she was supposed to disperse that salt to the city and into her home. She was never supposed to die as a pillar of salt; she should have lived as a useful pillar of salt in the city and her house. Lot's daughters were accustomed to being drunk, and they were accustomed to sexual immorality. If they had not been accustomed to these sinful behaviors, they wouldn't have so easily perpetrated the sin of incest with their father. Lot's daughters were plagued socially and psychologically with wickedness. They were emotionally, and spiritually unwell after leaving the place of contamination.

Imparting holiness and spiritual understanding in our children should be our top priority. Protecting our children from joining in the customs of the world around us is vital. A failure to properly protect children from wicked alliances and the normalization of evil can lead to them being plagued with spiritual, social, and emotional problems. It can keep them from properly identifying spiritual things and could ultimately destroy their lives.

When Eli was training Samuel to operate in the gifts of the spirit, he was tasked to provide leadership to Samuel. When God spoke to Samuel as a young boy, the first message he had for him was about his elder, Eli. God rebuked Eli and Eli's sons, and God pronounced punishment for wickedness in His house. Eli, like Lot, knew what was right before God, but he had not properly imparted this information to his sons. As a result, Eli's sons acted wickedly in the Lord's house.

First Samuel 2:12 explains, "Eli's sons, Hophni and Phinehas, were good-for-nothing priests; they had no faith in the Lord."

God describes Eli's sons as good for nothing, and this phrase is the same phrase we find in the passage on "losing our salt" as the people of the Lord. Eli's sons did not operate properly as priests. They should have operated on a spiritual level, bringing great spiritual impact to the surrounding people, as Lot's family should have done to the cities of Sodom and Gomorrah. However, Eli, like Lot, failed to train his sons into spiritual truths and into righteousness, so though he knew how to hear from God and how to interact with the spirit realm, his sons did not.

First Samuel 2:22 explains, "Now, Eli was very old, and he had heard everything that his sons were doing to all Israel and that they were sleeping with the women who served at the gate of the tent of meeting. So he asked them, 'Why are you doing such things? I hear about your wicked ways from all these people. Sons, the report that I hear the people of the Lord spreading isn't good! If one person sins against another, God will take care of him. However, when a person sins against the Lord, who will pray for him?' But they wouldn't listen to their father's warning—the Lord wanted to kill them."

Children need to learn to respect God and their parents from a young age. When children learn to ignore the commands of their parents and are treated as equals in the house, they grow up without proper honor for their elders. In today's American culture, many parents believe they are "friends" with their children. They refuse to properly instruct and discipline children into righteousness and truth, and they let the children feel like they are equal from infancy.

Lot's children didn't respect him or listen to him as a trusted elder and leader. Eli's sons felt the same way towards their father. Both groups of disobedient children felt they were smarter than their parents. They treated their parents with contempt and disrespect. Authority needs to be respected. Leadership is important because leaders help groups to progress forward. Children must learn to honor their parents, and if they aren't taught this during their childhood, they will grow up to be disrespectful.

The failure to instruct into righteousness and truth causes the next generation to become intimate with the world they were intended to reject and transform. To be sure children are safe from exposure to the plagues existing in the world around us, we must plan to train them to hear from God for themselves. We must train them in righteousness and never let them get too used to the traditions of the world.

We must ensure they don't get comfortable disrespecting and ignoring our warnings and our commands.

James 4:4 tells us, "You adulteresses [disloyal sinners—flirting with the world and breaking your vow to God]! Do you not know that being the world's friend [that is, loving the things of the world] is being God's enemy? So whoever chooses to be a friend of the world makes himself an enemy of God."

Hannah decided to dedicate her son to God. She decided to ensure he was raised up in the house of God. Samuel is compared to Eli's sons because although they were born into the line of priests, and they should have followed in their father's footsteps, they didn't. Samuel was born outside of the house, and his mom ensured he was brought in. Parents must decide to raise their kids outside of the world and in the house of the Lord. We must be committed to ensuring their spiritual future and destiny.

Scripture verifies the influence a parent can have on his or her child. Parents who raise their children in the world, even when they love the Lord, will not necessarily see their children experience salvation. We must impart spiritual truths to our children, and we need to ensure that they grow up with a reverence for God and His house. A love for God's house, means a hatred for evil found within the world. A love for God means honor and respect of parents. Ephesians 6:1–2 teaches, "Children, obey your parents in the Lord: for this is right. Honor thy father and mother; which is the first commandment with promise;"

Parents can take their children to Jesus. In Mark 9, a father took his child to Jesus to deliver him from a demon who wanted to take his life. This father's choice saved his child's life. Conversely, some parents have sacrificed their children to demon gods. These parents didn't save their children, they willingly gave their children to the demonic forces. These huge extremities between full reliance and submission to God vs. full reliance and submission to evil impacts the child, because children are vulnerable, and they need the protection and guidance of adults in their lives.

The Bible provides us with answers for dealing with every circumstance imaginable. God told us about the lives of people who experienced things we may experience today so we would have hope in all situations. Children who grow up with evil parents can be saved, and many are, because God loves them, even when their parents didn't. But sometimes children are destroyed indefinitely because their parents willingly handed them over to the devourer.

Even in the worst situations, God will heal and restore a man or a woman, an adult or a child who comes to Him for help. God wants to restore and deliver individuals and their families. He wants to help the person who is hurting and suffering because of the devil and because of sin. Second Corinthians 1:3–4 explains, "Blessed be the God and Father of our Lord Jesus Christ, the Father of compassion and the God of all comfort, who comforts and encourages us in every trouble so that we will be able to comfort and encourage those who are in any kind of trouble, with the comfort with which we ourselves are comforted by God."

In the Bible, Abraham was commended for his faith in God. Despite his faith, love and commitment for God, Abraham made mistakes with his own family. One of his mistakes corrupted the perfection of his family, hurting him, his children, and his wives. However, because Abraham was committed to righteousness, he continued to try to please the Lord. Abraham's faith in God enabled God to move on his behalf, and God provided help even in unhealthy, imperfect circumstances.

Christians can make mistakes in the flesh and still inherit their promises when their hearts are sold out to God. A willful decision to participate in sin is different than an accidental partnership with the flesh. God knows our hearts, and He knows when we are trying to serve him and we make a mistake, or when we are cold in our love and our commitment to righteousness.

Abraham allowed his wife to determine the course of their household. God holds men accountable for their wives and their children, and men are to spiritually lead the home. Lot's wife may have been saved if Lot had properly positioned his family spiritually, instead of allowing her to wander into the world for her identity. Abraham's family could have been spared the heartache, if Abraham had stood up to Sarah's carnal idea. First Corinthians 11:3 says, "But I want you to understand that Christ is the head (authority over) of every man, and man is the head of woman, and God is the head of Christ."

Choosing to conceive a baby in the flesh caused grief within their home because it was not God's intended plan. When God gave the promise to Abraham that he would be the father of many nations, he wanted Abraham to know his future, but he wanted him to wait. Abraham didn't need to scheme to create a new plan birthed out of the flesh because God's plan would have come to pass if Abraham and Sarah had been patient. The flesh and their impatience led them out of God's best for their life.

Patience is a fruit of the Spirit. We can be patient knowing God's will is going to come to pass, if we have seen and heard of the promises in the realm of the Spirit. We can know our patience will be met with a greater reward if the gift is from God. Romans 12:12 teaches, "Constantly rejoicing in hope [because of our confidence in Christ], steadfast and patient in distress, devoted to prayer [continually seeking wisdom, guidance, and strength]," Abraham believed God and He believed the promise, but He tried to make God's promise come to pass instead of waiting patiently on the spiritual manifestation of that promise.

As I was playing a game with my children this week and teaching them about self-control, I placed four candies in front of them and explained they could have one now, or they could wait and have all four when I got back.

I left the room for a few minutes, and when I got back, they were waiting patiently for all four of their candies. My kids are four and six years old, and they are mature enough to understand delayed gratification, so even when it was hard, they operated in self-control.

The more mature we are in Christ, the more we will be able to operate in the fruits of the Spirit. New believers need time to grow to their spiritual maturity. When my children realized they would have a better reward if they waited for me to get back, and that four candies were better than one candy, they decided it was worth waiting for. Understanding the reward provided them with motivation to wait for me to come back to the room.

However, if I had placed those same candies in front of my one year old and walked away, he would not have been mature enough to understand the delayed reward. He would have immediately eaten the candies because of his maturity level.

Mistakes made from spiritual immaturity are not the same as intentional sins. God knows when we are doing something evil or if we are simply immature and undiscerning about what we are doing. Abraham and Sarah exhibited a degree of immaturity in their understanding of God's promises. Believing they could expedite the fulfillment of His covenant, they attempted to assist God. Despite their earnest desire to please God and maintain faith in His promises, they sought to bring about the manifestation they had been assured.

God told Abraham his wife Sarah would be the mother of many nations. Abraham didn't see the manifestation of promise in the natural, but he didn't need to after he saw it in the realm of spirit. The spirit realm is more real than the physical one. The spirit realm is the basis for our entire worldly existence. Without the spirit realm, we would not be here, we would not exist.

Abraham and Sarah believed in the promise they received in the spirit, but they didn't have the spiritual maturity to wait for their reward. They believed God, but they were spiritually immature, and this led them to seek the reward on their terms, out of impatience and immaturity.

Galatians 6:1 tells us, "Brothers, if anyone is caught in any sin, you who are spiritual [that is, you who are responsive to the guidance of the Spirit] are to restore such a person in a spirit of gentleness [not with a sense of superiority or self-righteousness], keeping a watchful eye on yourself, so that you are not tempted as well."

Sarah's spiritual immaturity deterred Abraham and led him off course. Abraham should have remained in the leadership position and said no to Sarah. Abraham was more mature; he was wiser in his spiritual understanding. He needed to instruct Sarah into a place of righteousness because he was advanced in the spirit. Abraham received the spiritual promise much easier from the angels, showing us he was indeed more mature than Sarah, who laughed from disbelief in her heart.

Genesis 18:12–14 explains, "Therefore Sarah laughed to herself, saying, 'After I have become aged shall I have pleasure and delight, my lord (husband), being old also?' And the Lord asked Abraham, 'Why did Sarah laugh, saying, Shall I really bear a child when I am so old? Is anything too hard or too wonderful for the Lord? At the appointed time, when the season [for her delivery] comes around, I will return to you and Sarah shall have borne a son.' Then Sarah denied it, saying, 'I did not laugh;' for she was afraid. And He said, 'No, but you did laugh.'"

When we are advanced spiritually, we can see, hear, and experience things in the realm of the spirit that others cannot hear, see, or experience. God expects mature Christians to lead others because we are more mature spiritually and have the vision and understanding that they do not possess. A young child should never lead an adult.

Sometimes God positions us as the most mature person in the room, the city, or our family. God appoints leaders, as he appointed Lot, Abraham, and Eli. These men were to help train those under them into a deeper walk within the realm of the spirit. A failure to properly lead others, even when we are connected to God and hearing, seeing, and experiencing spiritual things, can have a detrimental outcome in the lives of those we needed to teach and lead. We can impact other's lives. We can change their futures!

Matthew 15:14 warns us, "Leave them alone; they are blind guides [leading blind followers]. If a blind man leads a blind man, both will fall into a pit."

Without our spiritual eyes being full of light, the entire body lies in darkness. Everyone needs spiritual vision to properly determine the course of his or her life. Spiritual, full-of-light people should never listen to those walking in the flesh or walking with limited vision in the realm of the spirit. To do so would be to follow blind guides, and it is foolish to follow someone who's blind when you have been given eyesight to see clearly.

Sarah was a blind guide to Abraham, because her eyesight was worse than his. She was leading Abraham, who had received supernatural insight, when he should have been leading her. Sarah was living through her flesh instead of her spirit. She couldn't see properly because she was following the flesh, which is inferior to the spirit. Abraham, who could see, should have been leading Sarah. He should have been showing her which way to go because he saw more clearly through the realm of the spirit.

Second Peter 2:7–8 teaches, "And if he rescued righteous Lot, greatly distressed by the sensual conduct of the wicked (for as that righteous man lived among them day after day, he was tormenting his righteous soul over their lawless deeds that he saw and heard)."

Lot could see more clearly than those around him. Lot was righteous, and he was keenly aware of the problems of the city. Lot was expected to use his sight to lead others. When God shows us the truth in the spirit realm, He shows us so we can receive something for our own lives, but He also wants us to use what we have been shown to impact others. God wants us to lead and help the blind, the lame, and the crippled. He wants us to show them the right way to go.

When we see people who are blind, we must have compassion and realize they need to healed and have their vision restored. Believers who are healthy should remain in control as a guide and never let a blind person guide us. Many people God places in our lives need us to see and to guide them, or they will fall into a pit. They need the Church to help them, or they will be plunged entirely into darkness, both now and forevermore.

Sarah's physical senses caused her to doubt God believing she could not conceive or deliver a child. When we rely on our physical vision, it hinders us in our faith. God does not need the natural world to carry out His plans. God is a spirit who created the natural world from the spiritual world, not the other way around.

Our natural world is subject to God. God is not subject to it. If something has been established within the realm of the spirit, it is more powerful than if it were established in the natural. This is often hard for people to comprehend, especially if they live through their carnal senses. But if we do not have God's insight and help to see the supernatural world around us, then we will live as physical beings, ignoring the supernatural world. We will believe the physical world is greater than the spiritual one.

God formed the world out of nothing. God doesn't need natural laws because the natural laws are subject to Him. When Jesus commanded the waves to be still, He was showing us that the world doesn't get to control the spiritual world. The spiritual world determines what happens within the physical world. Job 12:10 teaches us, "In His hand is the life of every living thing and the breath of all mankind."

Whenever people walk outside of God's plan, they follow a plan of their own mind, senses, beliefs, and desires. This carnal plan is a direct rebelling against God, because when people do not walk by faith, they are walking by sight, and without faith, and humanity cannot please God.

Sarah trusted the physical realm more than she trusted the spiritual realm so she devised her own plan from her flesh instead of from her spirit.

Isaiah 65:2 says, "I have spread out My hands all day long to a rebellious people, who walk in the way which is not good, following their own thoughts."

God doesn't force us to believe what we hear and see in the spirit. God will show us things in the spirit world, and at times, people still choose to walk by the flesh and ignore the promptings a of the spirit. We know Sarah received the promise from God. We know she received the spiritual message, but instead of believing it, she disregarded it and allowed it to become secondary to the messages she was receiving in the physical world.

Physical senses are helpful when we are navigating the physical world, but physical senses are never to dominate us more than our spiritual senses. Spiritual senses are primary senses, and physical senses are secondary senses. We can be tricked when we live in the physical environment, but when we are spiritually receiving and experiencing from God, we cannot be deceived.

Hebrews 3:19 tells us, "So we see that they were not able to enter [into His rest—the promised land] because of unbelief and an unwillingness to trust in God."

Rest in the physical realm comes from working in the spiritual realm. We work to receive from the Lord by using our faith. Once we work in the spiritual realm, we can rest in the physical world, because we know the spirit realm dictates the circumstances of the physical world. If we have done our part in the spiritual realm and we are using our faith, then we can rest knowing God's will is going to come to pass.

Fasting and praying at the beginning of a new year is spiritual work. We are choosing to sow within the spirit realm, knowing the work will produce an outward physical harvest. The spirit realm produces all physical things, so when we sow in the realm of the spirit, we will produce in the realm of the physical. When we tithe, and we expect the Lord to bless our food and our water and to return to us more than we sowed, we are working in the realm of the spirit, to receive rest in the natural world.

Using our faith is like using our physical muscles to work out. The more we work out, the stronger our faith will become. When we work in the spiritual realm, we don't have to toil and work in the physical realm, because God will ensure His word comes to pass on our behalf. But if we fail to use our faith, and we try to work out everything in the natural realm through our physical efforts, we will not fully experience the supernatural harvest and blessings God intends to give us.

We cannot force spiritual things to manifest from working through the flesh. We can cooperate with the Holy Spirit and God's spiritual system, or we can try to do it our own way. However, if we want to truly rest in God and we want to see the outward manifestation of our spiritual work, we must not resist the Holy Spirit and the system God created, even if it doesn't make sense to our natural minds. Acts 7:51 explains, "You men who are stiff-necked and uncircumcised in heart and ears are always resisting the Holy Spirit; you are doing just as your fathers did."

The Biblical definition of revelation is God's act of communicating unknown truths and facts about Himself He wants us to know. When God gives a revelation, we should believe it, not resist it. We should know God is wiser than we are. When we resist the Holy Spirit, we tell the Holy Spirit we know better than He does. When we receive a prophetic word from Heaven and we choose to ignore what we have seen, heard, or experienced because we feel we know more based on our physical revelation, we are resisting the Holy Spirit and showing Him dishonor.

In the book of Job, God asked men if they are all knowledgeable and wise. He was challenging humans to look at themselves and have an accurate and humble perception of themselves. Being puffed up with pride and thinking you know more than your Father in Heaven is foolish and disrespectful. We will never know more than God knows.

As our Father, He will always be superior in wisdom and knowledge, and we need to know our proper place in His house.

We have all seen a child who is disobedient to his or her parents. In our current culture, this attitude is propagated by Satan to teach children to exalt themselves over their parents. Plenty of television shows portray children who are wiser than their parents. Parents who should be respected as the leaders of the children are depicted as weak, stupid and at the discretion of their young children. Children exposed to these teachings will disregard their caretakers' authority. They will disrespect their parent's position as teacher, leader, and authority in the home.

God expects us to teach children to honor their elders and superiors. Satan teaches disrespect, contempt, and dishonor. God is our superior. He knows more than we know, and when we interact with Him, we should present ourselves in a way that demonstrates our understanding of our inferiority before Him. Coming to God as an arrogant, bratty child, assuming to know more than He knows is wrong and is the work of our enemy.

Plenty of children feel justified in disrespecting their parents. Children can come up with a plethora of reasons why they are entitled to their opinions or their way. Likewise, many of God's children feel justified in trusting their physical senses: sight, smell, taste, touch, and hearing. They feel they aren't doing anything wrong when they are not utilizing their faith God has given them. Feeling justified in our emotions or our disobedience doesn't mean we are truly justified or correct. We are only obedient and correct in God's eyes when we come under His rule, and we respect and submit to Him as Father.

Satan should have remained in his position within God's kingdom. He should have honored God as the superior being and given God honor because God created him. But Satan's pride and belief in himself as equal to God caused him to rise up against the One he should have submitted to. Satan was a beautiful, valuable creation. He was loved and important in the kingdom, but he was not and never will be superior to God.

Ezekiel 28:14–16 explains, "You were the anointed cherub that covers with overshadowing [wings], and I set you so. You were upon the holy mountain of God; you walked up and down in the midst of the stones of fire [like the paved work of gleaming sapphire stone upon which the God of Israel walked on Mount Sinai]. You were blameless in your ways from the day you were created until iniquity and guilt were found in you. Through the abundance of your commerce you were filled with lawlessness and violence, and you sinned; therefore I cast you out as a profane thing from the mountain of God and the guardian cherub drove you out from the midst of the stones of fire."

Like Satan, people were created by God. We have a special place in His kingdom, and we are given a role within his family. Realizing who we are in Christ is important because we can realize we are special, anointed and loved, as Lucifer once was. However, we need to proportionally understand that we are not God, and we will always be inferior to Him. If Satan can deceive us into believing we are equal to God or are to be served by God, he has trapped us into his plan of pride and personal conquest outside of our Creator.

We must trust God more than we trust ourselves. His revelation is the truth, and our revelation, when it isn't aligned with His revelation, is a lie. We must depend on God's revelation if we want to truly see and understand. Proverbs 9:10 teaches, "The [reverent] fear of the Lord [that is, worshiping Him and regarding Him as truly awesome] is the beginning and the preeminent part of wisdom [its starting point and its essence], And the knowledge of the Holy One is understanding and spiritual insight."

Sarah and Abraham didn't need to work to have their promised child. They needed to rest in the promise. God had already given them the victory because He gave them the promise. He had told them about the future through a prophetic word, so the future was a sure thing, regardless of the external circumstances in the natural world.

God's spiritual revelation to Abraham and Sarah should have been more real to them than their physical limitations. Sarah didn't need to work hard to make God's will come to pass; she simply needed to rest in God's word and receive the supernatural blessings accompanied with faith in the words of the Lord.

God desires for His people to rest and to work. There is time to work and time to rest. God established six days to work and one day to rest. Action is a demonstration of our faith and is necessary, but sometimes God wants us to rest in the promise He has given us for our lives. When we have done all we can do, and we know we are in God's will, we must stop working and rest, leaving the supernatural element to God and His power.

It may be tempting to try to make things happen without using faith when we know God has promised us something that seems impossible. In these situations, we may try to "help" God make His plan come to pass because of the limitations we see. The tendency to prioritize physical senses while neglecting our spiritual ones, inverts our perception. This reversal diminishes the power of God and His capabilities, and it places the humanistic worldview above the Lord. In these circumstances, people assume greater knowledge than God, demonstrating their doubt and behaving like disrespectful children.

God performs the supernatural element of His word when we enter His rest. Working in the physical world without working out our faith in the spiritual is in reverse and will always birth problems. If we believe we can do it without using our faith in God, we birth things outside of the spirit, when God wanted to give us the promise supernaturally through the work of the spirit. Hebrews 4:11 explains, "Let us therefore make every effort to enter that rest [of God, to know and experience it for ourselves], so that no one will fall by following the same example of disobedience [as those who died in the wilderness]."

Our flesh will try to convince us we are justified in our lack of faith in the promises. The enemy will try to steal our blessing, but when we receive a promise from God, we can choose to rest and know God will bring the promise, and sometimes we just need to be a little more patient, using our faith as a shield against the enemy.

Genesis 16 1–4 teaches, "Now Sarai, Abram's wife, had not borne him any children, and she had an Egyptian maid whose name was Hagar. So Sarai said to Abram, 'See here, the Lord has prevented me from bearing children. I am asking you to go in to [the bed of] my maid [so that she may bear you a child]; perhaps I will] obtain children by her.' And Abram listened to Sarai and did as she said. After Abram had lived in the land of Canaan ten years, Abram's wife Sarai took Hagar the Egyptian [maid], and gave her to her husband Abram to be his [secondary] wife. He went in to [the bed of] Hagar, and she conceived; and when she realized that she had conceived, she looked with contempt on her mistress [regarding Sarai as insignificant because of her infertility]."

Sarah quickly realized she had made a mistake by having Hagar conceive Abraham's child. Being dominated by the flesh will cause us to be blind to the realities of the spirit until it is too late to change our decision. Eve realized after she listened to the serpent that she had been deceived. Sarah realized she had made a bad decision after she was deceived into the behavior, and if we want to ensure we are not making bad decisions, we need to always trust the Lord more than our own perceptions or the word of an outsider.

Sarah's stepped out of her proper place as she attempted to control the people in her family. As she was led by the flesh, she hurt herself, her husband, and her maid. She continued to let her emotions determine her decisions in her relationships, even after realizing they were causing problems. Instead of turning from being dominated by her emotions, Sarah continued in her bad behavior. She continued to justify her actions and ultimately sent Hagar and Ishmael away from their home, because she was threatened by them.

Genesis 16: 5–6 tells us, "Then Sarai said to Abram, 'May [the responsibility for] the wrong done to me [by the arrogant behavior of Hagar] be upon you. I put my maid into your arms, and when she realized that she had conceived, I was despised and looked on with disrespect. May the Lord judge [who has done right] between you and me.' But Abram said to Sarai, 'Look, your maid is entirely in your hands and subject to your authority; do as you please with her.' So Sarai treated her harshly and humiliated her, and Hagar fled from her."

Sarah was harsh with Hagar. She was upset with Hagar for following her leading. Many parents are unhealthy and are dominated by irresponsible, emotionally based decisions. These parents punish their children for misbehavior after leading the children into a dysfunctional behavioral pattern. By failing to take responsibility and realize their personal impact on their children, the parents fail to understand how their own fleshly dominated lives contribute to the problems they see in their children. This leads them to becoming judgmental and harsh instead of being compassionate and loving, and children are punished for having a poor leadership example within the home.

If we want to see our children thrive, we must first look in the mirror and see what we are modeling. We must examine the leadership we have given them. The children in our homes are under our leadership and our care. God has entrusted them to us, for us to properly guide them into all truth. When we fail to examine our own sin and irresponsible behaviors, we will blame others and hurt those we are called to love, instruct, and help in their walk with the Lord.

Matthew 7:3–5 says, "Why do you see the speck that is in your brother's eye, but do not notice the log that is in your own eye? Or how can you say to your brother, 'Let me take the speck out of your eye,' when there is the log in your own eye? You hypocrite, first take the log out of your own eye, and then you will see clearly to take the speck out of your brother's eye."

God was present and He was a help even when this family experienced trouble. God cared about Hagar, and He pursued her, even when Sarah and Abraham rejected her. God saw the injustice done to Hagar, and He sent an angel to help her. God cares about the home lives of His people. He reached out to a family member neglected by the person who was supposed to protect her. God wanted Hagar to know she was not alone, even when she felt like she was.

Genesis 16:9–13 teaches, "The Angel of the Lord said to her, 'Go back to your mistress, and submit humbly to her authority.' Then the Angel of the Lord said to her, 'I will greatly multiply your descendants so that they will be too many to count.' The Angel of the Lord continued, 'Behold, you are with child, And you will bear a son; And you shall name him Ishmael (God hears), Because the Lord has heard and paid attention to your persecution (suffering). He (Ishmael) will be a wild donkey of a man; His hand will be against every man [continually fighting] And every man's hand against him; And he will dwell in defiance of all his brothers.' Then she called the name of the Lord who spoke to her, 'You are God Who Sees'; for she said, 'Have I not even here [in the wilderness] remained alive after seeing Him [who sees me with understanding and compassion]?' Therefore, the well was called Beer-lahai-roi (Well of the Living One Who Sees Me); it is between Kadesh and Bered."

God knew Sarah was demonstrating poor leadership and that she was unstable. God saw the harm done to Hagar and Ishmael as the result of Sarah's carnality. God never justified Sarah's wrong behavior in the scriptures. In fact, He showed compassion during Hagar's mistreatment, and He assured her she was going to be okay. God will meet people who are living in homes of dysfunction and abuse. He will comfort them and assure them that they aren't alone, even when they feel as if they are. God's presence serves as the sole source of hope for those who are enduring pain.

Although Hagar had ample justification to be guided by her emotions, she chose to be led by the spirit rather than by her flesh. Conversely, Sarah, who had every reason to express gratitude and follow the spirit, instead allowed herself to be governed by her worldly desires.

Hagar loved God and appreciated Him. She trusted God and showed great courage and faith in a heartbreaking circumstance. She was abused, mistreated, controlled, and abandoned within her home. Hagar and her son were left with no help from the ones who were supposed to care for them, but she persisted in her faith in God. She didn't blame God for the abuse of people, and because of her faith, God continued to help her and her son.

Genesis 17:17–18 says, "When Abraham fell on his face and laughed, and said in his heart, 'Shall a child be born to a man who is a hundred years old? And shall Sarah, who is ninety years old, bear a child?' And Abraham said to God, 'Oh, that Ishmael [my firstborn] might live before You!'"

Genesis 17:20 says, "As for Ishmael, I have heard and listened to you; behold, I will bless him, and will make him fruitful and will greatly multiply him [through his descendants]. He will be the father of twelve princes (chieftains, sheiks), and I will make him a great nation."

Abraham was 86 years old when Ishmael was born through Hagar. Abraham loved Ishmael, and asked God to help his son. God responded to his prayer of faith and love. Sarah wanted to remove Hagar and Ishmael from their inheritance and send them away from Abraham so they couldn't become heirs. Abraham suffered great loss when his wife Sarah banished his son Ishmael from his life. His heart was broken, but His son Ishmael received a blessing from God, because he interceded in prayer for his child's life.

Genesis 21:9–11 explains, "Now [as time went on] Sarah saw [Ishmael] the son of Hagar the Egyptian, whom she had borne to Abraham, mocking [Isaac]. Therefore, she said to Abraham, 'Drive out this maid and her son, for the son of this maid shall not be an heir with my son Isaac.' The situation distressed Abraham greatly because of his son [Ishmael]."

Sarah couldn't overpower God's decision to bless and care for Hagar and Ishmael. Sarah was used to doing things in her own effort, controlling the people in her life, but she learned she couldn't control God. God didn't allow Sarah to control him. God made a way for both children to be blessed and successful, against Sarah's wishes. All along, God didn't need Sarah to make His word come to pass, because His word will always come to pass, despite people's unbelief or attempts to stop it or alter it.

Genesis 21:12–13 says, "God said to Abraham, 'Do not let it distress you because of Ishmael and your maid; whatever Sarah tells you, listen to her and do what she asks, for your descendants will be named through Isaac. And I will also make a nation of [Ishmael] the son of the maid, because he is your descendant.'"

God doesn't need us to come from a certain family, or a certain cultural background. Hagar was an Egyptian, and she was not from the Israelite linage and family tree. Her son Ishmael was part Egyptian and part Israelite. According to the religious customs, he was ineligible for the blessing and the promise. Yet, Hagar and Ishmael's ancestral background didn't keep them from inheriting a blessing from the Lord. Hagar and Ishmael were blessed by God because of Hagar and Abraham's faith and relationship to Yahweh.

Many religious Jews and religious Christians are limited to see God's big plan for the world and are blinded by the law. They are often nearsighted and cannot see beyond the natural realm. They try to work for their blessing instead of resting through faith. They try to limit the blessing from coming onto those to whom God has given the blessing, because they don't feel some people are worthy of being welcomed into God's family.

Cultural bias contributes to people judging things by the standards of their own culture. A cultural bias leads people to be harsh and cruel instead of compassionate and sympathetic towards others who need to experience good things that are a part of their culture.

If we love our culture, we should promote our culture and share it with those who would benefit from what we have. Without realizing it, many religious people have tried to keep groups of people away from God, when God included these people in His family. We don't receive from God based on our family origin or based on our works; we receive from God based on our faith and our commitment to a relationship with Him.

Sarah should have walked by faith, because of her ancestral lineage. She had the blessing and promise of God, and she could have walked in it, not rejected it because of what she saw in the natural realm. Hagar walked by faith and obeyed the Lord, despite her ancestral background. She decided to trust God, and her faith, not her justification through the law, permitted her to receive from God. Inheritance from the Father comes from faith and dependence upon the Lord. Inheritance is not earned through works, the Father who sees gives it to those who believe!

Romans 4:13–18 says, "For the promise to Abraham or to his descendants that he would be heir of the world was not through [observing the requirements of] the Law, but through the righteousness of faith. If those who are [followers] of the Law are [the true] heirs [of Abraham], then faith [leading to salvation] is of no effect and void, and the promise [of God] is nullified. For the Law results in [God's] wrath [against sin], but where there is no law, there is no violation of it either]. Therefore, [inheriting] the promise depends entirely on faith [that is, confident trust in the unseen God], in order that it may be given as an act of grace [His unmerited favor and mercy], so that the promise will be [legally] guaranteed to all the descents [of Abraham]- not only for those [Jewish believers] who keep the Law, but also for those [Gentile believers] who share the faith of Abraham, who is the [spiritual] father of us all- (as it is written [in Scripture], 'I have made you a father of many nations') in the sight of Him in whom he believed, that is, God, who gives life to the dead and calls into beings that which does not exist."

Following God instead of our own desires, allows us to rest in God's perfect plan for our lives. It doesn't have to make sense to our flesh, because our flesh is subject to our spirits. If we ever find ourselves working to make God move to control God, fulfilling our own desires, timelines, or expectations, then we are sinning against God, and if we aren't careful, we will give birth to an Ishmael. Ishmaels bring suffering to the world, because they are born from sin and trust in the natural realm, not the spiritual one.

The birth of Ishmael caused hurt, instability, and suffering in Abraham's family. Sarah's obedience to her flesh perverted God's perfect plan for her entire household. Abraham's refusal to lead his wife hurt him and it hurt his kids. Hagar was never meant to endure the pain she endured at Sarah's hands. Abraham was never meant to experience the turmoil of losing one of his sons from his life, and Ishmael was never meant to endure the separation of his father.

We can only establish a healthy family through the Lord. Following the leadership of the Holy Spirit enables people to live in peaceful relationships with others, without abuse or harm. The Holy Spirit is the glue that keeps us from harming ourselves and others. Submitting to the Spirit's leadership produces a harvest of blessings that extend beyond us and reach into others' lives. As we agree with God and do what God says to do, even when it doesn't make sense to our flesh, we know our families will flourish.

Galatians 5:19–25 explains, *"Now the practices of the sinful nature are clearly evident: they are sexual immorality, impurity, sensuality (total irresponsibility, lack of self-control), idolatry, sorcery, hostility, strife, jealousy, fits of anger, disputes, dissensions, factions [that promote heresies] envy, drunkenness, riotous behavior, and other things like these. I warn you beforehand, just as I did previously, that those who practice such things will not inherit the kingdom of God But the fruit of the Spirit [the result of His presence within us] is love [unselfish concern for others], joy, [inner] peace, patience [not the ability to wait, but how we act while waiting], kindness, goodness, faithfulness, gentleness, self-control. Against such things there is no law. And those who belong to Christ Jesus have crucified the [sinful nature together with its passions and appetites. If we [claim to] live by the [Holy] Spirit, we must also walk by the Spirit [with personal integrity, godly character, and moral courage—our conduct empowered by the Holy Spirit]."*

Sarah didn't display the fruit of the Holy Spirit. Sarah showed a lack of self-control, irresponsibility, hostility, strife, fits of anger, jealousy, and other such things. She was spiritually blind, and she needed to be led into spiritual truth, not leading others.

If we want to operate in love, joy, peace, patience, kindness, goodness, faithfulness, gentleness, and self-control, we need the Holy Spirit's guidance. We need to follow the Spirit of God and reject anything outside of the word we have received from God. Whenever we face a discrepancy, God is right and we are wrong. Don't make decisions or live assuming you know more than God. Simply be obedient and trust God's integrity and character as the all-knowing parent who lives in Heaven.

Romans 8:14 says, "For all who are allowing themselves to be led by the Spirit of God are sons of God."

16

Adoption and Infertility

Adoption is a family process in which adoptive parents assume the responsibility of parenting a child not biologically related to them. The adoption process involves a filiation system where the legal status of the child is transferred from the biological parents to the adoptive parents. Adoptive parents go through proceedings to gain legal access to possess the child's rights. When biological parents cannot or will not fulfill their parenting duties to children, children need adoptive parents to raise them into adulthood.

Adoptions are legally binding agreements. Once a child has been adopted by new parents, the biological parents' rights and the responsibilities are annulled. Parents who choose to adopt a child willingly take on the responsibility and liability to raise the child appropriately. Adoptive parents become the child's parents and regard the child as their own. They raise, nurture, and develop the child with an unwavering commitment to the child's well-being.

Adopted children often grow into healthy functioning adults. The circumstances leading to a child being adopted are often traumatic, but, in many situations, adoption is the best option for the child, especially when the biological parents cannot perform parenting duties in a safe and effective way.

Many adoptive parents want to have children and are overjoyed to have a child of their own. Once a child is adopted, the parents are expected to perform the parenting duties of any other parent. Adoption is extremely successful when the adoptive parents are healthy and follow the Lord's guidance in raising the child. Relying on the Lord's guidance during parenting ensures that the child is taught right from wrong. This instruction will lead to a thriving, healthy, functioning child.

When Joseph adopted Jesus, God instructed him through his dreams of the best way to care for Jesus. God dealt with Joseph as Jesus's father on the earth, and He treated him as the responsible party for Jesus's safety and well-being. God consistently told Joseph what to do so he could protect Jesus. God will provide adoptive parents with the same supernatural help when they are open to it. He will show the parents exactly what they need to do to help their child.

Adoption is a powerful symbol of love. Adoptive parents do not *have* to adopt and care for a child, instead they *choose* too. They choose to adopt the child with joy and with a loving heart, letting the child become a member of their family. Adoptive parents love the child in the same way they would love their biological kin. This provides the child with a new identity and a new environment where he or she can grow and become the healthiest version of himself or herself.

Having a home and a healthy family allows children to feel loved and to develop properly. The initial biological relationship is only a small portion of the child's makeup. The larger portion of the child's identity is formed through relational bonds and interpersonal learning. The child's learning experiences matter more than the biological tie. Proper learning and connecting to healthy role models will shape the child's future far more than their biological attributes will.

Jesus was raised by an adoptive parent, and Jesus was the healthiest human to ever exist. Moses was also adopted by the pharaoh's daughter, and he was stronger in the spirit than many of the other Israelites who grew up in Israelite homes. Moses and Jesus were two adopted boys who became leaders of God's people. Being adopted didn't hinder them from experiencing overwhelming victory, because they were connected to God and God's house. A connection to God matters more than anything else.

Moses became a powerful leader despite childhood adversity. Moses's life exemplifies that it is possible for adoptive kids to be healthier and more successful than their counterparts, even when they have experienced problems. Children who are connected in their spirits to the Lord will reap the benefits of our Father in Heaven's love, leadership, and protection, even when everything on the earth is positioned to try to destroy them.

God expects all parents to take their jobs seriously by diligently working to provide for the needs of their children. It doesn't take a village to raise a child. God did not give the child to the village. God gave the child a mother and a father. The ultimate responsibility for the child's well-being lies in the hands of the parents. Parents need to remember the Lord has permitted them to perform the job they are doing, and they can do it efficiently when they rely on Him to help them.

Adoptive parents must understand they are spiritually called and equipped to handle their parenting duties. God will send people to help parents, but an overreliance on the world's support systems can harm the child. If the support and the professionals are performing their jobs in a secular, humanistic way and are positioned against God and His word, they are not helping but hindering the development of the child in their care.

Many professionals believe the lie that childhood trauma is irreversible. They believe adoptive children, or any other children experiencing crisis, are eternally damaged and less than children who have not been plagued with challenging circumstance. This demonic philosophy is then used as the psychological foundation for their treatment plans. Underlying all treatment, services, and recommendations is the lie of a doomed and less-fulfilling future.

If this lie of Satan is allowed to be planted into the hearts of children, the children will act it out. When a child's identity is linked to a lie, it will affect on their behavior and worth.

Although many professionals may not say they are agents of the enemy, when we examine the worldview they operate from, we can see they are blind to scriptural truths relating to healing and the full restoration of life. Scripture does not affirm that childhood trauma is a life sentence to bondage.

Treating a child as if he or she is damaged, disabled, or less than because he or she has experienced adversity will cripple the child, instead of strengthening the child. If a child has an identity rooted in a lie, he or she will falsely believe he or she will always suffer with pain. This causes such children them to settle in the pain instead of fighting against it. While the pain is real and a crisis happened, they do not have to indefinitely stay in it.

Trauma does not define one's identity. Our true identity and worth are determined by God. Experiencing traumatic events does not predetermine failure. When individuals come to understand their identity in Christ and recognize their role within God's family, they can overcome any challenges that life presents.

Paul and Silas were in prison. They were beaten and thrown into a nasty jail cell. In the natural realm, they were suffering in an undesirable situation, but Paul and Silas realized they could connect to God, even within a place of suffering. They realized they were connected to a heavenly source of love and protection, and this connection strengthened them and gave them joy when they should have felt no happiness or thankfulness.

The connection to God, and the positive expectation of their future, caused them to break out of prison. The supernatural power of God working through two men in a low place saved even the jailer in the prison.

Being connected to God is a supernatural occurrence. This connection can drive out the pain of the worst situations. It can heal, deliver, and set free even the most challenging of the suffering souls.

The enemy wants us all to believe we are weaker than we are. He wants to steal our strength. One of the ways he steals our children's future is through a confusion of their identity through the introduction of a sick-model identity. By repeatedly reinforcing the lie of sickness, disease, lack, and suffering, Satan tries to create a stronghold of lies within the child's brain, body, and spirit. If we want to tear down the fortresses of hell and take back the people the devil wants to steal, we must share the truth in God's word and stand on that truth no matter what the situation looks like.

Psalm 28:7 teaches, "The Lord is my strength and my shield; in him my heart trusts, and I am helped; my heart exults, and with my song I give thanks to him."

It is impossible to be full of joy if you believe the lie you are unloved and doomed to a lesser, unsuccessful future because of your biological parents' choices. A prophetic future of lack, doom, suffering, and hardship naturally brings depression, anxiety, and other problematic thoughts and behaviors. If we believe we are unlovable, unimportant, and that we will experience a life of adversity, we will act out the narrative presented to us. Believing there is hope for us and that we can overcome anything the enemy has thrown at us is the only hope that we will strive to be successful and victorious.

Children eventually lose the strength and the hope to fight in faith if they have only heard the enemy's prophetic lies. They must hear about the prophetic hope and positive future God has in store for His people for Satan's lies to be eradicated from their minds. If left unchallenged, Satan will produce a state of learned helplessness in a child through the victim cycle. Learned helplessness makes children believe the lie that they are incapable of changing or living a purposeful life, so they should not even try.

Learned helplessness is a psychological state in which individuals, after repeated exposure to uncontrollable negative events, believe they are powerless to change their situation even when they receive opportunities to do so.

Children who have experienced trauma are more vulnerable to learned helplessness, and Satan's ultimate plan is to use their trauma to enslave the children and control their futures. Being victorious through God is possible, regardless of the starting place or the pain we have experienced, and we must make sure children receive the opportunity to hear the message of hope, faith, healing, and restoration through Christ Jesus.

When a child has no hope or positive expectation of the future Satan steals the joy or strength and the shield of the child. Our shield is our faith. We cannot have faith when we do not hear the message of faith. This permits the child to become vulnerable to all evil. Parents must ensure that they never allow outside people to plant this lie in the hearts of their children, because this mindset is vile and sent from hell specifically to destroy a child.

Children who have experienced a crisis must be affirmed and know they are loved and have a great future ahead. They must know, even through suffering, that God is the healer and the comforter, who can give them a better life than they can imagine as they continue to resist the Satan's lies.

Philippians 3:11–13 teaches, "That if possible I may attain to the [spiritual and moral] resurrection [that lifts me] out from among the dead [even while in the body]. Not that I have now attained [this ideal], or have already been made perfect, but I press on to lay hold of (grasp) and make my own, that for which Christ Jesus (the Messiah) has laid hold of me and made me His own. I do not consider, brethren, that I have captured and made it my own [yet]; but one thing I do [it is my one aspiration]: forgetting what lies behind and straining forward to what lies ahead,"

The future is great for all who place their hope and their trust in Jesus. When we have experienced salvation through Christ, we are equipped to forget the things behind us and press into the future. Adoption into a new spiritual family is the beginning of life; it isn't the end! For many children who would have grown up in a dysfunctional, unloving, abusive home, the adoption process shouldn't be viewed as a curse, but as a new beginning and a chance to change and become a better version of the former self. It should be a fresh start, new hope, and a chance to live an even better life than before.

Many biological parents don't give their children up for adoption but are plagued with sickness, so they will transfer these problems to their children. The children who have healthy adoptive parents will fare much better than the children in the care of unhealthy biological parents. Adoption allows children to opt out of severe trauma within their biological families. Adoption isn't a disease or a curse. Adoption is often the environment a child needs to experience health.

The enemy can only take ground in our lives when we do not resist him and let him get close to our family and our hearts. Protecting our kids from the outside world and the enemy's voices is important. We can't trust everyone claiming to be our friends. We must see what lens, what future, and what spirit they prophecy with. If the prophecy isn't scriptural, it must be discarded and rebuked as witchcraft and rebellion against the Lord.

Leviticus 20:2 explains, "Moreover, you shall say to the children of Israel, 'Any Israelite or any stranger residing in Israel who gives any of his children to Molech (the god of the Ammonites) [as a human sacrifice] shall most certainly be put to death; the people of the land shall stone him with stones.'"

We often believe witches and witchcraft are only associated with women in pointy hats, riding on brooms and looking into crystal balls. However, the Bible paints a very different picture of witchcraft. Witchcraft is rebellion against God and His word through the explaining, understanding, and normalizing the voices of the evil spirits.

Many people let unclean evil spirits operating within the people of the world prophesy futures over their children. They allow these evil, ungodly men and women to tell them what their children's life is to be.

These men and women aren't wearing pointy hats or riding brooms. They are driving in cars and hold professional credentials, claiming to perceive and understand the future of a child the Lord has placed into your care—not theirs. Children who have experienced adversity and are already involved with the "systems" of the world often need to be completely separated from the "treatment" plans of those systems to be successful and healthy. Many people and the humanistic-based systems of the world reinforce sickness even when they claim to heal it.

Professionals who have been taught philosophy and treatment plans associated with doctrines rooted in the demonic will transfer sickness to the child. Counselors, for instance who affirm children to be justified in their emotions and behaviors because of their trauma will never heal the child. By teaching the child to accept sickness, the professional permits the weed growth trying to overtake the child.

Children with trauma need structure, accountability, and proper teaching even more than children who have never experienced trauma. Satan has already began shaping their minds and their identities through trauma experiences, thus it is even more important to drive those "weeds" out of the child's mind and identity through proper biblical teaching and cultivating. Validating the weeds does nothing but continue to allow those unhealthy thoughts and behaviors to grow and take over the child.

We can't normalize unhealthy behaviors and thoughts if we want to heal the person. We must replace unhealthy thoughts and behaviors with healthy behaviors and thoughts. It is not unloving to get rid of unhealthy thinking and behaving. The true proof of love is the confrontation of evil. Allowing weeds to overrun a house or a garden isn't loving; it is neglectful. A house that has been neglected will be overrun by pests, weeds, and complete filth and darkness.

When we love others, we will tell them the truth. Even if they don't like it, we will correct them and help them to be clean and whole again, because we know only the truth will set them free. When we rehabilitate houses or people, we need to first clean out the debris of the house. Only when the junk has been removed can new life restoration begin.

Properly discerning the child's needs through a spiritual lens and spiritual analysis will permit us to uproot and discard anything planted into his or her heart or mind. God will show us the strongholds and fortresses the enemy has placed in the child when we desire to know and when we operate under the Lord's anointing. A Spirit-filled parent, church leader, or other professional who is committed to understanding and raising a child to know and serve the Lord will be directed into the truth for the child's well-being. God wants to show caregivers how to target and destroy Satan's works.

The gods of many Americans come in the form of humanism, psychology, sociology, pharmaceuticals, and counseling. If parents are undiscerning and too trusting in the medical services provided to their adopted children, they can further immerse the child in sickness and disease when they are called to consecrate the child into the care of the Great Physician. Unwillingly, many parents, especially parents of children who have faced adversity, hand their children to the "Ammonites" or the people of the land who don't serve their God.

Adoptive parents, be assured in God's eyes you are the child's parents. When you lean into the supernatural help from Heaven, you can remove the trauma from children. God can take every part of trauma and pain and turn it into joy and dancing. He restores, rehabilitates, and sets on high anyone and anything connected to Him. Isaiah 61:4 explains, "Then they will rebuild the ancient ruins, They will raise up and restore the former desolations; And they will renew the ruined cities, The desolations (deserted settlements) of many generations."

Being double-minded and relying on the world brings defilement. A mixture of God's truth and the world's truth leads to a divided and perverted outcome. For an outcome to be pure and uncorrupted by Satan's schemes, there must be no tolerance of lies. There can be no unholy alliance with the enemy. We can sever ties with Satan and separate our homes and our children from the enemy, but we must first entirely separate from humanistic mindsets and self-understanding, choosing to believe God unwaveringly.

Water is polluted even when pollution comes in small increments. Pure water is pure because it hasn't been contaminated. Satan often pollutes the water, even water that appears to be pure. In doing so, he spoils the water we need to properly survive and grow. A little bit of pollution will corrupt the entire well. If we want to remain untainted, operating in fullness of health and life, we must refuse any compromise or any mixing with the pollution found in the worldviews of unbelievers.

Children are a blessing to their adoptive parents, and the adoptive parents are a blessing to the children. Adoptive parents who ensure their own hearts are right before they commit to raising the child will bless their child, and the child will also be a blessing to them. However, if there is an alternative or selfish reason for an adoption, those parents should resist adopting the child out of the protection of the child. Adoption should only occur when parents have a desire to protect and love another person. Adoption should always be done out of a helping heart instead of a personal fulfillment approach.

The love and the protection of an adoptive parent/child relationship must stem from an emotionally healthy place. Adoptive parents need to be sure they can give the child what he or she deserves from a parent.

Not all adoptions are beneficial to a child. In recent years, lesbian and gay couples have begun to adopt children. Built on an ungodly, sinful lifestyle, these parents begin their parenting journey as agents of the devil. Children raised in these atmospheres are being raised in a lifestyle that is against God and His word, and this is very dangerous for the child's future.

Rachel wanted to have biological children with her husband, and she desired to become a mother so much that she said she would rather die than to remain barren. Rachel watched women in her life conceive and have children of their own. This caused her to carry a burden of sorrow, shame, and sadness. Rachel was without hope and positive expectations of the future.

Genesis 30:1 says, "Rachel saw that she could not have children for Jacob, and she became jealous of her sister. She said to Jacob, "Give me children, or I'll die!"

We know Rachel prayed about her infertility, and the Lord heard her prayers. However, before God answered Rachel's prayers, Rachel violated God's perfect plan for her family. Instead of waiting for the Lord, Rachel decided she would become a mother through performing a work of the flesh.

Genesis 30:22 tells us, "Then God remembered [the prayers of] Rachel, and God thought of her and opened her womb [so that she would conceive]. So, she conceived and gave birth to a son; and she said, 'God has taken away my disgrace and humiliation.' She named him Joseph (may He add) and said, 'May the Lord add to me another son.'"

Like Sarah, Rachel had her husband impregnate another woman. The lack of spiritual maturity, understanding, and patience caused Rachel to behave out of her flesh and her emotions instead of waiting in faith. And although Rachel attained a son legally through her maid Bilhah, she did so outside of a covenant with God. Rachel chose Dan's name, and she received custody of him, but she did so out of God's will.

Rachel conspired to have Dan born into the world to fulfill her own needs and desires. She created life out of her selfishness and pride. Acting outside of God's plan, Rachel believed she could circumvent God and control her future. She tried to get something that did not belong to her, so she hurt people in the process. Rachel stole Bilhah's first son. She also stole the loving bond a child and parent should have from baby Dan, because she wanted to be personally validated.

Genesis 30:3–6 tells us, "She said, 'Here, take my maid Bilhah and go in to her; and [when the baby comes] she shall deliver it [while sitting] on my knees, so that by her I may also have children [to count as my own].' So she gave him Bilhah her maid as a [secondary] wife, and Jacob went in to her. Bilhah conceived and gave birth to a son for Jacob Rachel said, 'Now God has judged in my favor. He has heard my prayer and has given me a son.' So, she named him Dan [He Judges]."

Rachel looked through physical lenses and did not understand the spiritual implications of her choices. Rachel falsely believed the Lord gave her Dan, even when scripture doesn't validate this to be true. God did not willingly give Rachel a baby through her maid. Rachel stole another woman's future, body, and child, and even though she called the child her own, he was not hers to claim.

Surrogacy is becoming increasingly popular, especially in First World nations where medical capabilities allow people to conceive and bear children using another woman's body. Today, eggs and sperm can be implanted into a surrogate's body, and she can carry the child, deliver the child, and then allow the child to be separated from her for the couple's pleasure. Lesbian and gay couples, as well as straight couples, are increasingly attempting to normalize the use of surrogacy to produce children, even when this act is not blessed by the Lord.

Surrogate women are objectified, and surrogacy is a violence against women. "Sexual objectification occurs whenever a woman's body or sexual functions are separated from her personhood, reducing her to an object for consumption, rather than a human being with feelings, personality, intelligence, or needs." (Frederickson & Roberts, 1997). Today in America, it is becoming more common to use a surrogate, but we must teach young women and men the truth about surrogacy. Surrogacy objectifies and abuses women for money for another's distorted amusement.

Rachel didn't think about the impact she was having on Dan or on Bilhah. She didn't care about Bilhah, because she viewed her as an object to abuse for her own gain. Dan was also objectified, created as an object to be owned instead of a person to be loved. Dan's best interest was not to be born into a dysfunctional family, superficially created for a controlling woman's personal fulfillment. Rachel was willing to harm anyone, including a baby, to make sure she got what she felt entitled to get. Her behaviors were not those of a God-fearing woman.

Narcissistic personality disorder is characterized by a pattern of exaggerated feelings of self-importance and an excessive need for admiration. Narcissistic people have a diminished ability to empathize with other people and their feelings, and they often disregard others entirely to ensure they receive what they feel they deserve. Narcissists destroy other people's lives because they feel they are more valuable than other people. Narcissists want to control and determine others' futures as they use them to get whatever they desire.

Rachel was a narcissist. She didn't care about the feelings, needs, or lives of anyone else, because she only cared about herself. Narcissism is a spiritual disease first, and it manifests as a social emotional disease second. Narcissism is rooted in the desire to feed personal desires as opposed to spiritual ones. Galatians 6:8 teaches, "For he who sows to his own flesh (lower nature, sensuality) will from the flesh reap decay and ruin and destruction, but he who sows to the Spirit will from the Spirit reap eternal life."

If Rachel had waited on God, she would have been given Joseph when it was God's timing, and she wouldn't have harmed anyone else in her family. Rachel didn't need to hurt anyone else because God planned to bless her with her own baby. Rachel should have denied herself and submitted herself to God and waited on His perfect timing for her baby's arrival.

When we become new creatures in Christ, we die to our former selves. Dying to the former biological family and joining the new, spiritual family is the best thing that could happen to us for our growth. It is the only chance we have at living an abundant life on the earth now and in the future in Heaven. Dying to the cravings of the flesh is a sign of a spiritual birth in a person's life; without the old person dying, the new person cannot exist.

Luke 9:23 says, "And He said to all, 'If any person wills to come after Me, let him deny himself [disown himself, forget, lose sight of himself and his own interests, refuse and give up himself] and take up his cross daily and follow Me [cleave steadfastly to Me, conform wholly to My example in living and, if need be, in dying also].'"

People who participate in surrogacy objectify and abuse a woman and a child. God sees surrogacy as a disgrace and a disgust. Young women need to be warned about these types of predators, so they can perceive when they are being violated in the name of modern medicine. Selfishness, stealing, and envy are all characteristics that the employing surrogate parents have. These behaviors are not the fruit of the Spirit of God.

Those who advocate the use of surrogacy are misguided. They can pretend to be good, but their fruit speaks for itself. Don't eat their bread, share in the corruption, or take anything from these types of people. Proverbs 23:6–8 says, "Do not eat the bread of a selfish man, Or desire his delicacies; For as he thinks in his heart, so is he [in behavior—one who manipulates]. He says to you, "Eat and drink," Yet his heart is not with you [but it is begrudging the cost]. The morsel which you have eaten you will vomit up, And you will waste your compliments."

Theft is never the way God brings "blessings" into His people's lives. When something is stolen, it is not blessed by the person who stole the item. God doesn't endorse stealing. God expects thieves to pay an account for what they stole. Many people will stand before God one day and give an account for their wicked behavior relating to surrogacy if they do not repent and have their sins cleansed through the blood of Jesus.

In First Samuel 5:1, the Ark of the Covenant was stolen during a battle. The enemies placed the ark next to their god Dagon. The next morning Dagon was on his face, and the fear of God caused them to return the Ark of the Covenant.

As the enemy steals children and attempts to use them as commodities to be trafficked or abused, God will avenge them. God hates it when humans are treated as inanimate objects. Humans are even more important to God than the box, a symbol of the Ark of the Covenant. How much more then will God avenge the blood and the damage of the ones who are being abused by wicked people?

Many narcissistic people feel an exaggerated sense of importance. And because they feel entitled to a baby, they are a direct danger of harming the innocent child they are adopting. Trafficking human beings as objects to be consumed is a mark of the enemy. Even when these acts are legalized in the American courts, they are not blessed in God's kingdom. Rachel believed God was blessing her when she received Dan, but that does not mean God truly was blessing her evil actions. Merely believing we are justified in the acts of evil doesn't mean the acts are truly pure or blessed by the Lord.

Rachel hurt many people, and she felt justified in doing so. She did not show a sense of repentance for her sins and her violations against others. Rachel was spiritually blind and didn't properly comprehend God's truth. She refused to see the truth, even when she was presented with it.

Rachel was jealous of and in a competition with her sister, Leah. Scripture identifies both jealousy and competition as unholy fleshly characteristics. Rachel's jealous spirit caused her to act in ways that were ungodly. She didn't consider others more significant than herself, and she wasn't humble before God or people, because she considered herself to be of utmost importance.

Philippians 2:3 teaches, "Do nothing from rivalry or conceit, but in humility count others more significant than yourselves."

Rachel's selfish ambition blocked to her spiritual vision. She did not see her situation from a healthy spiritual lens because she was self-absorbed, operating out of her flesh nature, instead of her spiritual one. Rachel had grown accustomed to being accommodated as the most valuable of her family. As she grew up, she was favored by her father, and as an adult, she was favored by her husband, Jacob.

James 3:16 explains, "For where jealousy and selfish ambition exist, there will be disorder and every vile practice."

Rachel felt entitled to a baby because she believed she was superior to Leah. Rachel carried so much selfish ambition that she used another woman to see that her desires were met. God wanted to deal with Rachel's sin and her heart before He opened her womb. He wanted to teach her humility, patience, and true love through a full reliance on Him.

Genesis 29:16–20 says, "Now Laban had two daughters; the name of the older was Leah, and the name of the younger was Rachel. Leah's eyes were weak, but Rachel was beautiful in form and appearance. Jacob loved Rachel, so he said, 'I will serve you [as a hired workman] for seven years [in return] for [the privilege of marrying] Rachel your younger daughter.' Laban said, 'It is better that I give her [in marriage] to you than give her to another man. Stay and work with me.' So Jacob served [Laban] for seven years for [the right to marry] Rachel, but they seemed like only a few days to him because of his love for her."

God tried to prepare Rachel for motherhood through a season of infertility. God wanted to give her a baby, but before she could be a good mom she needed to change her unhealthy reliance on herself. Being a mother requires a profound level of self-sacrifice. It is difficult to nurture, protect, and care for a baby effectively while adhering to a self-centered worldview. God wanted to remove the weeds from Rachel's spirit, healing her inner woman, so He could continue to bless her outwardly rewarding her to be a mom.

Rachel refused God's emotional healing plan, and she hurt others out of her refusal to personally heal. Today, many people hurt others because they are not healed and restored from their own problems. Instead of owning the deficiencies they try to cover them up. Proverbs 28:13 says, "He who conceals his transgressions will not prosper, But whoever confesses and turns away from his sins will find compassion and mercy."

Rachel wanted her way, and she exalted herself above her Creator, trying to get what she felt she deserved. She didn't humble herself before her Creator. Rachel followed in Satan's footsteps, as it was Satan who also felt entitled to more. He felt he was being kept from a privilege, and he believed he was able to tell God what to do, instead of being told what to do and humbling himself in his position before God.

Romans 12:3 warns, "For by the grace [of God] given to me I say to everyone of you not to think more highly of himself [and of his importance and ability] than he ought to think; but to think so as to have sound judgment, as God has apportioned to each a degree of faith [and a purpose designed for service]."

Rachel's husband was spiritually wise, and he acknowledged that God was keeping Rachel from conceiving. Jacob discerned the root of the problem properly because he saw in the realm of the spirit. Jacob confronted Rachel of her arrogance against God, and when he did, Rachel lashed out at him for his loving rebuke. Rachel threw a temper tantrum, like many narcissists do when they do not get their way. She became mad at Jacob for trying to instruct her into the truth of God, instead of humbling herself to the reality of the situation.

Proverbs 9:8 says, "Reprove not a scorner, lest he hate you; reprove a wise man, and he will love you."

Genesis 30:2 says, "Then Jacob became furious with Rachel, and he said, "Am I in the place of God, who has denied you children?"

God is watching family dynamics. God cared about Leah's mistreatment and lack of love. He saw and responded to Leah's suffering by blessing her with children. Being a mother provides women with a sense of love, connection, and importance. Outside of Leah's children, no one in her life appreciated her, and God cared that she was being neglected by others. God didn't want Leah to be alone and suffering. He wanted her to know she was important, so He blessed her with many children.

Genesis 29:31–35 says, "Now when the Lord saw that Leah was unloved, He made her able to bear children, but Rachel was barren. Leah conceived and gave birth to a son and named him Reuben (See, a son!), for she said, 'Because the Lord has seen my humiliation and suffering; now my husband will love me [since I have given him a son].' Then she conceived again and gave birth to a son and said, 'Because the Lord heard that I am unloved, He has given me this son also.' So she named him Simeon (God hears). She conceived again and gave birth to a son and said, 'Now this time my husband will become attached to me [as a companion], for I have given him three sons.' Therefore he was named Levi. Again she conceived and gave birth to a [fourth] son, and she said, 'Now I will praise the Lord.' So she named him Judah; then [for a time] she stopped bearing [children]."

Leah named her children to magnify the Lord. She was thankful that God saw her pain and blessed her for her suffering. Leah looked to the Lord for strength, validation, and help. She was used to being unloved, mistreated, and used by the world. Leah had a contrast between God and the world. She knew God was blessing her womb and her life.

God teaches us about healthy and unhealthy jealousy through the narratives of Leah and Rachel. Healthy jealousy is the result of feeling like someone or something is in our proper place. In healthy jealously, we become jealous because we are kept from receiving the love that is ours to receive. God wanted Leah to be loved and respected by her dad. He wanted her husband and her sister to care about her, and He saw they were withholding the proper love and admiration she deserved to receive from them.

Leah was righteously jealous, because her jealousy stemmed from wanting to be protected, loved, and cared for in a proper and godly manner. Leah was jealous of the love she didn't get because others continued to violate her, use her, and mistreat her when she had the God-given right to be loved. Leah was valuable, and her life mattered to God, but the people around her rejected her and mistreated her for their own gain. Because of the mistreatment by humans and her humble heart, God took notice of her and helped her.

Deuteronomy 4:24 explains, "For the Lord your God is a consuming fire, a jealous God."

God wants us to love Him. God deserves our love, and when we fail to give it to Him, He has a healthy jealously. God doesn't want us to care about the world or other people more than we care about Him. He doesn't want us to treat Him as unimportant or less than anyone or anything else in our lives.

Many adopted children or children from dysfunctional families feel jealous of the love they don't receive from others. They feel righteously jealous because they are hurt that they didn't receive the love they were supposed to have. God understands this pain and rejection. He understands feeling jealous and sad about the loss of connection, love, and relationship with those who should want to be in a relationship with Him.

Leah's father didn't safeguard her best interests. He didn't protect and honor his daughter. Parents who are involved in dangerous, sinful lifestyles, and who give up the rights of their children don't provide the child with the love they should have. They don't safeguard their children's best interests, and this is painful. However, we can have hope knowing our God sees and understands. We can believe God will provide us with more because of the pain and the neglect of those who were meant to love us.

Many adoptive children may at times feel unloved and unseen by their adoptive parents, especially when their adoptive parents adopted them with impure motives. If parents couldn't have children and adopt a child because they feel they are owed one but feel the adopted child is not as good as a biological child, then the child will see that he or she is the parents' second choice. This causes the child to feel rejected and unloved, knowing the parents wouldn't have him or her if they could have children on their own.

Jacob didn't intend to marry Leah; he intended to marry Rachel. Jacob was only with Leah because Rachel was not available. Leah knew she was not Jacob's first choice. She knew he didn't really love her or want her, but he kept her out of an obligation.

Adoptive children are at times treated with contempt by their siblings in their adoptive home. Many adopted kids struggle to feel accepted by their brothers and sisters. Leah felt her sister was unkind, treating her poorly and with contempt. Leah knew her sister's heart was not right towards her, and this hurt her because she wanted her sister to love and respect her. Rachel should have cared about Leah, and she should have treated her with compassion, love, and care, instead of being jealous of her.

When a child has been adopted, parents need to work on the sibling relationships in the home. They cannot tolerate or normalize any mistreatment in the sibling relationship. Biological children must be taught to respect and love the adopted child as a rightful member of the family. Children who have been adopted need to know they are not inferior to a member of the family unit, and they are just as much apart of the family as a biological child.

If we don't receive the love we want to receive, we must remember that God notices, cares, and repays for the love stolen from us. Like Leah, all of us can lean on God even if we are not properly cared for by our families. When we lean on God as our source of life, He will love us, even when no one else around us seems to notice our suffering. God continued to bless Leah with her own children. God kept Leah close to His heart, and He provided even more than she wanted because she didn't allow the mistreatment to change her humble, God-fearing, loving heart.

Leah wanted others to love her, and although this wasn't wrong, she finally realized after God continued to bless her, that her identity to God was more important than her identity in others' eyes. God wants us to receive our validation from Him first before receiving anything in the natural world. He wants us to know we matter to Him and that His love is enough, even if no one else notices or cares about us.

Genesis 29:35 explains, "She conceived again, and when she gave birth to a son she said, 'This time I will praise the Lord.' So, she named him Judah. Then she stopped having children."

Until the birth of Judah, Leah was thankful to God, but she was still largely focused on others' rejection. She didn't fully comprehend her value to God because she still focused on needing her family to love her. God was divinely jealous of her desire for and her admiration of the men and women around her. He continued to woo her into His loving presence. Eventually, Leah got the message that God and His love was sufficient.

Rachel had unhealthy jealousy. She craved something that was not hers. Rachel wanted natural things God had not yet given her, and she tried to steal her way into the blessing. Rachel didn't deserve to have her sister's children, and she was wrong to feel entitled to them. Her infertility was the result of a spiritual deficiency, and she could have handled her infertility through a spiritual connection with the Lord.

Whenever we lack something in the natural, if God hasn't given it to us yet, it doesn't mean He won't or that He doesn't want us to have it. We may need us to simply receive more spiritual revelation. God wants His children to be fruitful and multiply. He wants to give women children, and if we are struggling with infertility, we can go to God and believe He will help us to conceive and bear children out of humble faith, not out of obligation and entitlement. God heard and answered Rachel's prayer it just wasn't on her timeline.

When we become jealous of other people's gifts and blessings, we are coveting and sin against the Lord. Trying to take something that doesn't belong to us won't help us. If we want to be righteous, we must receive things through faith by accessing them in the spirit, and then we will be blessed in what we receive. Proverbs 10:2 says, "Treasures of wickedness and ill-gotten gains do not profit But righteousness and moral integrity in daily life rescues from death."

God is always looking for new children to add to His family. He wants everyone to come into His house and experience true love and to live an abundant life. As we are adopted into God's family, our old family ties are severed, and we become legally attached to our new family. The biological relationship doesn't dominate us anymore because our new family's identity is more influential than the family we came from. We are born again, and we are joined to a heavenly family, full of other brothers and sisters who share our faith and our Heavenly Father.

Ephesians 1:4-5 teaches, "Even as He chose us in Him before the foundation of the world, that we should be holy and blameless before Him. In love He predestined us for adoption to Himself as sons through Jesus Christ, according to the purpose of His will."

God works with us, removing the weeds and fifth from our past lives. He restores us and makes us brand new. In the first few years as a believer, we grow. We begin to separate from our past and attach ourselves to our new future. God understands when we are immature and need His help. He sees when we need more insight, and He works with us to give us the things we need for optimal health. If we have been mistreated, neglected, or unloved by people, and we have not received things we are meant to have, God will ensure we are repaid and that we will receive more than we could imagine.

God gave His best, His Son Jesus Christ, to receive us into His family. He believes we are valuable and worthy, and He wanted to rescue us from the unhealthy family system we were born into. He knew we would be destroyed if we were not pulled out of our former home. He knew the only way we could be well is if we joined His family. Matthew 13:45-46 explains, "Again, the kingdom of heaven is like a merchant in search of fine peals, and upon finding a single pearl of great value, he went and sold all that he had and bought it."

For thousands of years, God has experienced what it feels like to be rejected by people who are supposed to love Him. Some people have always refused to acknowledge His existence, even when He has tried to have a relationship with them. God came to earth as a baby, and He entrusted Himself into the arms of people who had to care for Him and nurture His physical body. Jesus walked by people on the street every day whom He created, and those people denied Him, mocked Him, and refused to acknowledge His value.

God knows what it feels like to be abandoned and unloved. He knows what it feels like to be unseen by people who should appreciate who you are. God knows what it feels like to be completely abused and even put to death by the people who should have recognized your value. Even with the rejection, pain, and disrespect, the Lord counted it all worth it, so He could have a family of people who really loved Him—people who didn't have to choose Him, but they did.

Our adoption into God's family is beautiful. He chose us when He didn't have to. He gave Himself so we can experience a healthy family and true love.

Like any adopted child, we get to decide if we will accept His love! Will we give Him our whole hearts and be thankful for the new life that we have received? Will we gladly join our new family and reject the pain of the past instead of holding on to it? Or will we focus on the people and the things we don't have, rejecting the Father's love because we fixate on what we don't have instead of what we do. Our hearts matter: they influence the outcome of our lives and our families' future!

17

Embodying Christ

Believers are in God's army. All of us, upon our confession and allegiance to Jesus Christ, are enlisted against enemy forces. To be successful in the war against Satan, we need to go through basic training, receiving knowledge about who God is, and what His mission is. If we are going to be able to advance God's kingdom, we must know the internal operations of the war and what we are expected to do.

Believers must know how to fight and how to seize and conquer the enemy forces against them. God's word, whether spoken or written, protects us from all the attacks of our enemy, Satan. The word of God is a weapon protecting us from harm. God's word stops Satan from penetrating his plans and purposes into our life. Satan can't harm us when we are in alignment with God.

We must be able to see, hear, and operate in the realm of the spirit to be victorious over our flesh or evil spirits. Revelation is our provision. In all wars, planning and provision are vital for success. Without the necessary plans and provisions, soldiers can be conquered. God wants us to receive our provision. He has given us everything we need to keep the enemy at bay, but we need to learn how to use the things we have been given.

A gun in the hands of a person who doesn't know how to aim and fire doesn't provide the protection it was intended to. Likewise, a person who doesn't know who they are in the spirit, or what they have in the spirit, may have the weapons, but he or she doesn't know how to use them in the war. To be precise and effective in our spiritual walks, we must learn and train in the spirit. We need to learn how to use the weapons of war God has given us as His Church.

Matthew 6:9–11 teaches, "Pray, therefore, like this: Our Father Who is in heaven, hallowed (kept holy) be Your name. Your kingdom come, Your will be done on earth as it is in heaven. Give us this day our daily bread."

We are instructed to pray always for God's will to be done on the earth as it is done in Heaven. To manifest our provision from Heaven, we need to take ground against the enemies' troops and plans by aligning with the plans and pursuits of God. If we do not know God's will or plans, then we can't align our plans to match it. But when we know what God wants done, and we partner with Him to do His work, we will receive our supernatural, abundant supply.

A lack of revelation and wisdom prevents us from knowing where we should be, or what we should be doing. If we aren't sure where the supply room is, we can't receive the supply we need to continue the journey. We need to ask the Lord what we are to be doing and where we are to be doing it. We need to know where we are and where we are going. By communing with God and getting our orders, we learn where we are and where we are going.

God will give each person marching orders. He has an assignment or mission for each of us. When we know what we are to do, and where we are to do it, we will begin to receive supernaturally from Heaven. God won't leave us without help if He has called us to a place. He will always provide for us in the places where He leads us.

I began to experience supernatural abundant supply from Heaven when I obeyed God's orders and stayed home as a mother. When I aligned with God's will and His plan for my life, I began to experience the Lord's supernatural provisions. If we try to go our own way and we walk the way we feel we should go, then we will wonder why we haven't received anything from the Lord. We should understand that we won't receive when we aren't in the right location.

God has a place for us. He has an exact location we need to be to receive the blessings He has for us. Elijah was fed by the widow because he went to the place where the Lord told him to go. If we are not following the Lord's leadership, and we are asking the Lord to bless our plans instead of partnering with Him to see His plans for our life fulfilled, then we will only prosper in a natural—not supernatural—way.

Our first portion of prayer should focus on ensuring we are heading in the proper direction, so we can guarantee the proper spiritual reinforcement from Heaven. Direction and heavenly provision position us for victory in any given situation, whether our finances, our health, relationships, or anything else we are looking for. As we pray, we must remember to pray the way we were instructed to pray.

The Bible clearly notes a right and wrong way to pray if you want to see supernatural results! We need to pray to see God's will done on the earth. God's will, not our will, must be the centerpiece of our prayer points. God promises us to give us more than we even ask for if we seek first the kingdom. As we put God and His kingdom first, we know we will have what we need, and we will have an overflow too!

Matthew 6:7-8 explains, "And when you pray, do not heap up phrases (multiply words, repeating the same ones over and over) as the Gentiles do, for they think they will be heard for their much speaking. Do not be like them, for your Father knows what you need before you ask Him."

If we are always asking God to meet our needs, we are praying incorrectly. God has already promised to meet our needs. He has promised to give us our provision. When we pray, we need thank God for the provision He has already given us. We need to realize God has already provided us with the things we need. All things we need are already available in the spirit realm, but we need to learn how to draw them out.

If we have a million dollars in our bank account and we don't know how to get it out of the bank, it will be difficult, if not impossible, to get the money out of the account. Even with the provision, we could struggle unnecessarily because we don't know how to access because we are blocked from accessing the funds in the account.

Satan wants to block us from knowing what we have in Christ. But we often block ourselves from getting the provisions because we don't know what we have in our accounts as believers.

If we are always praying for our needs, we are not focused on kingdom needs, and this is why God tells us to understand that we are not to consider or worry about our needs. We can focus on the higher purpose, God's purpose. In doing so, we will receive everything we need and even things we want. God's kingdom, when it is exalted and placed first within our lives, will always supernaturally provide more than enough for us and others around us. We can operate on a higher standard than in the world. We can walk in the realm of the supernatural.

As soldiers, we don't need to worry about our food and clothes. Any enlisting army provides the necessities. Our mission is to put our focus and energy on the task and the job we have been given. We need to pay attention and use strategy from Heaven on how to take ground against the opposing forces. As we place our focus on the war against Satan and the souls and lives of those who need deliverance, help, and assistance, we will receive an abundance of everything the world works tirelessly to achieve.

Matthew 6:12–13 says, "And forgive us our debts, as we also have forgiven (left, remitted, and let go of the debts, and have given up resentment against) our debtors. And lead (bring) us not into temptation, but deliver us from the evil one. For Yours is the kingdom and the power and the glory forever. Amen."

In part two of our prayers, we pray to keep our hearts pure against hate or resentment of others. When we let Satan plant pain and resentment towards others in our hearts, we allow those things to steal our focus. We give Satan the opportunity to distract us from the goal at hand. Satan's mission against the Church is to suppress or stop the advancement of the kingdom. He wants to limit and distract the troops to keep them from taking territory from him.

God wants us to focus on the kingdom and limit distractions, because distractions allow the enemy to remain in the places God wants to drive him out of. Satan uses distractions to prevent us from fully focusing on God's mission. He wants to wound us, often through other people, so we cannot focus on the proper mission.

God instructs us to forgive and to move on from the attacks of the enemy. He wants us to not be fazed by Satan's wounding. When we are offended and feel sorry for ourselves, we will not be able to advance against the kingdom of darkness anymore, because we will be distracted from our heavenly mission. When Satan tries to wound us through other people, we can realize we are not wrestling against the person, but an Antichrist spirit.

Don't allow the devil to use people to stop you from advancing. Don't give the devil the opportunity to see you weak, sad, and vulnerable from his attack. If Satan has tried to use a person to harm you, pray for the person and forgive the person. This is the spiritual way to win the war against the demonic. We wrestle not with flesh and blood, but with spirits who want to see us defeated and limited in our progression. The attacks are personal, and they are from hell, so resist them and rebuke them, not giving the enemy a foothold into your life.

As we obey God's specific instructions regarding prayer, we see God's supernatural force activated in our lives. When we pray as God told us to pray, this moves the devil and all the intended attacks out of our way, and it allows us to move against him as defensive soldiers taking back what is ours. We need to realize that we have what it takes to be successful against Satan and his demons. We have everything we need in our spiritual arsenal, and the Lord has given us a blueprint and a strategy that works every single time!

God's words are our nutrition we need to fuel the body for success. God's word is not limited to the Bible, even though God often encourages us using scripture. God can speak to us in different ways. He doesn't speak to His people in one way exclusively. God uses angels, dreams, visions, auditory, visual, or anything else He deems necessary to ensure we get our daily bread. More than anything, God wants to communicate with us, commune with us, and help us to see His mission and His assistance in every aspect of our lives.

We should never be caught up in wondering how God will provide what we need. We should simply focus on the truth that He will. God will give us help, and He will give us marching orders. He will tell us what to do, and we will hear a voice saying, "This is the way to go, walk in it." God isn't the author of confusion. He won't hide and confuse us about the path we need to walk on. All believers have an internal operating system connected to Heaven, and we are programmed to receive God's instructions.

The foods we eat and the liquids we drink are the basis of our health and our strength. If we indulge in the wrong foods, this prevents our bodies from optimal performance. Eating the enemy's food is detrimental because the enemy forces plan to poison us and make us sick to make sure we are weaker than we should be. In wars, enemy forces often poison food and water sources, because they know if they can pollute the water and the food, the soldiers are weaker than if they had been eating pure and healthy food.

Eating heavenly bread and drinking the pure water of life guarantees we are strong, healthy, and able bodied in the spirit realm. Good, uncontaminated nutrition requires self-control. If we are going to feed our spirits, we must say no to the foods that are not meant to be part of our diet. Some foods weaken the body and the spirit, and other foods sustain and strengthen them. Realizing our part to play with our self-control and decisions helps us to take responsibility for the things we allow to come into our bodies and temples.

John 6:48–51 says, "Jesus said, 'I am the Bread of Life [the Living Bread which gives and sustains life]. Your fathers ate the manna in the wilderness, and they died. This is the Bread that comes down out of heaven, so that one may eat of it and not die. I am the Living Bread that came down out of heaven. If anyone eats of this Bread [believes in Me, accepts Me as Savior], he will live forever. And the Bread that I will give for the life of the world is My flesh (body).'"

Jesus Christ is the pure bread. He sustains and provides us with all we need to survive and thrive. The enemy will extend an invitation for us to dine at his table. He will offer us polluted rations, hoping we will be deceived and take a bite. But when we stay focused on Jesus, and we are accustomed to pure food and water, we will identify the corrupted food and will push it back from our plates. By staying pure and loyal to our mission, we show our spiritual commitment, and we remain strong.

In hospitals or other medical facilities, people are often conjoined with infusion pumps (IVs). Infusion pumps are medical devices that provide people with needed fluids, medications, or other nutrients that aid in their protection and healing. IVs are given to patients intravenously, so the needed nutrients are provided quickly through the veins. Veins are blood vessels that transport blood from the several regions of the body. These vessels work to impact the heart.

If people are conjoined to Jesus Christ, they are connected to an IV that never runs out. Jesus provides us with all the fluid, medication, and other nutrients we need to be successful in life and in battle.

When Jesus went back to Heaven, He sent His Spirit, the Holy Spirit, to live in us and to connect to us. He sent the Holy Spirit to be our IV. The Holy Spirit is our source of help and nutrients, providing us with the constant supply of spiritual assistance. Our connection to the Holy Spirit infuses life into our hearts.

The baptism of the Holy Spirit is mandatory for a constant spiritual supply. Without the baptism of the Holy Spirit, we are living without our IV in the battle. The baptism of the Holy Spirit is separate from our water baptism and our conversion to Christianity. Scripture affirms the men and women in the upper room needed the Holy Spirit to perform the kingdom work against Satan. Acts 2:33 says, "Exalted to the right hand of God, he has received from the Father the promised Holy Spirit and has poured out what you now see and hear."

In the upper room, the men and the women were believers, and they believed in the reality of Jesus's life, ministry, and death and resurrection. If they did not know these things, they would have never waited many days to receive the gift from Heaven Jesus had promised to give them. Believing in Jesus Christ is the first step of salvation. Without believing, one cannot go onto step two, which is to be baptized in water.

Matthew 3:16 explains, "As soon as Jesus was baptized, he went up out of the water. At that moment heaven was opened, and he saw the Spirit of God descending like a dove and alighting on him. And a voice from heaven said, 'This is my Son, whom I love; with him I am well pleased.'"

Jesus was baptized in water, and He told us to also baptize people who believe in Him. Water baptism is a symbol of our new life and our new birth. When we are baptized, we display to others what we believe, and demonstrate what has happened on the inside. Being baptized is the symbol of being born again. As we go under the water, we show we understand that the old man dies, and the new man, the man of the spirit is born.

Being born again is a requirement to enter a covenant relationship with God. As we confess our belief in Jesus, we pledge to die to our old sin nature. This alliance to God and His kingdom permits us to enter a heavenly covenant relationship with our Creator. We become new creatures, leaving behind the customs, and the behaviors of our nature. As we are born again, we lose the pattern of sin, the mark of sin, and the control of sin, and we pledge ourselves to Heaven.

However, there is a third part of our salvation experience we need to carry out the mission and the purposes of God's kingdom. To fulfill our call as soldiers and empowered Saints in the kingdom, we must receive the baptism of the Holy Spirit. Many Christians fulfill the first two parts of their enlistment. They sign the papers, they accept the call, but they lack in the spiritual equipment department. If Christians don't receive baptism of the Holy Spirit, they don't have their full spiritual armor and are not fully prepared to fight their enemy.

Acts 8:9–20 says:

But there was a man named Simon, who had formerly practiced magic arts in the city to the utter amazement of the Samaritan nation, claiming that he himself was an extraordinary and distinguished person. They all paid earnest attention to him, from the least to the greatest, saying, "This man is that exhibition of the power of God which is called great (intense)." And they were attentive and made much of him, because for a long time he had amazed and bewildered and dazzled them with his skill in magic arts.

But when they believed the good news (the Gospel) about the kingdom of God and the name of Jesus Christ (the Messiah) as Philip preached it, they were baptized, both men and women. Even Simon himself believed [he adhered to, trusted in, and relied on the teaching of Philip], and after being baptized, devoted himself constantly to him. And seeing signs and miracles of great power that were being performed, he was utterly amazed.

Now when the apostles (special messengers) at Jerusalem heard that [the country of] Samaria had accepted and welcomed the Word of God, they sent Peter and John to them, And they came down and prayed for them that the Samaritans might receive the Holy Spirit; For He had not yet fallen upon any of them, but they had only been baptized into the name of the Lord Jesus. Then [the apostles] laid their hands on them one by one, and they received the Holy Spirit.

However, when Simon saw that the [Holy] Spirit was imparted through the laying on of the apostles' hands, he brought money and offered it to them, Saying, Grant me also this power and authority, in order that anyone on whom I place my hands may receive the Holy Spirit. But Peter said to him, Destruction overtake your money and you, because you imagined you could obtain the [free] gift of God with money!

In the books of Acts, the believers needed to have the apostles place their hands on them, imparting the baptism of the Holy Spirit, despite previously receiving and believing the good news about the kingdom of God and the name of Jesus Christ. Believing the good news, and being baptized in water were the first two requirements needed for their conversion to Christianity. However, the baptism of the Holy Spirit, the filling with the fire of God through the laying on of hands, was a separate and third step in fulfilling the call of Christ.

All believers need to believe, be baptized in water, and then receive the Holy Spirit to be properly spiritually empowered and equipped. The baptism of the Holy Spirit allows us to do the supernatural in the kingdom of God. Without the baptism of the Holy Spirit, we are not endowed with the proper amount of spiritual power required to exert force against our enemy, Satan. The firepower of heaven is within the baptism of the Holy Spirit.

If you have not received the baptism of the Holy Spirit, and you are a believer, it is never too late to receive it. Once you ask the Lord for it and you seek it out, the Lord will pour it out on you, and you will never be the same again. The baptism of the Holy Spirit is free. God wants to give it you, and to receive it, you must only ask Him for it and believe you will get what you have asked for! Once you receive it, you will know you are full of the Spirit. You will exhibit evidence of the change.

First Corinthians 10: 2–5 says, "And all [of them] were baptized into Moses [into his safekeeping as their leader] in the cloud and in the sea; and all [of them] ate the same spiritual food; and all [of them] drank the same spiritual drink, for they were drinking from a spiritual rock which followed them; and the rock was Christ. Nevertheless,

God was not well-pleased with most of them, for they were scattered along the ground in the wilderness [because of their lack of self-control led to disobedience which led to death]."

Being led by the Spirit of God and having the Spirit of God burning inside of our spirits must be combined with the willful control of our flesh. Until we get to heaven, we will live in our flesh bodies, and we must make our flesh nature subordinate to our heavenly nature. Each day, we must make a conscious decision to put to death the old nature using our spiritual self-control to ensure we are acting out of the spirit and not out of the flesh.

All of us need to be filled with the Holy Spirit continuously. As a cup begins to diminish if we are drinking it, we must continue to fill the cup up to remain in a position of overflow. Ephesians 5:18 teaches, "Do not get drunk with wine, for that is wickedness (corruption, stupidity), but be filled with the [Holy] Spirit and constantly guided by Him."

When people drink wine or other strong drinks, they need to continue to drink to remain drunk. Drinking a little wine or alcohol lasts for a little while, but over time, the effects of the drink begin to diminish. Alcohol is the devil's counterfeit Holy Spirit. To be drunk on the new wine of Heaven, and to experience the full effects of the Holy Spirit, a person must drink and continue to drink. The more we drink the new wine, the more we will experience the effects of what we are drinking and consuming.

If we want to be filled with the Holy Spirit and the power of God, we must continue to drink. The more we drink, and the potency we seek, the more we will be filled. If we want to be drunk, we should desire the most potent form of the drink. Not all people or things carry the same level of anointing or potency. The Holy Spirit is like a drink, He is available and accessible to those who go after Him, and desire Him in the purest and most potent form. God will fill us to the level we are willing to partake.

God will not force us to comply or to be filled with His Spirit. Walking by the Spirit of God is a choice. If we choose to have one glass of wine at dinner God, permits us to do that, but if we choose to become dependent and require more to survive, then He will meet us there as well. We determine how much of the Holy Spirit we need in our lives. We determine how much we drink and which level of Spirit we drink at.

In a war, it is wise to have all provision and knowledge. Without proper provision and knowledge, the soldier is at risk, even if his comrades are not. A soldier in the field without a gun or without his armor, won't survive or advance against the enemy in the same manner as the soldier beside him who is prepared and protected. The commanding officer didn't want the ill-prepared soldier to die or be defeated, but if the soldier refuses to use what he has been given, the commanding officer can't do anything else to help him.

God wants us to use the things He has given us to use. He wants us to arm ourselves daily against the schemes of our enemy. He doesn't like seeing any of His children overtaken by the enemy. But if we as the soldiers refuse to cooperate with the tactics and provisions we have been granted, then we are the problem, not the enlisting army. As insubordinate and rebellious soldiers, we harm ourselves and others on our side because we are not obeying authority and orders.

Knowledge of the Bible provides us with insight into the mind of God as well as with insight about the strategies and purposes of the enemy. In a war, it is essential to know how your militia will advance and be successful. This information of the plans, purposes, and tactics to be used against the enemy forces equips us to fight courageously and effectively. When we fail to prepare ourselves for battle, God is disappointed because we were defeated even as the stronger troop.

While we are living on the earth, we should never be asleep and content with being ignorant or ill-prepared against our enemy. Scripture assures us the enemy preys on those who are unprepared, unaware, and in slumber. Satan roams the earth looking for people who are easily defeated because they are not alert and engaged in the war against him. Don't be distracted, and don't be asleep. Pay attention and remember that you already have the victory and the provision you need to win this battle and the next if you simply believe and receive the help from God.

Isaiah 56:10 says, "Israel's watchmen are blind, They are all without knowledge. They are all mute dogs, they cannot bark; Panting, lying down, they love to slumber."

God is looking for His people to stand strong and fight against the enemy forces. He is looking for people who will do His work! Will you stand up and be brave? Will you determine to take ground for God's kingdom? The choice is yours, but you will be on the battlefield regardless of whether you are a weak and defeated soldier or a strong, brave, and empowered one. Ezra 10:4 declares, "Stand up, for it is your duty, and we will be with you. Be brave and act."

Novices are not experienced and are new to a field. When we are born again and first accept Jesus Christ as our Savior, we are novices. Being a novice or a newly enlisted and low-ranking solider in God's kingdom doesn't last long when the new believer is provided with the proper training and information, and exerts personal commitment and effort. God promotes men and women quickly when they are committed and loyal to Him.

If we want to be promoted like David or Samuel, we must have a loyal and honest heart towards the Lord and His kingdom. We must respect others in kingdom authority positions and learn the ranks.

Training is twofold. We must learn to respect those in authority positions above us, by humbly learning from the people God gives us to train us. As we are learning, we must only eat what we are permitted to eat and learn to recognize the two military powers: good and evil. We must also begin to discipline our spiritual bodies through exercise and movement. As we learn to use the tools of the Holy Spirit, we learn to operate in the realm of faith and the realm of the supernatural.

Soldiers need to exercise to be fit and strong. Faith is the spiritual exercise we need to fight against Satan. We can build up our faith. We can work out in the spirit regularly and learn to use faith to push back everything in our path. Jude 1:20 teaches, "But you, beloved, build yourselves up on [the foundation of] your most holy faith [continually progress, rise like an edifice higher and higher], pray in the Holy Spirit,"

When we are building muscle strength in the gym, we are constantly adding weight so we can get stronger. As we add new weight we are pushed to a new level and a new limit outside of what we are comfortable with. In the realm of the spirit, we are to increase our capacity and our ability to use our faith. Faith must be developed, grown, and continuously utilized and pushed if to continue to grow and develop.

The proper use of faith is to use it for things that are otherwise unattainable. We need to push ourselves to do things we couldn't otherwise do. If we can attain something in the natural, and it doesn't require us to use our faith, then our faith will never grow from the experience. The only way to strengthen ourselves in faith is to use the faith to reach for things outside our of our comfort zone or capacity in the natural realm.

The stronger we become, the more we will be able to overcome. If our food has been uncompromised, our faith has been utilized, and our arsenal is full and loaded, then the enemy forces will never able to defeat us. When we lose a battle in the realm of the spirit, it isn't because God wanted us to lose, it is because we were lacking in one area, and the enemy used our weakness against us. If we want to remain untouchable and undefeatable, then we must prepare for the battle we are in, and we must remain alert and awake through the quickening of the Holy Spirit.

Never stop training and never stop feeding yourself with the proper food you need to survive the war. Seasons of weakness and suffering are not biblical. God doesn't want us to take time off and to become weaker in our faith or in our diet regimen. Just like one week of vacation can steal our physical stamina and our physical fitness, one week of off in the spirit realm can steal spiritual strength and determination from us. David was taking time off from the battle, when he engaged in a sin with Bathsheba. Taking time off from the battle, caused David to be wounded and distracted.

We destroy and take over the enemy's fortress and camps by force. To forcibly take anything from Satan, we must be violent and intentional. We must know the mission, the tactics, and the plans of the enemy, ensuring we never are caught off guard because we are the ones raiding and occupying his camps, not the other way around. Destroying the fortresses of Satan is our mission. It is the call of all believers.

Matthew 11:12 says, "From the days of John the Baptist until now the kingdom of heaven suffers violent assault, and violent men seize it by force [as a precious prize]."

As Christ's body, we are to perform the duties of Christ. The head cannot operate without the body, and the body cannot operate properly without the head. Jesus Christ needs us to do His work, just as much as we need Him to do ours. A fit and healthy body requires both nutrition and exercise. To ensure that Jesus's body is working in optimal condition, we must be willing to do the spiritual work of faith, and the spiritual work of diet control and refusing compromise. Only then can His body be at its optimal performance on the earth.

If we have never been to the gym and lifted weights and we try to bench press two hundred pounds on our first set, we will not be successful, even if we try with all our might. It isn't possible for someone who has never done cardio to run ten miles straight.

Likewise, a person who has never used his or her faith before may have a hard time achieving spiritual things right away, because the person is weak in his or her faith and understanding of spiritual things. It takes time to train our physical bodies, and it takes time and effort training in the spirit realm to become a spiritually equipped, high-ranking warrior.

As we know the time is running short, we must start today in our training. Train today in the realm of the spirit, so you can become stronger and fully equipped to do the battles and assignments you are called to do. If we compromise in the flesh or refuse to activate our faith, it is detrimental to the whole body of Christ and to the headship of Jesus. Realizing this is the first step to beginning the journey of transformation.

When we finally come to grips with our lack of accountability and responsibility in our physical bodies, we are positioned to begin to see progress in the gym. Until we realize how out of shape and incapable our bodies are, we will never begin the journey to transformation. God wants us to be healthy in all areas of our lives. To be healthy spiritually, physically, and psychologically, we must put in the work, and we must be consistently committed. Realize where you are weak and plan to become strong; don't settle or become friends with weakness.

When David fought the lion and the bear, he was training to one day face Goliath. Without the important season of training, David would have been underequipped to face a giant of Goliath's size. A little faith can do tremendous things, but a man or woman who has exercised and built their trust in God's word can do even more! It was supernatural for David to take down lions and bears as a young boy, and his little faith moved the mountains in his life.

Don't believe you can't do mighty things for God, even in the very beginning. If you want to do even more, you must realize it is up to you to determine how your race turns out. God put you in the race when He saved you from your old nature. He picked you up and put you on the right track, but for the car to be in the optimal condition, you must take care of it, and you must do the work required to see the car perform at its best. Without personal spiritual work, you can't win, even when you have been given every potential to do so.

In my first and second pregnancies, I didn't work out or pay any attention to the condition of my body. I ate a lot of junk food, and

I inconsistently worked out. These choices led me to an unfulfilling pregnancy and an unfulfilling birth experience. Taking responsibility for my choices and my ignorance was necessary for me to begin my third pregnancy in a different way. My good choices, combined with my faith, prepared me for my home birth victory.

If I had failed to take responsibility for my pregnancy, I would have continued to blame everyone else for why I didn't have the results I wanted during a pregnancy. While it is true that the medical professionals and others in our lives often take advantage of us and contribute to our downfall, ultimately, we allow them to do so if we don't stand up and take our proper authority. We choose what we allow. We determine the outcomes out of life.

As the medical professionals often try to take a place of authority over their patients, even when they don't have the right to do so, Satan will take control over us when he is permitted to. But God's laws, when they are acted on protect us, because the law says Satan cannot take control of our lives and cause us indefinite harm if we understand who we are in Christ Jesus. God has given us infinite amounts of power and authority, and if we understand our covenant rights, we won't allow Satan to take away our freedom. We won't sit by idly letting anyone else make the decisions or determine the outcomes for our lives.

As we take our authority and our position in Christ and combine our spiritual identity with our personal accountability, we can do all things through Christ. Jesus Christ is the One who gives us our starting place of health and strength. He is the backbone of success, prosperity, and supernatural abundant life. He came to help us get back the things the enemy stole. He died so we wouldn't have to suffer any longer, even during our short stay on the earth.

Hebrews 2:14–15 declares, "Therefore, since [these His] children share in flesh and blood [the physical nature of mankind], He Himself in a similar manner also shared in the same [physical nature, but without sin], so that through [experiencing] death He might make powerless (ineffective, impotent) him who had the power of death—that is, the devil—"

Jesus Christ died for us to make the devil's plans impotent. He lived the life of a man and He died as the sacrificial lamb so we wouldn't have to live under the dominion of the devil. The devil is impotent in our lives. He is helpless, powerless, and unable to effectively harm us if we have been born again and baptized in the Holy Spirit. The devil is not our Father. God is.

If you need to experience supernatural help from Heaven, then do your part and plug into the supernatural. Be willing to admit you aren't where you need to be and then make a plan to get stronger, healthier, and more able bodied in the realm of the spirit. It is easy to blame the devil, but if you are a believer and aren't seeing victory, then the devil isn't the problem; the problem is you and your contribution to the spiritual body you live in.

During certain seasons of my life, I stopped working out and my body became weaker and unable to do things I could previously do effortlessly. If you push yourself to be better, you will only get stronger. The same is true for spiritual things. When we use our faith and we trust God's word, eating the best of the land from God's table, we become capable of more. But we must never stop training and relying on God. To stay strong, we need to stay focused and committed to our spiritual health. We need to keep training always!

Jesus is coming back for His Church. He will remove us from this world and give us a new world where we will be able to live with Him forever. But as citizens of Heaven, all of us can experience Heaven while we live on the earth. We taste, see, hear, smell, and touch spiritual and supernatural things today to remind us we are a part of another world and another kingdom that is very real and alive, outside of the one we live in now.

There is more out there than what we see, and when we are willing to participate in it, we will experience it now, right where we are. God allows us to partake in the heavenly kingdom while we live on the earth. He rescued us from the suffering and the curse of this world so we wouldn't have to endure the same things the world endures while we await His return. Because God loves us, He sent His son to redeem us, to purchase us, and to keep us from the curse of the law and the evil one. If we are willing and obedient, we will eat and drink the good of the land now and forever.

As people learn a new language, they learn it best by being fully immersed in the culture. When we are growing in Christ, we learn about God by being fully immersed into His Church, with His people and His presence. Learning takes time, but God knows if we are doing our best and if we are giving Him our all. He knows when we are committed to learning, growing, and healing. He knows when we are fully immersed in His kingdom.

The devil stands taunting the Church with the same lies that Goliath used to taunt the Israelites and pharaoh used to enslave God's people. Yet, the devil and his kingdom don't have the power, authority, and control over the child of God. The devil could send 10,000 chariots and they would all be washed away in the sea. God stands with us, commanding the enemy to "Let my people go!"

If you have these strongholds within your mind, the enemy has tried to trick you into a helpless position where you aren't a threat to him. I pray now for the removal of any strongholds in the minds of the people. I cast down the strongholds in the name of Jesus. I command liberty, freedom, and fresh vision. We aren't weak, helpless, or prey. We aren't enslaved to anyone or anything. We carry the highest power. We are the Church of Jesus Christ.

One time, when all three of my children were very sick, experiencing severe wheezing and vomiting. I tried fasting, and I prayed constantly, asking God for help. My youngest son was only a few months old, and my daughter was coughing unlike anything I had ever experienced. I searched the Bible, I sang praise songs, and I stayed up pacing the halls, speaking in tongues and praying fervently for God's protection and grace upon my kids.

When this attack occurred, I was just beginning to understand the divine healing protection for my own life and for my children's lives. I did not have a deep revelation of it, and even though I believed God didn't want us to be sick, my faith in fighting against sickness and disease had not yet been built up. I fought for the rights I knew belonged to us, and I gave it everything I had, but I was not where I needed to be in my faith to resist this attack of the enemy.

After three days, God revealed to me that He didn't want me to beg Him for help. God wanted me to realize that through faith, we were already protected, saved, delivered, and made well. He promised me He was with us, and He was our protector and our deliverer.

During that sickness, I grew in my faith because I used my faith. I gave the fight every single part of me, and I contested for the rights I knew we had. When we begin it is harder to get the weight up but overtime it will become easier if we keep using our muscles to gain our spiritual strength. Don't wait until you need to utilize your muscles to begin activating them. We can use our muscles every day and keep ourselves prepared for a fight when the devil brings one our way. Build your faith now, so you can take on anything the enemy tries to send against you or your children.

God allows mothers and fathers to be the gatekeepers of their children. In the kingdom, gatekeepers were guards that protected cities, temples, or other important buildings. Gatekeepers were given their job so they could designate who could and couldn't enter the city or the dwelling. They were permitted to watch and maintain order and safety behind the walls of their entrusted location.

As gatekeepers of our children, we can determine what comes in and what doesn't. God has given us a job to guard the special temples of our kids. Until children are old enough to begin fighting for themselves, they need their parents' help. They need responsible, properly equipped gatekeepers to keep them safe from their enemy. Satan wants parents to let him in their kids' lives, and he hopes the parents are weak, asleep, or apathetic in their position, so he can gain access.

If we are nothing else in the kingdom of God, then we as mothers are gatekeepers of prized possessions. We have children who are important to God and to His kingdom. God has gifted us with our kids so we can value them and guard them, ensuring the enemy doesn't have his way in their lives. The position of a gatekeeper over children is essential. I believe it is one of the best jobs there is. Do your job and do it well; there is a reward for serving God and protecting His mission and His people.

Psalm 84:1–12 (emphasis mine) says:

How lovely are Your tabernacles, O Lord of hosts! My soul yearns, yes, even pines and is homesick for the courts of the Lord; my heart and my flesh cry out and sing for joy to the living God. Yes, the sparrow has found a house, and the swallow a nest for herself, where she may lay her young—even Your altars, O Lord of hosts, my King and my God.

Blessed (happy, fortunate, to be envied) are those who dwell in Your house and Your presence; they will be singing Your praises all the day long. Selah [pause, and calmly think of that]! Blessed (happy, fortunate, to be envied) is the man whose strength is in You, in whose heart are the highways to Zion. Passing through the Valley of Weeping (Baca), they make it a place of springs; the early rain also fills [the pools] with blessings.

They go from strength to strength [increasing in victorious power]; each of them appears before God in Zion.

O Lord God of hosts, hear my prayer; give ear, O God of Jacob! Selah [pause, and calmly think of that]! Behold our shield [the king as Your agent], O God, and look upon the face of Your anointed! For a day in Your courts is better than a thousand [anywhere else]; I would rather be a doorkeeper and stand at the threshold in the house of my God than to dwell [at ease] in the tents of wickedness.

For the Lord God is a Sun and Shield; the Lord bestows [present] grace and favor and [future] glory (honor, splendor, and heavenly bliss)! No good thing will He withhold from those who walk uprightly.

O Lord of hosts, blessed (happy, fortunate, to be envied) is the man who trusts in You [leaning and believing on You, committing all and confidently looking to You, and that without fear or misgiving]!

Reference Page

Allied Market Research. (2021). Baby Infant Formula Market Size, Share, Competitive Landscape and Trend Analysis Report, by Type, by Ingredient, by Distribution Channel : Global Opportunity Analysis and Industry Forecast, 2022-2031.

Bell, A. F., Erickson, E. N., & Carter, C. S. (2014). Beyond labor: the role of natural and synthetic oxytocin in the transition to motherhood. *Journal of midwifery & women's health*, 59(1), 35–108. https://doi.org/10.1111/jmwh.12101

CDC Wonder. *National Overdose Deaths from Select Prescription and Illicit Drugs*. National Center on Health Statistics. [Google Scholar]

Cheyney, M., Bovbjerg, M., Everson, C., Gordon, W., Hannibal, D., & Vedam, S. (2014). Outcomes of care for 16,924 planned home births in the United States: the Midwives Alliance of North America Statistics Project, 2004 to 2009. *Journal of midwifery & women's health*, 59(1), 17–27. https://doi.org/10.1111/jmwh.12172

Declercq, E. R., Sakala, C., Corry, M. P., Applebaum, S., & Herrlich, A. (2014). Major Survey Findings of Listening to Mothers(SM) III: Pregnancy and Birth: Report of the Third National U.S. Survey of Women's Childbearing Experiences. *The Journal of perinatal education*, 23(1), 9–16. https://doi.org/10.1891/1058-1243.23.1.9

Fredrickson B. L., & Roberts T. A. (1997). Objectification theory: Towards understanding women's lived experience and mental health risks. *Psychology of Women Quarterly*, 21, 173–206.

Gibson, C., Medeiros, K. E., Giorgini, V., Mecca, J. T., Devenport, L. D., Connelly, S., & Mumford, M. D. (2014). A Qualitative Analysis of Power Differentials in Ethical Situations in Academia. *Ethics & behavior*, 24(4), 311–325. https://doi.org/10.1080/10508422.2013.858605

Healy, M., Nyman, V., Spence, D., Otten, R. H. J., & Verhoeven, C. J. (2020). How do midwives facilitate women to give birth during physiological second stage of labour? A systematic review. *PloS one*, 15(7), e0226502. https://doi.org/10.1371/journal.pone.0226502

Lieberman, E., & O'donoghue, C. (2002). Unintended effects of epidural analgesia during labor: a systematic review. *American journal of obstetrics and gynecology*, 186(5 Suppl Nature), S31–S68. https://doi.org/10.1067/mob.2002.122522

(n.d.). The Legal Infrastructure of Childbirth [Review of *The Legal Infrastructure of Childbirth*]. *Harvard Law Review*, 134:2209. Retrieved July 20, 2024, from file:///C:/Users/18048/Desktop/134-Harv.-L.-Rev.-2209%20(1).pdf

Medical Education in the United States and Canada; a report to the Carnegie Foundation for the Advancement of Teaching

Milner, J., & Arezina, J. (2018). The accuracy of ultrasound estimation of fetal weight in comparison to birth weight: A systematic review. *Ultrasound (Leeds, England), 26*(1), 32–41. https://doi.org/10.1177/1742271X17732807

Muro-Valdez, J. C., Meza-Rios, A., Aguilar-Uscanga, B. R., Lopez-Roa, R. I., Medina-Díaz, E., Franco-Torres, E. M., & Zepeda-Morales, A. S. M. (2023). Breastfeeding-Related Health Benefits in Children and Mothers: Vital Organs Perspective. *Medicina (Kaunas, Lithuania), 59*(9), 1535. https://doi.org/10.3390/medicina59091535

Murphy R. J. (2023). Depersonalization/Derealization Disorder and Neural Correlates of Trauma-related Pathology: A Critical Review. *Innovations in clinical neuroscience, 20*(1-3), 53–59.

Murray, S. R., Shenkin, S. D., McIntosh, K., Lim, J., Grove, B., Pell, J. P., Norman, J. E., & Stock, S. J. (2017). Long term cognitive outcomes of early term (37-38 weeks) and late preterm (34-36 weeks) births: A systematic review. *Wellcome open research, 2*, 101. https://doi.org/10.12688/wellcomeopenres.12783.1

Osmundson, S. S., Min, J. Y., & Grijalva, C. G. (2019). Opioid prescribing after childbirth: overprescribing and chronic use. *Current opinion in obstetrics & gynecology, 31*(2), 83–89. https://doi.org/10.1097/GCO.0000000000000527

Porter, M. (n.d.). *VCU's Egyptian Building commemorated with Historic Marker*. VCU News. https://www.news.vcu.edu/article/VCUs_Egyptian_Building_commemorated_with_historic_marker

Reardon D. C. (2018). The abortion and mental health controversy: A comprehensive literature review of common ground agreements, disagreements, actionable recommendations, and research opportunities. *SAGE open medicine, 6*, 2050312118807624. https://doi.org/10.1177/2050312118807624

Sperlich, M., & Gabriel, C. (2022). "I got to catch my own baby": a qualitative study of out of hospital birth. *Reproductive health, 19*(1), 43. https://doi.org/10.1186/s12978-022-01355-4

Sumrall, L. (1982) *The Gifts and Ministries of the Holy Spirit.*

van Zuylen, M. L., Ten Hoope, W., Bos, E., Hermanides, J., Stevens, M. F., & Hollmann, M. W. (2019). Safety of epidural drugs: a narrative review. *Expert opinion on drug safety, 18*(7), 591–601. https://doi.org/10.1080/14740338.2019.1617271

Vaxxed: From cover up to catastrophe. Childrens Health Defense. (n.d.). https://live.childrenshealthdefense.org/chd-tv/videos/vaxxed-from-cover-up-to-catastrophe-movie/

A Message from the Author:

I have experienced profound healing and liberation from the torment of illness through God's grace. My life has been transformed for the better, and I am eternally grateful for the healing work that Jesus Christ has accomplished within me. There was a time when I was burdened by mental anguish, physical pain, and a sense of spiritual separation from God. However, upon accepting Jesus as my Savior, I came to understand the reality of God's divine healing power. The more time I devoted to His presence, the more my perspective on every aspect of my life changed.

It is not God's intention for sickness and disease to govern our lives. Throughout His ministry, Jesus devoted a significant portion of His time to healing the sick. He desires to bring healing to you today in whatever form you may need. Jesus genuinely cares for your well-being, while Satan seeks to deceive you into accepting illness as a norm. The adversary aims to instill passivity regarding our health. In contrast, God calls us to confront Satan and to steadfastly claim our right to wellness.

The Bible offers pure and perfect knowledge; it is a source of truth that provides deliverance and hope, even in moments when all seems lost. God liberates us from the inherent sinful nature with which we are born, as well as from the challenges we face in a world fraught with sin and evil. When we partner with Him, God empowers us to achieve, to succeed, and to overcome. He grants us the authority to become more than we could ever hope for or imagine on our own. Through our rebirth and adoption into God's family, we undergo a transformation from a state of brokenness and despair to one of perfection and restoration.

As born-again Christians, we are transformed into new creations, endowed with capabilities that surpass those of the average individual. The Church of Jesus Christ possesses a supernatural arsenal to combat adversarial forces, a resource unavailable to the world. We can triumph in life's battles because God has already granted us victory through Christ. Today, let us actively utilize our spiritual weapons. By embracing the truth, we can engage in the good fight of faith and achieve prosperity in all things.

About the Author:

Ashton is an American child behavioral specialist, educator, evangelist, wife, and mother. She holds a Bachelor of Science degree in Psychology and a Master of Education degree in Counselor Education. With experience teaching in both private and public educational settings, Ashton has worked with individuals across a broad spectrum of developmental stages. Additionally, she has functioned as a counselor under the supervision of Licensed Professional Counselors, providing support to both children and adults. As an author of various publications, Ashton showcases her knowledge and expertise. She engages with both children and adults, imparting the teachings of God's word through her adaptability and understanding of diverse developmental needs. For additional information, related books, and further resources, please visit: **BohannonBoutique.com**

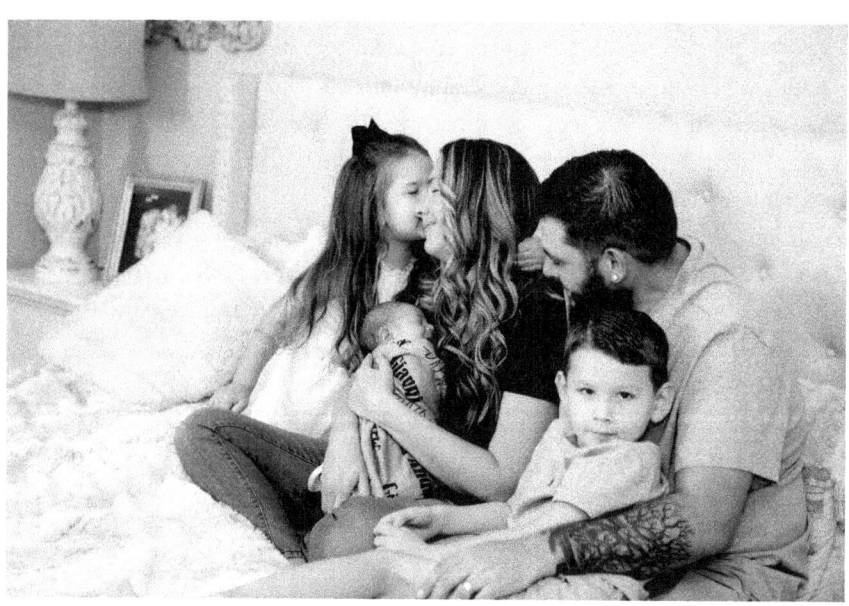

www.ingramcontent.com/pod-product-compliance
Lightning Source LLC
Chambersburg PA
CBHW050518100526
44581CB00001B/24